THE
BOOK
OF
SEX

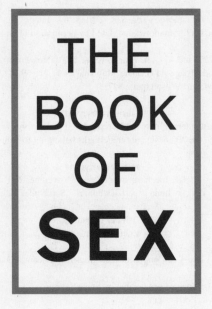

THE
BOOK
OF
SEX

Edited by Steve Salerno, Rodale for Men

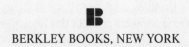

BERKLEY BOOKS, NEW YORK

A Berkley Book
Published by The Berkley Publishing Group
A division of Penguin Putnam Inc.
375 Hudson Street
New York, New York 10014

"Hot Dates" are reprinted from *The Century of Sex*, edited by James R. Peterson and Hugh M. Hefner copyright © 1999 by Playboy Enterprises International, Inc. Used by permission of Grove/Atlantic, Inc.

Photos by Jorg Badura (pages 161, 227, and 411), A. Bracho (page 217), Greg Federman (pages 101, 133, 153, 167, and 211), Elisabeth Greil (page 47), Ludo (page 417), Dale May (pages 1, 21, 69, 87, 179, 297, 375, and 383), Robert Whitman/Graphistock (page 121), and Kurt Wilson (page 347).

PRINTING HISTORY
Rodale Inc. hardcover edition / November 2001
Berkley trade paperback edition / September 2002

Visit our website at
www.penguinputnam.com

Library of Congress Cataloging-in-Publication Data

The book of sex / edited by Steve Salerno.
    p.   cm.
    Includes index.
    ISBN 0-425-18678-4 (pbk)
    1. Sex instruction for men.   I. Salerno, Steve.
HQ36 .B63   2002
306.7—dc21

                2002018478

PRINTED IN THE UNITED STATES OF AMERICA

10 9 8 7 6 5 4 3 2 1

Introduction

Were you aware that you have a vagina? This may not come as a surprise if you're a woman, but considering that we wrote this book for men, that particular fact could indeed have you glancing downward. It's true: Every man has a dangling piece of flesh on his bladder that would have turned into a real vagina had not testosterone turned him into a male in utero. Bet you didn't know that.

All men have gaps in their knowledge about sex, women, their own bodies, and even the plumbing that makes it all come together. The consequences of those gaps vary from minor unease (such as being the only guy in the locker room who doesn't get the joke) to major anxiety (such as your first time with a woman who confesses that in the past she was sexually abused) to serious legal problems (such as coming to work one day and learning that a former co-worker has filed suit against your employer because of an offhand remark you'd forgotten about. . . . And by the way, you're fired). What's more—though nobody likes to admit it—some of us suffer from the most distressing gap of all when it comes to sex: How do we get our fair share of it?

Hence, this book. It covers every major and minor sex-and-relationship issue you face as a man, from the familiar to the forbidden. It will give you more knowledge about this most fascinating of subjects than you ever thought possible. And between the sheets, knowledge truly is power.

Not to pat ourselves on the backs—well, maybe just a little—but we believe *The Book of Sex* to be the final word on the subject. If it's got to do with sex, it's in here. We're not much interested in telling you *what* to do—after all, what gets your motor running may cause someone else's engine to stall out. We simply want to let you know what's on the complete inventory of mankind's most intriguing activity. You'll need to make your own selections.

With this book as your road map, you'll never again get lost in sex's pleasurable-yet-puzzling terrain. You won't even have to stop to ask for directions. You'll know what's out there—even if some of it seems way, way out there.

Armed with info from the most authoritative, up-to-the-minute sources, we'll walk you through the nuances of flirting, dating, courting, mating, breaking up, dating again. You'll learn how to read her secret signals. How to flirt with flair instead of phoniness. How to tell when she's ready for dinner and a drink with you . . . or for much more. We'll give you sample dialogue for some of life's most awkward moments so you'll never again be afraid to approach a woman because you're thinking, "I don't know what to say. . . ."

We'll teach you the subtle-yet-profound difference between style, which is good, and slickness, which isn't. You'll learn what your abs may have to do with the quality of your sex life. You'll learn what to look for in a younger woman—and how to find out if that younger woman is maybe a little *too* young. You'll also learn the many benefits of dating an older woman. We'll give you tips to help you get the woman you really want, whatever her age.

When it comes to serious naked time, we'll recommend sex techniques that will keep her calling your name and dialing your phone number long after the lovemaking ends. You'll never worry about being compared to past lovers—not even if she is the sort to make comparisons—because you'll know how to do things those guys never even imagined. And if the time comes when you don't want her to call you anymore, we'll tell you how to handle that too. Neatly.

Already married, you say? Great. We'll give you advice that will help take the stress out of your marriage and put the spice back in. We'll have the two of you doing things that would make you both blush if only you weren't enjoying them so much.

Of course, just as important as giving you new information is dispelling the old beliefs that are dead wrong. Do you know why a gift of red roses or racy lingerie may fall flat? Why body odor may be a good thing after all? What she loves most about you? (And no, it's not what you think.) Do you know why the morning after may be more important—yes, even to you—than what happened the night before?

Breeze through the book, and you'll see that we organized it alphabetically, like an encyclopedia. That's to make it easy for you to find entries on a particular subject. But we also added cross-references at the end of most items to lead you on to related topics you may not have thought of. Say, for instance, you're looking for info on the singles scene. In that particular entry, we give you a number of solid tips for making

the most of your hunt for companionship. And at the end, we direct you to related information on Internet dating. It's all there right at your fingertips.

Along the way, we'll present running features on milestones in sex history, sex in song, sex in other cultures, and sex at its outer limits as well as a true-or-false quiz that will keep you guessing—and smiling. (So the next time your pregnant wife complains about having to carry a baby for 9 months, you can tell her to be thankful she's not an Asian elephant, whose gestation period lasts for 20 months. Well, on second thought, it may not be wise to compare a third-trimester, potentially violent woman to a pachyderm. But you get the idea.) You'll hear about some of the craziest places where people have had sex, some of the strangest legal cases involving sex, and some truly off-the-charts sexual customs.

The bottom line is, whether you're trying to create the magic or get it back; whether your relationship is on the way in, on the way through, or (we're sorry to hear) on the way out; this book will be your faithful companion, your personal guide to a more passionate and satisfying life. It's been said that the journey itself is more important than the final destination. We agree wholeheartedly—especially with the pit stops we have planned for you. So buckle up, friend, because you're going for a ride.

—Steve Salerno
Executive Editor
Rodale for Men

THE
BOOK
OF
SEX

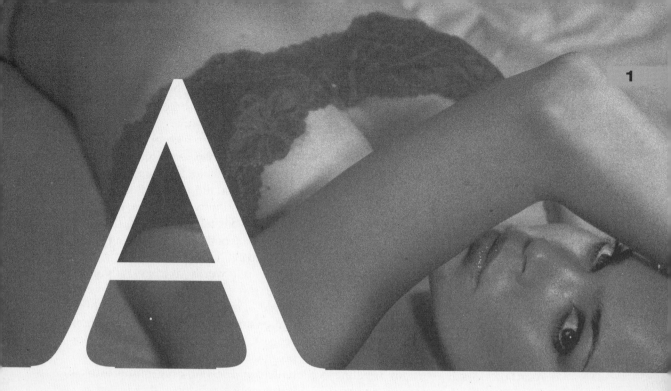

abnormal

"Is this abnormal?" That's a common question about sexual urges and behavior. It's also a pointless one. Next time it comes to mind, realize that there are many different standards by which a sexual practice can be judged "abnormal" or "normal." Is it statistically common? Then masturbation, for example, is normal. Is it biblically sanctioned? Then masturbation is abnormal. Approved of by today's medical experts? Then masturbation is very normal. Is it legal? In private, yes; in public, no. Clearly, masturbation can be normal or abnormal, depending on how close you are to Jerry Falwell's sphere of influence at the time.

With so many competing arbiters of what's normal, you're never going to get any one definitive answer. So, when you're deciding whether or not to participate in some sexual activity, there are more useful criteria than what others are doing or what they think about that activity. Does it give you pleasure? How does your partner feel about it? Is it safe? Are you being pressured into doing it? How do you feel about it after you do it? Does it harm anyone? Is it good for your relationship? These are more productive questions than "Is it abnormal?"

Also see: kinky, paraphilias, perversions, taboos

abortion

Medically speaking, it's the termination of a pregnancy by the premature expulsion of the fetus from the uterus. That means abortion, per se, is much more common than you may think, since miscarriages are really spontaneous abortions.

The surgical procedure that more

than one million American women voluntarily undergo each year is called a medical abortion. The deliberate termination of a pregnancy is, has always been, and will always be a tough issue. It's one of those topics, like politics and religion, that you can't get into without leaving somebody on edge (if not downright furious). Indeed, it involves both politics *and* religion. People get killed over abortion—and many will tell you it involves a form of killing in its own right. So we won't presume to tell you how to feel about it. We're merely going to equip you with knowledge, in case you and a woman with whom you're involved ever have to face this difficult decision.

The overwhelming majority (about 90 percent) of medical abortions are done within 10 weeks of conception and are 10-minute procedures performed in a doctor's office. They essentially consist of removing the fetus with a vacuum suction device through the dilated uterus. Ending more advanced pregnancies—between 12 and 20 weeks—is more difficult, with increasing risk of complications. Terminating pregnancies beyond 20 weeks requires chemically induced premature labor in a hospital setting. Medical abortion is considered a very safe gynecological procedure; 10 times as many women die from full-term pregnancies as from induced pregnancy terminations.

abortion pill

The abortion-inducing pill known as RU-486 (mifepristone) gives a woman a choice within a choice about ending a pregnancy. It was developed in France in 1980 and has been used by some 620,000 women in Europe, China, and Israel. The U.S. Food and Drug Administration approved mifepristone in September 2000, making available for the first time in this country an alternative to surgical abortion. So a woman who opts to end her pregnancy can bypass anesthesia, surgery, and abortion clinics for a simple series of pills administered by a doctor. She has more accessibility and privacy. And if you're the one taking her to the doctor, it enables you both to avoid crossing picket lines and get home in one piece.

The pill works like so: A woman makes three trips to a doctor in a 2-week period. First, she is prescribed three mifepristone pills to block the action of progesterone, a hormone necessary for pregnancy. Two days later, she takes two tablets of a second drug, misoprostol, a hormonelike substance that makes her uterus contract to expel the embryo. After 12 days, she returns for a follow-up so the doctor can be sure she's no longer pregnant.

A woman considering RU-486 needs to know the following: First, she can take it only up to 7 weeks after the start of her most recent period. Second, not all doctors are qualified to administer the pill. They must be able to accurately determine the duration of the pregnancy and that it is not ectopic, and they must be able to perform a surgical abortion or have another doctor available who can do so if one becomes necessary. Some physicians may opt not to prescribe the drug, citing personal or ethical reasons; the patient may have to insist on a referral. (And *insist* may be the perfect word, with some doctors.) Third, she's likely to experience side effects. The most common are bleeding, cramping, nausea, headache, vomiting, and diarrhea. One percent of women need surgery to stop heavy bleeding, and 5 percent still need surgical abortions to remove remaining fetal tissue. If the pill doesn't work at all, the patient will be urged to get a surgical abortion rather than continue the pregnancy, because the pill can cause birth defects.

Though the abortion pill is less invasive than surgery, for some women it can be just as emotionally traumatic. If your partner decides to use it and you're not opposed to her choice, by all means be there for her when it's over.

Also see: morning-after pill

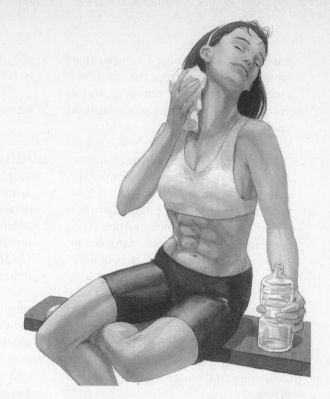

abs

Next time you need something to think about during sex, try noticing how involved your abdominal muscles are in the proceedings. Pelvic thrusting just wouldn't be the same without them, would it? You'll also see that your abs are key for countless other subtle movements and body shifts you make during the act. Throw in their role in supporting your back, and you've got some pretty sexy reasons for improving them.

It's not that sex needs to be a show of strength. And it's not that taut abs are a prerequisite for pleasure. But anything that enhances enjoyment is worthwhile, and stronger abdominal muscles definitely do that.

You don't have to get fancy about your gut work. A basic regimen of crunches will suffice for starters. Simply lie on your back with your knees bent, your feet flat on the floor, and your hands cupped behind your ears. Contract your abs to lift your shoulders (not your back) as high as you can. Hold for a second, then ease yourself back. Repeat without resting. The trick is to stay with it, so start out easy with three sets of 10 repetitions and slowly work your way up to three sets of 20. And don't forget to check with your doc before starting any new exercise regimen.

You'll feel the difference soon enough. So will she.

Also see: athletic sex, beefcake, body fitness, exercise, male body, muscles, weight loss

abstinence

This straightforward-sounding word means different things to different people. To some, it's the absence of sexual intercourse. To others, it's the absence of any kind of sexual contact with another person. Still others even include sexual contact with themselves. However you define it, there's a decent chance that you'll experience it from time to time, whether as a welcome time-out after a bad relationship, a physical separation from a monogamous mate, a religious observance, or just a case of being unlucky in love—the dreaded losing streak.

Voluntary or otherwise, temporary abstinence isn't going to hurt you. You won't forget how. Your plumbing won't rust. Prolonged abstinence, however, may cause some problems. Many urologists believe that ejaculation is beneficial to the prostate and the many glands in it that produce ejaculatory fluid. And since the penis is made up of vascular tissue and erection is a vascular event, a prolonged lack of erections may damage this tissue. So there really is something to the old "use it or lose it" theory.

There are some benefits to abstinence, too, as hard as that may be to believe. It's the only foolproof strategy for avoiding sexually transmitted diseases and unwanted pregnancy.

Just remember the words of sex educator Debra W. Haffner: Vows of abstinence are hard to keep; they fail more often than condoms do.

Also see: celibacy, dry hump, frequency, impotence, safe sex, sex—lack of, virginity—hers

AC/DC

A jocular and somewhat passé slang term for bisexuality or someone who is bisexual. The idea is that he or she can plug into either kind of current. No wonder it's outdated.

Also see: anima and animus, switch-hitter, yin and yang

adultery

What Jimmy Carter committed in his heart. And what one other recent president committed . . . well, just about everywhere. *Adultery* is a word that's been loaded with moral and legal overtones since the Ten Commandments were chiseled. You tend to hear it in the same paragraph as phrases like "Thou shalt be smitten down" or—maybe worse—"My lawyer will be getting in touch." It even comes from a Latin root for "polluted" or "defiled."

All this negativity creates a lousy context for any useful discussion of the all-too-human issue of cheatin'. See the entry for *affairs*, at right.

Also see: boredom, danger, risky sex, variety

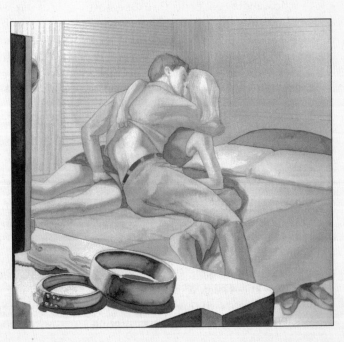

affairs

Is a quick one with the stripper at your buddy's bachelor party an affair? How about ongoing intimacy with a woman friend whom you care about but never go all the way with? Weekly motel sex with that pert party girl in accounts receivable? That *has* to be an affair, doesn't it?

No right or wrong answers here. Couples are all over the map when it comes to defining infidelity. What matters is that you and your wife or partner share the same definition of betrayal. We're not going to referee this one for you, either. You two must be able to clarify—out loud—the ground rules of your monogamy. And then live by them.

That "live by them" part isn't always so easy, is it? One excuse guys tend to like is the scientific theory that the human male is anthropologically hardwired to spread his seed for the sake of the species. Another is our sex-saturated pop culture, with its mixed message that (a) marriage is what you strive for but (b) the single life is where all the fun is. Finally, there's just so damn much opportunity to stray these days, with men and women intermingling more and being more overtly sexual.

What's a married or attached guy to do? Simply recognize that, though lust affects us all, actual infidelity is a choice. An affair doesn't start just because there's an attraction, no more than a bank robbery starts because you have bills to pay. An affair starts because you deliberately give in to the impulse. Look, we all want to eat more doughnuts than are good for us, but most of us consider the consequences, and we pass. And then we don't hang around the doughnut shop

too much. Well, same thing with that knockout bartender who's been coming on to you.

But say you do stray, and then you end it. Do you tell your partner? Used to be the answer was straightforward: Confess, exorcise the demons of secrecy, and work on your relationship. That's still often a good course of action, but these things aren't always so cut-and-dried. Ask yourself why you would tell. Is it merely to assuage your guilt? Or is it for a more constructive reason, such as resurrecting intimacy with your partner? Then weigh your motives against the consequences of telling. Will the two of you be glad in the long run? Or will the revelation do more harm than good? Sorry, but nobody can walk you through this one.

If you suspect that she's the one having an affair, ask her. Calmly present your case, remind her how you'd feel if she violated your mutual agreement, then listen to what she says in reply. She may have a perfectly credible explanation for whatever aroused your suspicions. If she does, you need to swallow hard, take her in your arms, and go on as if nothing had happened. *Don't tell her that everything's fine and then go snooping around or otherwise looking for trouble.* You told her that you accepted her explanation, remember? Let it go—until or unless you stumble on more incriminating evidence.

Once an affair is revealed, the issue isn't going to fade away on its own. Sometimes it's a marriage buster. Most of the time it's not. Either way, you have an obligation to investigate what happened, why it happened, and what it means. Like every other stage of an affair, the aftermath must be approached with a grown-up's sense of responsibility, and with all eyes wide open.

Also see: commitment; Don't ask, don't tell; guilt; marriage—open; midlife crisis; trust—rebuilding; wandering eye

afterglow

The euphoric feeling that settles over you and your lover after orgasm is a priceless opportunity for the two of you to bask in the closeness that satisfying sex promotes.

Clinically speaking, afterglow coincides with what's called the resolution stage of the sexual response cycle, where your mind and body begin to return to normal after orgasm releases the exquisite tension that started building with arousal. But you're not back to normal yet. You're still in that highly pleasurable altered state of sex, without the distractions of arousal. You don't have to do much to enjoy it.

Except stay awake—for her sake. This is when you let her know that you appreciate her for more than just that foundation-rattling orgasm she gave you moments earlier.

We know what you're thinking: After sex, you're too drowsy to be convincingly romantic. You have to be up at daybreak for that meeting with your boss. Hell, if you could muster any sort of strength, you'd get up and put your mud-caked sneakers in the garage so you wouldn't have to hear about them again in the morning.

None of this changes the fact that your woman may want to snuggle. In fact, most women famously hate it when you succumb to the temptation to fall asleep after coming.

They don't act this way just to annoy you. For both sexes, in fact, postcoital habits are pretty hardwired. A man's body resets to a resting state within 2 minutes. You want sleep. She takes much longer to wind down, typically 15 or 20 minutes. During this time, she wants cuddling.

So oblige her.

Make an effort to think of afterglow as an energy that surrounds you after orgasm. The trick is to experience that energy, and a good way to do it is to tune in to the breathing that's going on—yours and hers. Remember, being in the moment is everything.

You'll snuggle, of course, and possibly stroke each other lightly. You may still even be inside her. Sounds that may or may not resemble words might escape from your mouths. But the real intimacy here is happening on the nonphysical plane, if you will. It's a deep, other-worldly connection with another human being that can feel more wonderful than orgasm. (We are not making this up.) Guys just like you report that the interactions with their partners during afterglow can be as gratifying as the more energetic aspects of sex, adding a new, intensely connected dimension to their relationships.

Further, she'll appreciate you more. She knows that you're overriding your own nature, so she'll likely be sweeter and more understanding of *your* foibles.

There's even a chance that she won't bring up the filthy sneakers.

Also see: afterplay, intimacy

afternoon delight

More than a nooner and nothing like a quickie, an afternoon delight is to sex what a daytime doubleheader is to baseball: long, slow, and delicious, with more bang for your buck and always the prospect of extra innings. Sex in the afternoon has it all over the usual late-night edition anyway. You have more energy. You're less likely to sleep afterward. You've got the aesthetics of natural light. And you run no risk of missing Letterman's monologue.

You need to approach an afternoon delight as an unfettered indulgence in all things sensual. Block off the entire period from lunch to dinner, arranging things so that no interruption is possible. Hide, if you must, in a hotel room. And make sure that you both have nothing, absolutely nothing, to do before sunset except enjoy each other over every one of those hours. Take your time before intercourse, during intercourse, and after intercourse. In fact, this is the kind of afternoon where you never stop making love, whether you're actually in coital contact or just relaxing in the Jacuzzi. The world belongs to just the two of you, if only for one drawn-out afternoon.

Also see: appointments, quickies, workaholism

afterplay

No, we don't mean watching the game highlights on *SportsCenter.* And by the way, though it's not called after*work,* if she hasn't yet joined you in the land of bliss, you do indeed have some work cut out for you. Even if the Big Unit is temporarily on the DL, you owe it to your partner to use alternative methods to bring her, too, to that happy place known as orgasm. Or at least make sure that she's fully satisfied with her lusty layover. She won't feel very playful if she's uncomfortable from not having climaxed.

But assuming that the sex was mutually good and both of you emerged from afterglow feeling a bit frisky, this is the time to nurture your intimacy and move the pleasure in new directions—by goofing around.

So tickle each other like little kids, or trace your initials on each other's tummies. Words of love? Well, compliments are fine, but a lighthearted tone is what you want—not contrived lines or a loaded pop quiz like "How was it for you, babe?" Activity? Feed each other peeled grapes. Take a bubble bath together. Do anything that feels good, as long as you do it together.

Afterplay is a kick for its own sake, but it also helps settle the two of you into a nice, relaxed groove. If she's a fairly new partner, that's going to pay dividends the next time the two of you get it on.

Which could be sooner than you think, since afterplay sometimes leads to a new round of, well, play. (Oddly, when this happens, you don't seem to worry much about that early meeting.) Then you can both fall happily asleep.

aging

Getting older doesn't ruin your sex life. But it does change it. Whether that's a good thing or a bad thing is up to you.

Consider these major physical changes that usually describe sex after 60: It takes longer for you to get an erection. You need more direct stimulation to do so. Your erection is likely to be less firm. Your urge to ejaculate is less pressing. The duration of your ejaculation is shorter. Your orgasms are less intense. Your semen is expelled with less force, and there's less of it. Your refractory period is longer.

Now, instead of panicking, ask yourself how much it really matters. Is there some rush to get an erection? Does having your genitals directly stimulated by your partner sound like a bad idea? (See? Don't you feel better already?) What's more, as long as your erection is firm enough to get the job done, who cares? And who cares how much semen comes out or how far it's shot? In fact, one of these changes—the less-pressing urge to ejaculate—is a *goal* for a lot of guys, not a problem.

Seniority is a plus in other ways. For one, your technique is likely to be more intimate, more varied, and ultimately more enjoyable. Best of all, you're probably better able to satisfy your partner.

The worst change? One day, it hits you that you're still looking at college coeds but they've been looking right through you—or giggling at your comb-over—for years. Talk about mortal blows!

Also see: erection difficulties, heart conditions, impotence, medications, menopause—yours, midlife crisis, orgasm—delayed, prostate cancer, prostate enlargement, testosterone replacement therapy, young women/older men

ahhh

Said to be the simplest, purest sound a human can make. Thus, it's an expression of joy that has announced, accompanied, or commented upon countless orgasms.

Perhaps because of its simplicity and depth of emotion, it's also the vowel sound in the word *God*. This is true in languages and religions throughout the world: Among the many deities whose names are invoked both in prayer and in physical passion are Krishna, Rama, Buddha, Siddha, Jehovah, Yahweh, Allah, and Kami Sama. It's been joked that in the throes of sexual ecstacy, even atheists scream out, "Oh, God!" It's not hypocrisy. It's just that "Universal truth!" or "Life energy!" doesn't quite cut it.

Let this phonetic insight inspire you to ponder the spiritual aspects of sex. After all, we're talking about the physical and emotional merging of two beings that can actually create a third being. There's definitely a lot of "ahhh" to that.

Also see: come, grunting, moaning, orgasm, spiritual sex

AIDS

The mother of all sexually transmitted diseases is caused by the human immunodeficiency virus (HIV), which slowly eradicates the immune systems of its victims until they are killed by opportunistic infections known collectively as acquired immunodeficiency syndrome, or AIDS. Since the first documented AIDS victim died in 1959, HIV has infected some 47 million people worldwide. In America today, between 800,000 and 900,000 people live with the virus, and about one-third of them don't even know they have it.

With AIDS, of course, came the realization that sex could kill you, even if you weren't fooling around with a gun zealot's wife. We've gotten away from that fear a bit as drug treatments have been developed to suppress the virus. Magic Johnson seems as robust as ever, despite the passage of more than 10 years since his diagnosis.

But here's the hard truth: Sex can still kill you. And there's no cure. And being a man makes you a prime target: In all parts of the world except sub-Saharan Africa, there are more men than women dying of AIDS.

Yes, there are drug cocktails that can treat you. Yes, they can bash down HIV to nearly undetectable levels. Yes, there are new, improved drugs on the horizon. Just don't confuse this with a cure. If you're unfortunate enough to contract HIV, you'll probably be on those very expensive drugs for a lifetime. And that lifetime—however long or short it may be—could include side effects, like sky-rocketing cholesterol counts and hypertension, that can leave you at high risk for coronary disease and strokes. Oh, and you'll still be able to pass the disease on to others.

So that's the scary stuff—now for some perspective. From a purely statistical standpoint, consider yourself fortunate if you're a North American nonintravenous-drug-using heterosexual male. Individuals in that category constitute only about 4 percent of new AIDS cases each year in the United States. In the 1990s, that translated to between 2,500 and 3,200 straight men annually.

The Centers for Disease Control and Prevention estimate that 60 percent of HIV-positive men in the United States were infected through homosexual sex, 25 percent through injection drug use, and 15 percent through heterosexual sex. Of newly infected men, approximately 50 percent are black.

It's a far different story in other points on the globe. As of this writing, 80 percent of new AIDS cases worldwide were transmitted via heterosexual intercourse. In sub-Saharan Africa, AIDS is the leading cause of death.

Why hasn't that happened in the United States? Here's where it gets complicated. Experts are quick to point out that it *could* happen. Luckily, there are a handful of things mitigating in our favor. We use condoms more regularly (though not consistently enough). We're also less likely to let other STDs go untreated. Herpes, gonorrhea, and chlamydia greatly increase your chances of catching the virus if you sleep with someone who's HIV-positive. That's because any inflammation increases the odds that the virus will enter your system. Unfortunately,

Hot Dates 1871 The Comstock Act made it illegal to mail information about abortion, birth control, or sex. By 1900, the law had resulted in the destruction of 98,563 items for "immoral" use of rubber.

Foreign Affairs
To this day, large numbers of young girls in India and throughout Africa, including in Egypt, are forced to endure clitoridectomies, in which their clitorises and most of their external genitals are cut away. Advocates say it dissuades virgins from premarital sex and douses women's desire for extramarital affairs once they've wed. **Our guess is that it doesn't make the women feel too amorous toward their husbands either.**

In Extremis
For a female bedbug, sex can be something to die for. The male bedbug breaks the shell of the fe-

True or Phallus?
Female black widow spiders kill and devour their mates after sex.

BAWDY BALLADS "If I Can't Sell It, I'll Keep Sittin' on It (Before I Give It Away)," *Georgia White*

continued on page 16

poor people living in places without ready access to appropriate antibiotics, such as sub-Saharan Africa, are much more likely to go untreated.

The disease is also more easily spread if there's a high amount of the virus in an infected person's system. North Americans are more likely to be treated with virus-suppressing drugs that others elsewhere in the world can't afford. While an infected person taking the cutting-edge drug cocktails can still pass on the disease, the odds of his doing so are considerably lower.

You know how to reduce your own risk. Maintain a monogamous relationship with someone who has been tested. Use a condom at all times with anyone whose HIV status you don't know. Avoid prostitutes: Their incidence of AIDS is much higher. Be aware that, along with intravenous drug use, the riskiest practices are penetrative sexual acts, including anal and vaginal intercourse and performing oral sex. (By the way, contrary to some urban legends, it's unlikely that you'll get AIDS from being on the receiving end of oral sex.)

And finally, make your sexual health a part of your yearly physical. Docs often won't ask unless you bring it up. If you have multiple partners, get yourself screened for STDs at the same time that you're having your cholesterol levels checked. Most tests consist of urine and blood samples. Testing is important because with some STDs, such as chlamydia, you may not have any outward symptoms. And as we mentioned, untreated STDs increase your risk of catching HIV from an infected partner.

Also see: fears/phobias, nonoxynol-9, prison, safe sex, STDs

airhead

For flyboys who've seen military action, it's the term for a landing area in enemy territory. For those seeking another kind of landing, *airhead* is probably the lowest rating on the intelligence scale that a prospective sex partner could earn, since it implies that there's nothing but air where a brain should be. How much this matters is up to you, of course, but be aware of two things: One, there's nothing gender specific about the term; 'nuff said. And two, even if it's true that airheads are easier to score with, you still have to talk to them afterward.

Also see: bimbo, communication, partner

alcohol

For all the attention it gets, the marriage of alcohol and sex comes down to two simple properties that you already know about. One is that alcohol lowers anxiety and inhibitions, which can help sexual things happen. The other is that it depresses the central nervous system, which can prevent sexual things (such as erections) from happening. So an oft-recommended approach is to drink moderately enough to enjoy the upside without the downside.

Fine. But here's another approach you can try: Separate sex from alcohol so that you can explore the former without the distraction of the latter. Yes, you can drown anxiety with booze, but you'll have a better time if you create a situation where there's no sexual anxiety to drown. In the long run, unaddressed inhibitions will limit your sex life.

In the short run, alcohol sabotages more than erections. It also screws up the skills you use for great sex. When you drink, you sacrifice control of your body. Your ability to communicate suffers. Your sensitivity to your partner's needs is shot to hell. And you smell funny.

This is not to suggest that you swear off alcohol or that sex after a shared bottle of wine is never a good idea. Just take a closer look at what really goes on when you fuel your sex with booze. You may decide that you'd rather drink with the guys and concentrate on other things with the ladies.

Also see: anticipatory anxiety, bars, drugs

Alcoholics Anonymous

Alcoholics Anonymous (AA) meetings are for sharing feelings, not phone numbers. Though it's no secret that plenty of men and women get together somewhere along those 12 steps. Now, alcohol abuse is not a recommended strategy for getting dates. And we're not suggesting that you go to AA for the babes. But all those meeting-generated couples bring up at least three good points to keep in mind if you're currently partnerless. One is that you don't need a drinking environment to meet women. Another is that *any* place where men and women interact is fertile territory. And finally, honesty and openness—which is what AA is all about—are more powerful attractants than sexual posturing and high-pressure come-ons.

Also see: bars, meeting women

anal beads

For true lovers of anal play only. Beads range in size from that of marbles to that of Ping-Pong balls, and they are attached to a string. Here's the idea: At some point

during your sexual encounter, you lube them up and slide them one by one up a rectum, hers or yours or both. Then you go about your erotic business, whatever that may be. At or near orgasm, you slowly pull them out—bumpety, bumpety, bump. Some people find this exquisite.

Not surprisingly, the sensation that makes anal beads so pleasurable for some is exactly what makes them uncomfortable for others. The nerve-ending-rich anus is so sensitive that the pressure from the little balls can simply be too much. Even a lot of anal bead veterans can't stand to pull them out right at climax; they either wait till things settle down a bit or time the extraction for just before orgasm.

If you want to go for it, make sure that your anal beads are made of silicone, with a silicone-coated string. The cheaper plastic jobs often have sharp or rough spots, the last thing you want. Plus, silicone is much easier to keep clean. To stay on the safe side, get two sets of beads—his and hers—so you're not sharing the beads or the bacteria they may pick up. As with any kind of anal sex, use lots of water-based lubricant. Make sure to wash the beads thoroughly between usages. And always check that the knot at the end of the string is tied, so the beads won't come off and necessitate an embarrassing explanation at the emergency room.

Also see: ben wa balls, boredom, kinky, klismaphilia, lubricants, rectum, rimming, sexual aids, sodomy, sphincter, suppositories

anal plug

Though it sounds rather like a plumbing device, an anal plug (or butt plug, if you prefer) is a sex toy, designed for pleasure.

It's more or less pine-tree-shaped for easy insertion into the anus, dildolike but much smaller. The key feature is the wide base that keeps the whole thing from getting swallowed into the rectum. Anal plugs come in various shapes and sizes and are available in either rubber or silicone. We recommend silicone because that type lasts longer and cleans up nicely.

An anal plug provides ongoing stimulation while you go about your sexual business, either alone or with company. Since it stays put on its own, your hands are free for other pursuits.

Start with the smallest one you can find at a sex shop. Use lots of lubrication. Forget about poking it in and out; letting it just sit there and react to your body movements will be action enough, at least at first. And until you're accustomed to it, keep it in for only 5 minutes or so. Once you're used to the sensations, you can leave it in for as long as is comfortable. If you find that you're clenching your muscles to keep it in place, remove it or you could develop anal-sphincter problems.

Our advice? Leave the marathon sessions to veteran butt pluggers, who've been known to wear them to the office. . . . Food for thought next time your secretary seems to be smiling her way through a staff meeting.

Also see: boredom, dildo, kinky, klismaphilia, rectum, rimming, role reversal, sexual aids, sphincter, suppositories, variety

anal sex

The opening of the rectum is loaded with nerve endings, making it a sensory-rich venue for sexual play. Since you and your partner each have one, the opportunities for anal pleasure are doubled. Sexual contact can be limited to the outer area or proceed into the canal itself and, in your case, all the way up to the prostate. Anal intercourse—penetration of the anus with the penis—is only the best known of an array of anal activities. The stimulation can also come from a finger, a tongue, or a sex toy.

Anal sex is more common among heterosexuals than you may think. Probably at least one in four straight men has tried it. Some male/female couples find anal play exquisite. Some avoid it because they consider it nasty, while others do it precisely *because* they find it nasty. Still others think it enhances sex because it fits into a role-playing or power game.

Of the millions of opinions about anal sex, only two matter—yours and your partner's. If the two of you like it and feel fine about it afterward, do it all you want.

But do it right. You can't just slide in the back door one night on a whim. As with any new sexual foray, the two of you should reach an understanding ahead of time. Decide what anal variation you might like to try first. Then, if you're going to insert anything, have plenty of water-based lubricant on hand; the anus doesn't self-lubricate, so friction can be too painful without it. Take it slow. Probe, don't thrust. Keep checking in with each other. How does it feel? Pull out—slowly—if there's any sharp pain.

You can move from the vagina to the anus, but you can't go back again: The anus hosts bacteria that you don't want to introduce elsewhere. And not only should you always wear a condom during both anal and vaginal sex, you should wear a *different* one for each activity.

Finally, to make the experience that much more pleasurable, consider mutual bathing as mandatory foreplay and afterplay, with special attention paid to the featured orifice.

Also see: hygiene, lubricants, pederast, rectum, rimming, role reversal, size—ass, size—penis, sodomy, sphincter

androgyny

The possession of both male (andro) and female (gyn) characteristics. Medically speaking, that can describe a hermaphrodite, the anomaly of the animal (and human) world that boasts both male and female genitals. Androgyny, then, can put a whole new twist on the idea of solo sex.

The way you hear the word used around the sexual scene these days has more to do with appearance than with anatomy. Androgyny is a look, especially a lesbian look that's neither femme nor butch. But androgynous fashion isn't exclusively the domain of homosexuals or bisexuals. In fact, there's no evidence that it says anything about sexual orientation. Tomboys, for example, adopt a look that's both traditionally male and recognizably female, and therefore neither. Yet most tomboys are heterosexual.

Also see: cross-dressing, femme, gender bender, hermaphrodite, transvestism, yin and yang

anima and animus

Psychology pioneer Carl Jung's Latin labels for the female (anima) and male (animus) sides of the human soul. Anima is sensitive, receptive, emotional. Animus is active, aggressive, independent. That's hardly news, but here's the kicker: Everybody has both. In fact,

anima usually refers specifically to the feminine side of a man. It's the shadow existence of even the most macho guy. Whatever else you got, you got anima.

Don't fight it. Celebrate it. Embrace your anima. Jung believed that a man becomes whole only when he integrates his anima and animus. Modern sex therapists believe pretty much the same thing—that your sex life is more fulfilling when you allow your feminine side to participate. That doesn't mean putting on a bra or changing your sexual preference. But it does mean paying attention to and acting on your more feminine impulses when they arise. This could be as simple as allowing yourself to be more tender and loving toward your partner. Or it could be telling her that you want her to "do" you or hold you down or even slip a finger inside you. Whatever your pleasure, sex can be more fun if you don't limit yourself to traditionally masculine behavior.

Also see: AC/DC, hermaphrodite, heterosexuality, role reversal, yin and yang

animals

Think your woman should be more of an animal in bed? Sure, it would be great if she (and you, too, for that matter) were less inhibited, louder, more inclined to sniff and lick and grunt. But sex that's literally animalistic is something you don't want.

Here's why: Most animal sex behavior is stereotyped, meaning that animals do only what they're genetically programmed to do—no more, no less. Zero creativity. No fun. Boring. And with just a few exceptions, females in the animal kingdom can (or will) copulate only when they're ovulating and fertile. We humans are virtually alone in our capacity to get it on anytime and anywhere. Would you really have it any other way?

Unlike animals, we're free to have sex for reasons other than reproduction—reasons like intimacy, emotion, pleasure, fun. Because we're human, sex is charged with meaning for us. And that's exactly what eroticism is: sexuality with meaning. Animals are sexual but not erotic. We're both, with limitless possibilities for sexual pleasure available to us.

So you don't want your woman to be more animal-like in bed. You want her to be more human.

Also see: bestiality, love

anticipatory anxiety

You've just hung up the phone after she's agreed to go out on a date next weekend, and you're already "feeling around" for an elusive hard-on. Or maybe you're on that date, but you come too soon—shortly after they serve the salad at dinner. Despite their apparently antithetical results, both of these problems stem from the same root causes: Too much thinking. "Am I going to be able to get the job done?" Too many questions. "Will I please her?" "Geez, is this as big as it's going to get when she's in the room?" Too much worrying. "I'll think of baseball.... I'll think of Marge Schott.... And then I'll think, 'Oh, baby, it's outta here! Grand slam!'"

What anticipatory anxiety actually "anticipates" is none other than that gunshy troublemaker, performance anxiety, and its trigger-happy kid brother, premature ejaculation. So you've got another term, but the same old problems.

And you'll continue to have them as long as you keep thinking of sex as a performance. The good news is that since anticipatory anxiety hits early, you've got time to do something about it now and have great sex later. Keeping in mind that she, too, may be anxious, steer the conversation toward the upcoming sexual activity. Go ahead and tell her that you're nervous. That may be the last thing you'd think of doing, but you're much more likely to elicit an anxiety-lowering response from her by talking about your concerns than by fooling her into thinking that they don't exist.

Keep talking. Tell her how you'd like to feel while making love to her (carefree, close) and how you don't want to feel (pressured). Then get her to reveal her feelings about having sex with you. Knowing her true desires is less stress-provoking than dreading expectations that she may not even have.

A nice bonus is that all this verbal foreplay can be pretty thrilling in its own right. But you're really doing it to see your looming bedmate as what she really is: a sexual partner, not an audience. Without an audience, there's no performance to be anxious about.

Also see: alcohol, clumsiness, performance anxiety, premature ejaculation, self-esteem, shyness, spectatoring

aphrodisiac

There's no such thing, but there are plenty available to you. Contradictory? Only because the word *aphrodisiac* is thrown around so wildly. Is an aphrodisiac something that improves your physical sexual functioning? Then Viagra is certainly an aphrodisiac for men with erection problems (as is good health for everybody). Is it something that makes sex more likely? Alcohol qualifies, then, insofar as it reduces the inhibition that may stand between attraction and consummation. Is it anything that makes sex a better experience? If so, this book is full of aphrodisiac possibilities, from A to Z. Or is it something that makes you feel sexy? Again, tons of things work for one person or another. For you, it may be confidence. For her, it may be chocolate.

But let's get real here. The aphrodisiac that man has been searching for throughout history isn't any of those things. It's a potion that will make a particular woman want to have sex with you and only you, right here and right now. *That's* what's had folks grinding up rhinoceros horns and extracting sheep testicles all these centuries. We're here to tell you that such a thing doesn't exist, will never exist, and shouldn't exist.

Sex is too complex to be distilled into a single potion. Sexual desire alone involves physical, psychological, social, cultural, and situational components, and no two people combine those components in the same way. Even if some mad scientist were to come up with a formula that would influence all those factors simultaneously, he would have to learn about the specific target's sexual makeup and customize the potion. Good old-fashioned courtship or seduction would work a lot faster.

The best aphrodisiac advice is like the best financial advice. To have money, you can work steadily, spend frugally, save faithfully, and invest wisely. Or you can try to win the lottery. To have sex, you can pay attention to who she is, learn what she wants, make her comfortable with you, and then go about creating the conditions most likely to lead to her arousal. Or you can hunt for an aphrodisiac. The first strategy may not always

work. But the second probably never will.

Also see: arousal, courtship, oysters, power, seduction, sexual attraction, Spanish fly, travel as an aphrodisiac, yohimbine

appointments

For sex, that is. With your wife or girlfriend. Strange as it sounds, appointments are highly recommended for any couple whose once-frequent interludes of passion have given way to work, kids, and more work.

Sure, scheduled sex sounds cold and calculated. It's like lumping lovemaking in with the business lunches and dentist visits. What about romance? What about spontaneity?

Here's a better question: What about all those sexless weeks slipping by because, by the time you fall into bed, both of you are too beat to do anything but sleep? Not much romance or spontaneity in that state of affairs, is there? But it is indeed common these days—the price we pay for being so damn successful.

Do yourselves a favor. Overcome that reflex resistance to the idea of sex appointments. Put down "Sex with So-And-So" at least once on your week's agenda—and make sure So-And-So does the same thing. Any time that works is a good time, but beware the late-night date. That's the fatigue-filled default hour for sex that probably led you to unplanned abstinence in the first place.

Having trouble making an open slot for sex time? Then do the following: Set aside your daily planners, both of you. Take a deep breath. Ask yourselves (with appropriate alarm), "What has happened to our priorities?" Turn back to your daily planner and proceed until you've nailed down the appointment. Make a mutual vow to keep it.

What you'll find is that the whole idea of sex appointments isn't so cold and calculated after all. Anticipation is part of sex, and you now have something specific to anticipate. You may even react as you did when the two of you were dating—dreamy, nervous, practically drooling with expectation. This is logical, since a date is exactly what you've made. Try it.

Also see: boredom, fatigue, sex—lack of, variety

arguing

The two of you actually have more to worry about if you *don't* argue.

Any couple who are together longer than a few dates are going to see in each other things that they don't like. And they're going to find holes in their relationship that need filling. If you never argue, either you're burying these issues or you just don't give a damn. Burying the issues creates time bombs. Worse, not giving a damn means your relationship has already bombed.

So go ahead, argue. But do it right. You want your conflicts to be infrequent, productive, and civilized. Learn to constantly and comfortably communicate about your relationship. Chew over potential problems before they grow into fodder for open warfare. Also, analyze the anatomy of your arguments. Couples tend to bicker over recurring themes, like control, power, or freedom. Each argument may seem unique, but strip away the superficial triggers and you'll probably find you're rehashing the same things time and again.

In a perfect world, you'd come out of your tiff with improved mutual understanding and progress toward solving the underlying conflict. Alas, if you're typically imperfect, neither one of you thinks any progress has been made until the other is in 100 percent agreement with your way of thinking.

Hot Dates Circa 1900 "Sex education" pamphlets warned against masturbation and told teens to suppress their sexual thoughts by thinking of their mother's pure love, or sitting with their testicles in ice water.

continued from page 9

Answer:
True. But not every time. Like most things involving females, it's a mystery what makes Mrs. Spider decide to take her mate's life.

male and deposits sperm in special pouches in her itty-bitty body. If she mates with more than a half-dozen males, she'll probably succumb to her wounds.

Even kinkier: **The males are switch-hitters** in the sex game, with special organs to accept the sperm of other males. So a female may receive not just the sperm of the male with whom she mates but also that of his homosexual partner.

LEGAL BRIEFS
A Wisconsin couple sued a bakery, alleging that after their three-tiered wedding cake failed to arrive at their reception, they were too stressed to consummate the marriage.

The groom claimed that the marriage remained unconsummated for 3 days, while his bride added that **she didn't "actively" participate in sex for 2 weeks**.

BAWDY BALLADS "Get on Top," *Tim Buckley*

continued on page 23

One useful trick for overcoming such unproductive tendencies is the no-accusation rule: You both try to couch your statements not so much in terms of what the other person is doing but rather of how you feel about it. The theory here is that "I'm feeling hurt by what's been going on" is more likely to get through her protective shields than "You're hurting me." This ploy needs to be obeyed in spirit, not just in letter, since there's not much difference between "You're a jerk" and "I feel that you're a jerk."

Another good strategy is for each of you to repeat what the other has just said before responding to it. This not only forces you to listen to and (ideally) understand what she says but also *proves* to her that you're listening and trying to understand.

Problem is, the heat of battle may not be the ideal time to try out communication techniques. Table the discussion as soon as you agree that it's getting you nowhere. There's no law that says you have to solve this thing today. At least the problem is now out in the open. Sleeping on it is a lot better than a premature, false—and therefore doomed—resolution. Go ahead and take it up again tomorrow, with cooler heads. Just make sure you do resume the discussion so neither of you feels that your concerns are being ignored.

One last tip: Repeated fever-pitch anger or any actual violence indicates a problem that goes way beyond whatever you're arguing about. Get help. Professional counseling or a discussion with a trusted physician, clergyman, or friend is a good idea.

Also see: communication, divorce—avoiding, making up, violence, withholding

aromatherapy

It combines ancient wisdom and recent research in its use of fragrances for healing or just improving your quality of life. The idea is that the scent from highly concentrated essential oils (usually distilled from herbs or flowers) helps your olfactory membranes to create subtle but positive internal changes.

Given the cozy relationship between scent and sex, you might expect aromatherapy to claim to help in the bedroom. It does. Here are some of the top sex-enhancing scents of the last few thousand years.

The ancient Greeks considered the licorice smell of anise to be sex-conducive, and it still ranks high among both men and women in scent-preference surveys. Ginger was the Persians' scent of "burning desire." As for rose, there must be some reason why it's inspired love through the ages. Jasmine is associated with the night, when passions bloom. More clinically speaking, it's thought to increase your awareness of your surroundings by promoting the brain's electrical waves. Sandalwood, which aromatherapists say mimics the human scent, is all the rage these days, much as patchouli was in the 1960s.

Essential oils are strong; the ones we mention shouldn't touch your skin in an undiluted form. The general recommendation for dilution is 15 to 18 drops of the essential oil to 1 ounce of a carrier oil, such as sweet almond, olive, or vegetable oil.

You can find essential oils at health food stores; and when you buy them, you'll see that there are lots of ways to get the scent working in a room, including scented candles, incense sticks, steam devices, fancy diffusers, and simple spray bottles. Have some fun with this, and make sure that your partner is into it. If you just spring it on her, she'll get the aroma part right away but miss the therapy implications. She also may hate the smell, a problem that could have been avoided with some agreement at the outset.

Also see: fragrances, pheromones, scents

arousal

Arousal is the body's sexual response, the one that gets a penis erect and a vagina lubricated. Being turned on implies a physical *and* psychological state, but the two operate independently and don't always join forces. You can feel sexual desire without it leading to physical arousal. And vice versa—for instance, you can get erect from rubbing up against a table without, we assume, desiring sex with the table. What's more, there are degrees of arousal. You can be aroused enough to get an erection yet not aroused enough to sustain it. And women who aren't sufficiently aroused are unlikely to enjoy intercourse; they may even find it painful.

This is why extended foreplay is such a good idea. But be clear on what's really going on. You're not arousing her per se; you're helping her experience her own arousal. So taking signals from her usually works better than calling all the shots yourself.

Your own arousal? Well, everybody has certain "arousal conditions"—about themselves, about their partners, and about their environments.

You may, for example, need to feel 100 percent awake to get in the mood; sleepy sex may just not do it for you.

That's a condition about yourself. One about your partner may be a certain body type. One about your environment might be a need for complete privacy. And that's how you can enhance mutual arousal: by putting a little thought into what your respective conditions are and then creating them as much as possible.

Also see: atmosphere, erection, foreplay, preference

athletic sex

In the movies, there are just two kinds of good sex. One takes place in gauzy slow motion, with a syrupy musical score and sheets that never slip from their strategic placement. The other is a hyperactive gymnastic routine. He spends a lot of time carrying her around the room, knocking over furniture but never becoming uncoupled. She, in turn, bounces on top of him like he's a trampoline. We assume they're satisfied afterward, but we *know* they're exhausted.

Sex that's more like the latter than the former is sometimes called athletic, which is not to be confused with rough sex. Athletic sex can be a lot of fun for those whose tastes (and conditioning) run that way. What it shouldn't be is some sort of standard for measuring passion. There's nothing inherently more gratifying about physically demanding sex. It's just one way of going about things. And it's fine. But if your aim is to score sexual-prestige points by putting on an impressive physical display, you may be missing the best of what sex offers.

Also see: exercise, rough sex, standing positions, sweating, wild women

atmosphere

It comes down to three little words: *time*, *place*, and *person*. If you're annoyed, tired, drunk, or otherwise incapacitated, it's the wrong time. It's the wrong place if it's haunted by unwelcome associations, too dirty for your tastes, insufficiently private, or otherwise uncomfortable. And if it's the wrong person, all bets are off. So repeat that mantra—time, place, and person—as you seek an environment suitable to getting in the mood.

As for creating a seductive atmosphere. . . . Music, scents, flowers, art, lighting, pillows, videos—you have a million ways to go but only one important piece of advice to follow: Do it *your* way. Don't create atmosphere just because you think she'll like it. You have to be into it too. Don't do anything just to impress her. And don't overdo it. An atmosphere created for the sole purpose of manipulating her into having sex risks backfiring big-time. An atmosphere that sincerely reflects your own sensuality sends the right message—and it's sure to please at least one of you.

Also see: fantasies, flowers, fragrances, mood

attraction

Though *sexual* attraction is complicated, what makes you attractive in a more general sense isn't. Now, don't scoff at the idea of nonsexual attraction. For one thing, a platonic female friend can be the best sexual confidante and counselor you'll ever find. Plus, even the hottest couples need something besides sexual interest to sustain them. And finally, being connected with other human beings—male and female—is just plain healthy. They can't *all* be sexual partners.

What makes you attractive may not be what you expect. First off, you have to want to be attractive. Women sense when a man is open to the idea of attracting others, and they respond to it. That's why it makes sense to dress up a bit on a date. It's not just that you look better but that you send the L'Oréal-esque message that she's worth it. Women like that, just as you like that quality in them.

Just know where the line is drawn. When self-possession becomes self-centeredness, the attraction meter plummets. For example, the immature guy calls attention to his own pecs to attract a woman. The attractive guy calls attention to *her* eyes. (No, he doesn't call attention to her "pecs"—at least not right off.)

A woman is also attracted to a man with whom she can feel relaxed (even if, ironically, she's excited by him at the same time). And she is least likely to relax with a guy who comes off as obsessed with his own agenda, be it his job, his snowboarding, his gun collection, or his desire to have sex with her. Don't be that guy.

Also see: dating, meeting women, preference, self-esteem, sexual attraction

B

back

You don't think of it as a key body part for sex . . . till it hurts.

A bad back restricts your mobility, making sex a chore. It can also erase your erection (as any pain has a way of doing). And the sad fact is, 8 out of 10 men do have back problems at one time or another. For some, it's most of the time. If that's you, your first order of business is to acknowledge that chronic back pain or stiffness is interfering with your sex life. Forget about trying to hide the obvious—from yourself or your partner. Talk about it. She'll probably appreciate the information and happily take up the challenge to help make things work better. And she can indeed help.

Of course, you can help yourself too. To rid yourself of one major cause of chronic lower-back pain, take your wallet out of your back pocket. When you sit on it, it tilts your pelvis and puts stress on your sci-

atic nerve. Carry it in your front pocket or in your coat or suit jacket. Better yet, leave it home and let her pick up the tab.

Since that alone probably won't completely solve the problem, take an aspirin or some other anti-inflammatory about an hour before you plan to have sex. Then, spend some of that hour in a hot tub. Finally, stretch for 3 minutes or so before going into action. To stretch your lower back and hips, lie on your back, hold the back of your right knee with your right hand, and pull toward your chest. Hold the stretch for 30 seconds. Switch legs and repeat. Your partner can help by putting her hand on the front of your calf, just below your knee, and gently pushing your knee to your chest. When you feel the stretch, let her hold it for 30 seconds, then have her release. Switch legs. Next, have her push both of your knees to your chest, for a full stretch across your lower back. This is one time when a small amount of wine can help loosen you up, in more ways than one.

Invite her to start off the erotic touching with a gentle back massage. Then, when it's time for more energetic play, the two of you can seek back-saving positions. First, lie flat on your back. The floor is a good sex surface—it won't shift and bounce like a bed. Put a folded towel under the small of your back to maintain a natural arch. Stick a pillow under your knees to take pressure off your lower spine.

From there, you can gently engage in any sexual activity that doesn't require you to exert yourself. Try massage or oral sex. In fact, this is a great position for sixty-nine. When you're both ready, she can flip around and straddle you from above. Make sure she takes it slow; even if you're the passive partner, sudden movements on her part that cause you to move jerkily can still prompt screams—and not the good kind.

If you tire of the woman-on-top position, she can sit or lie on a bed or chair that puts her pelvis at penis level when you're kneeling in front of her. You can enter her comfortably while betwixt her legs. This position allows you to control the pace without putting stress on your aching back.

Hard as it is to see anything good in a bad back, think of it as an opportunity to explore new sexual pleasures. Your search for back-friendly positions is also a search for new joys. And toning down the pace and athleticism is more than a boon for your back. It also opens the door to calmer, more meditative and intimate sexual satisfaction for both of you. Keep all that in mind, and you just may come out ahead on the deal.

Also see: athletic sex, body fitness, disability—overcoming, exercise, massage, sixty-nine (69)

bars

They're often associated with the dark side of sex: empty gratification, disease, danger. Even the heartiest of party guys hesitates to brag about having met his fiancée in a bar. And singles bars suffer from the ultimate reputation killer: They're out of style.

But don't swear off saloons as mate-meeting sites. In fact, bars offer a key advantage in the hunt for romance. Call it context clarification. If you sense subtle signals from a woman nearby, there's a better chance that they indicate sexual interest if you're sitting in a bar than if you're in a medical clinic.

Of course, there are bars and there are bars, so do a little context control yourself. Frequent an establishment where the kind of woman you're seeking feels comfortable and where the atmosphere is conducive to approaching people. You're not going to find Ms. Right at a seedy dive full of retching drunks (at least, not unless you get turned on by holding her hair while she hurls). Nor will you get anywhere at a staid lounge where everybody wants to be left alone.

As for singles bars . . . Despite their passé rep, they've adapted rather than perish. Poke around, and you'll find that lots of today's trendy clubs offer something suspiciously close to what singles bars once offered: a theater in which to play out the human mating dance. It's just that the owners and patrons—no dummies, they—avoid the discredited term *singles bar.*

And what about the reasons those bars got discredited in the first place? Well, we're smarter now than in 1980 (albeit just as horny). We know that safe sex is always best and that HIV and other sexually transmitted diseases don't particularly care whether the two of you met in a bar or a church. We know that getting to know your partner for more than a few hours means safer, not to mention more satisfying, sex.

And we know that keeping your alcohol consumption to moderate levels is not only less deadly but also more fun. Lushes don't usually get very far with the opposite sex (and sometimes can't get very far, even if given the chance). If going to a bar guarantees that you'll get blitzed, find another way to meet women. Try an Alcoholics Anonymous meeting, for starters.

Also see: alcohol, eye contact, flirtation, meeting women, one-night stand, pickup lines, signals, singles scene

beard burn

Straight men aren't often on the receiving end of a sandpaper beard, so we seldom appreciate how much it hurts. And you know when it bothers a woman the most? During oral sex. Her thighs are soft. Her thighs are sensitive. And her thighs are getting scratched at a time when she should be focused on the pleasure she's feeling in between them. It doesn't matter that you're aware of your 5-o'clock shadow and you promise to be careful. You can't be careful enough. Besides, careful is the last thing you want to be. You should be able to let yourself go crazy without worrying about your cactus face getting in the way.

This one is a no-brainer: Leave the 2-days'-growth look to the empty-headed teen idols who started it. Either shave it smooth or grow it out. (Once it reaches the true beard stage, facial hair is far more tolerable. It's the stubble that makes women homicidal.) And if you're clean-shaven and planning on getting lucky tonight, shave again in the afternoon. It's a small price to pay for unbridled sex—and to avoid having your ears yanked off just as you're getting into it.

Also see: give head

beauty

There's no denying it: Physical beauty is desirable in sex. When was the last time you fantasized about making it with Barbra Streisand? What's that you say? You think Streisand is really hot? Or you know someone else who does? That brings

Hot Dates 1901 Dr. Prince Morrow, who conducted a study of venereal disease, estimated that some 75 percent of New York City men had been infected with gonorrhea and that 5 to 18 percent had syphilis.

Seemed like a Good Idea at the Time...

Of all the many ingenious items devised to help men put more lead in their pencils, the Male Electronic Genital Stimulator has to be one of the most embarrassing. It's a small, battery-operated gizmo with external controls that allow a man to regulate the amount of current he sends to pudendal nerves in the lower spine; a malfunction of these nerves can cause sexual dysfunction. The device's main drawback? A guy has to insert it into his anus before—and leave it there during—intercourse.

True or Phallus?

Saltpeter—potassium nitrate—inhibits sexual desire.

BAWDY BALLADS "Hot, Wet, and Sticky" *Galaxy*

continued on page 30

us to our point. There's no such thing as absolute beauty, sexually speaking. What you consider perfect beauty in a woman is really just a perception, and it's influenced by lots of factors. Biology, for example, bases beauty on facial symmetry, a sign of healthy support for the gene pool. Culture, on the other hand, creates its own norms of beauty, such that a total babe in one society couldn't get a date in another. (Most of the Western world is blessed with commercial mass media that make sure we never forget what our norms of beauty are.)

The upshot? If you insist on a certain standard of physical attractiveness, you're cheating yourself. When sizing up potential sex partners, there's a better payoff in focusing on whatever features have erotic potential for you than there is in seeking status points via some overall beauty goal. Translation: If she has a really nice ass, concentrate on that instead of worrying about the ever-so-slight bump on the bridge of her nose. And often, once you hit it off with that less-than-perfect-but-not-so-bad someone, an amazing thing happens: She becomes gorgeous. A man in love sees his partner a lot more positively.

Remember, beauty is a perception—and a perception based on love or sexual attraction is as legitimate as any other.

Also see: attraction, body shapes, interracial sex, legs, preference, sexual attraction, sexy, size—ass, size—breasts, size—nose

beds

The best bed for sex is the kind with clean sheets. As long as it's big enough for two, everything else is a matter of taste. Let sleep-quality factors determine mattress firmness and frame type. What matters for sex is that your sheets, blan-

kets, and comforter are sensuous, inviting, and—we'll say it again—clean. Bachelors, take note.

Now, turn your attention to the room that your bed is in. Sex therapists suggest that you try sex outside the bedroom, which you do sometimes. Sleep experts urge that you reserve the bedroom for sleep only, which you also do sometimes. But your bedroom is still where most of the action takes place. So do yourself a favor and eroticize the environment. Get rid of your torn, scratchy polyester sheets, and invest in a few sets of soft and silky linens. Place a night table or two close to the bed for easy access to birth control, lubricants, and whatever other little extras you use in your love life. And get the exercise equipment and television out of there, along with the old newspapers and dirty laundry.

Yeah, yeah, we understand that there's no place else to put the weight bench. We also agree that late-night movies in bed are one of life's indispensable luxuries. And it's true that for a lot of couples with good sex lives, all that background clutter doesn't matter when push comes to shove. But it's still a good idea to reestablish sex as the highest and best use of your bedroom and to at least consider the possibility that all the extraneous stuff may be interfering with intimacy.

Whatever you decide, *wash those sheets*.

Also see: biological clock, body oils, boredom, hygiene, pubic lice

beefcake

Male cheesecake, with the emphasis on brawn and virility over the pretty-boy look. Beefcake exists in the flesh (for example, Chippendales dancers), but, like cheesecake, it's more associated with commercial photography. A beefcake model exudes testosterone and a sculpted physique but not much depth of character. He's a boy toy. The relatively new beefcake craze means women now have what men have long had: lots of idealized images of the opposite sex to lust after. It also means that men now have what women have long had: media-imposed standards of aesthetic sex appeal that are impossible to live up to.

Also see: abs, body fitness, muscles, stud muffin

beer

Prepare for some sacrilege here. We'd like to humbly suggest that you forgo the brew in any situation that might qualify as a sexual prelude, especially with a new or prospective partner. Yes, we know that it's a man's inalienable right—protected by the Magna Carta, the U.S. Constitution, and properly interpreted Scripture—to drink beer whenever and wherever he may please. We know that nothing else goes quite as well with Mexican or German food. And we know that there are some suds-loving women in this world who can outquaff the Oakland Raiders. Still, we're guessing that you like sex at least as much as beer. Try to separate the two.

Here's why. First of all, beer is alcohol, an overrated icebreaker that often puts up more obstacles to good sex than it breaks down. But even assuming that there are benefits in a pre-passion aperitif, beer doesn't cut it. It makes you stupid. (We can't back that up with any hard evidence, but look around the next time your pals are busting it up during Monday Night Football). It makes you

burp. It makes you run to the john. It makes your breath smell like the corner taproom. Most of all, beer sends her the wrong message. It tells her that being with her is no different from hanging with the guys. It tells her that your time together is just another reason to drink beer. Justly or not, ordering a cold one when you're alone with her might create the impression that she doesn't "have it"—and that maybe you don't, either.

We're not suggesting that you pop for a $12 cognac just to impress the lady. And we're not intimating that you adopt some entirely phony suave persona. Look at it this way: You're a combination of personalities. You're one way with the guys, another way with your parents or in-laws, still another way with kids around. All of those different yous are just compartmentalized, slightly modified versions of the total you. We're suggesting that you access a version of yourself that communicates a simple yet important thought: "Being with this woman is special."

So order something you can share—a bottle of wine, champagne, some sake—anything but a pitcher of brew. Or suggest something exotic that you'd like the two of you to try. If you really want to go off the deep end, go for the ultimate sacrilege: Skip the drinks altogether. Look into her eyes and say, "Tonight I'm on the wagon because I want to concentrate on you completely, with all my senses. I'm having jasmine tea."

Actually, you may end up calling for a shot of whiskey anyway, to revive her after she faints upon hearing such a thing. That's something you can tell your buddies about over a few beers.

Also see: alcohol, Alcoholics Anonymous, bars, drugs

begging

It would not be imprudent to say that men generally prefer dogs over cats. Women, in turn, are fonder of cats than of dogs. There are likely many reasons for this, but we're only interested in one: begging.

Dogs beg. Incessantly. Cats do not. Instead, they haughtily turn away, tails in the air. And women flock to them. See the parallel?

When you paw at a woman for a little nookie, you appear, to her, very much like a slobbering dog. And unless she's into Saint Bernards and peanut butter, that's turn-off city.

Besides, it's wholly beneath you. It assumes that women want sex less than men do and that men must always initiate the action—two stereotypes that we'd dearly love to break.

If in the past you've found yourself pleading too much, we have a solution for you. Employing it requires some gumption, but it has major payoffs over the long haul. It's simply this: Stop initiating sex. For now. Be as charming, playful, and affectionate as you can be, but do not let your actions cross over into the sexual.

You're going to have to take matters into your own hands for a while, so to speak. Do it without making a big, pouty deal out of it. A few weeks may go by, maybe even months. So be it. Keep glad-handing on a regular basis; don't let the frustration build too much, or you'll get ornery and start wandering over that line we told you not to cross.

After a while, she'll be the one initiating sex. Let her. But hang with your game plan a bit longer. One time does not make a habit. Get her accustomed to coming to you. Hey, it's fun being a cat.

Also see: boredom, communication, desperate, flirtation, horny, masher, masturbation, mood, rejection—sexual, seduction, turn-ons, withholding

ben wa balls

Though supposedly handed down to us by the wise keepers of oriental tradition, they're great for a gag gift but not much else. This pair of hollow metal balls, neither quite an inch in diameter, have smaller balls inside. A woman is supposed to insert them into her vagina so that when she goes about her daily activities, the inner balls move around inside the hollow outer balls, causing subtle vibrations that will send her into paroxysms of pleasure. Or so we're told.

If some jokester gave you a pair as an anniversary present, your significant other can insert them as an exercise in vaginal sensory perception or muscle control. And she can leave them in there as a little added attraction during intercourse, though we don't recommend deep thrusting if she does. Otherwise, just give 'em to your cat to play with.

Also see: anal beads

best friend's wife

What kind of a guy would make it with his best friend's wife? You know the answer to that one already.

But we'll tell you something that maybe you didn't know: The thought is going to cross your mind someday, if it hasn't already. This is true even if—especially if—the two of you enjoy that chummy kind of friendship where sex is so far from either of your plans that you think nothing of being in otherwise sexually charged situations.

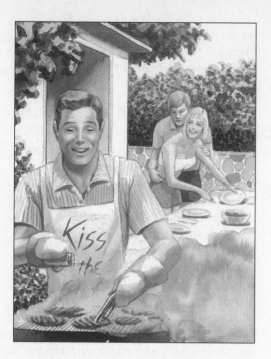

So, there the two of you are, watching TV in their bedroom while your main man is working late. Or there you are, in the time-share condo while he's out on the slopes. You've enjoyed just hanging out a thousand times with no complications . . . until one day, there's an unexpected shift in the atmosphere. Suddenly, you see her less as your buddy's wife and more as a woman.

You want her. And she might very well want you too.

Realize first that the desire itself is understandable. Neither of you is to blame, and neither of you is doing anything wrong. Unplanned-for moments of mutual lust make sense in this context since the two of you are together so much. The usual strategy for avoiding unwanted sexual complications—staying the hell away from her—is still the best advice, but it may not be an option here. At least not all of the time.

So what do you do if that day comes along when you're unavoidably together and you think you see that certain light in her eyes? Just follow Nike's advice in reverse: *Don't* do it. You are 100 percent responsible for what happens, no matter what she does. A real man doesn't say, "I couldn't help it" or "It just happened." Tell her, "Look, I'd love to, but I'm not going to." If you mean it, you'll say it like you mean it, and that will be the end of that. All three of you will be glad you took charge of the situation. Look at it as an opportunity to solidify your friendship—with her and with him (whether he knows it or not).

Also see: affairs, boss's wife, discretion, fantasies, guilt, horny, jealousy, lust, risky sex, sexual attraction, sloppy sex, swinging, travel ruins relationships, trust—rebuilding, wife's best friend, winking

bestiality

Sex with an animal is very common in mythology and is not all that rare as harmless sexual fantasy. You can find it in some of the raunchier pornography. In real life, though, cross-species sex is strictly taboo.

Which is not to say that it doesn't happen. It does and has throughout history. One of the shockers of biologist Alfred Kinsey's sex research was the revelation that plenty of good old American farmboys were molesting the livestock or practicing animal husbandry with their embraceable ewes. And a few 1950s housewives, Kinsey found, were taking care of their pets in ways that

June Cleaver never imagined. Today, advocates of "the zoosexual lifestyle" plead their bizarre case on the Internet and justify their actions as being based on a powerful love of animals. They've failed to convince the growing animal rights movement, however, which condemns bestiality (or zoophilia) as "interspecies sexual assault."

Our take: Do we really need to have this argument? Let's just forget about fooling around with the fauna. Have your sex with human beings.

Also see: compulsive behavior, fantasies, paraphilias, perversions, pets, pornography, sex therapy, sodomy, taboos, zoophilia

bidet

An ingenious hygienic device that you sit on as you would a toilet, while adjustable jets of water cleanse your genitals and anus more thoroughly and enjoyably than any amount of messy wiping. Given its obvious pre- and post-coital usefulness, it's a little strange that the bidet (which, while French, is pronounced along the lines of the Australian greeting "G'day") hasn't caught on in the United States.

You can have a freestanding bidet installed near your toilet (if you have the space) or have the jet devices added to your standard commode (if you don't). Also, some of the more froufrou hotels may offer a suite with a bidet in the bath-

room. Or you could always move to France.

Also see: anal sex, French, hygiene, klismaphilia, rimming

bimbo

The reigning queen of female stereotypes. Some beer-sotted boors use the term as a putdown of women in general, but it usually means something pretty specific. A true bimbo is clueless but doesn't know it. She's also gorgeous and well-aware of it. From a guy's point of view, she's the sexual equivalent of cotton candy.

But here's the weird part: Plenty of men are gung-ho for such a dish, to the exclusion of more fulfilling fare. And it's not always because they're as dumb as the bimbos they go for. Though beauty and brains may be the ideal combination

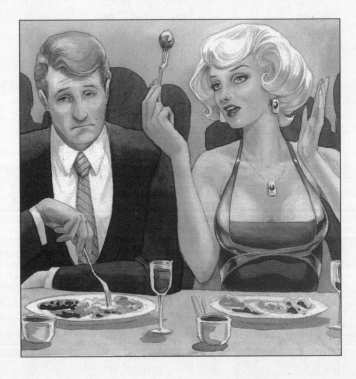

that *you* seek in a woman, for certain guys the brains just get in the way of the beauty. This may be a throwback to the bad old days when women were relegated to sex-object status, but who's to judge the druthers of others?

So if you want to star in "I Married a Bimbo," don't be swayed by political correctness. Just be prepared to pay the price. That price may include loneliness. It may include a lack of intellectual stimulation from your partner. It may include zero emotional intimacy. And it may include constant insecurity, as richer blokes make their moves. Worth it? Your call.

By the way, not too long ago *bimbo* was slang for a guy—just any guy. As the term began to be applied to the female gender, it initially implied a lady of loose morals before coming to connote a brainless bombshell. And now, of course, you'll hear about male bimbos, or himbos—that is, hunks of slow-witted beefcake, the masculine equivalents of bimbos. We've come full circle.

Also see: beefcake, jealousy, Madonna/whore complex, trophy wife, young women/older men

biological clock

This term is used to describe two different physical phenomena. One is the immutable biological fact that the human female's ovulating days are finite, ending with menopause around age 50. Furthermore, having children after age 40 or so puts a woman at a higher risk for pregnancy complications. Since many modern women don't even think about having children while in their 20s, their 30s may be marked by a sense of urgency about making the big motherhood decision. Their biological clocks are ticking. This

can be a real struggle for them, and you'd do well to take it seriously.

The other biological clock is just as real, but there's more you can do about it. This clock is set to your internal body rhythms, also called circadian rhythms, and it determines your peak hours of the day—including what time is prime time for sex. It's an issue if, say, you're a morning kind of guy and she's hottest at the midnight hour. But these are preferences, not requirements. We're willing to bet that if you prefer sex in the morning, that doesn't mean you hate it at night. So work it out, you two. Try this: Get in bed together a half-hour earlier. You'll have more energy to oblige her nocturnal desires. Then, wake up a half-hour earlier, giving her more time to adapt to your A.M.-oriented biological clock. Hey, do this right and you could have twice as much sex.

Also see: aging, appointments, fatigue, fertility

birth control

See: contraception

birthdays

If she's a new lover—or you want her to be—find out early when her birthday is. You don't need to be surreptitious about it: This is not information that women usually withhold (at least not till they reach middle age, when many prefer to avoid the subject entirely). Once armed with a date, you have left the simple matter of what to get her. . . . Okay, it's not so simple. Rare is the decision that produces more stress and sweat than a birthday present for the woman with whom you're sexually involved.

Make it easy on yourself. Forget about knocking her off her feet with the world's most original birthday present. Stay away from anything elaborate, esoteric, comic, or potentially embarrassing. Just focus on pleasing her and giving her what she likes. If you have no idea what that may be, you can't go wrong with the classics: red roses . . . jewelry . . . a meal at a fine restaurant. Really nice (not funny or schmaltzy) birthday cards are also much appreciated.

Classic gifts became classic because they've never failed to please. So let the wisdom of the ages do your work for you, and enjoy the special day.

Also see: flowers, lingerie, surprises

bisexuality

Also called bi or, more accurately, ambisexuality, this connotes being sexually attracted to both men and women. But if you really want to understand bisexuality—in others or, perhaps, your-self—don't think of it as any one kind of behavior. For example, it's a mistake to assume that simple arithmetic means bisexuals can't be monogamous. Many are very monogamous. And there are many ways to express bisexuality. Some bisexuals, for example, fall in love with only one gender and sleep around with the other. Others fall in love with whomever they fall in love with, man or woman. Some have sex exclusively with men for a few years, then switch to women, and continue to seesaw. Others mix it up as they go along. Some go through a bisexual phase and then stick to heterosexuality or homosexuality for the rest of their lives.

What's more, the whole matter of bisexual "identity" isn't all that cut and dried. There are men and women who have sex with both genders but would never identify themselves as bisexuals. And there are those who are big on claiming bisexual orientation without really practicing it. There are guys who

---

Hot Dates 1909 When Paul Ehrlich discovered a drug that could combat syphilis, the remedy was denounced for "encouraging sin."

---

continued from page 23

Answer:
False, even though for many years it was put into dormitory food at boys' schools and juvenile facilities.

Foreign Affairs
The men of one tribe in Uganda make their dongs long by suspending stones from the tips, beginning at puberty. Just as bodybuilders add weight to various exercise routines as they grow stronger, these tribesmen attach more weight as their penises grow stronger—and longer. **Many a guy will walk around with a 20-pound weight swinging from his thing.** A shaft of 18 inches is not uncommon.

Alas, as it stretches, it also becomes skinnier. Some men are so "successful" that they can tie their tools in knots.

In Extremis
The American opossum has the shortest gestation period of any mammal. It gives birth 12 to 13 days

---

BAWDY BALLADS "Good Rockin' Daddy," *Etta James*

continued on page 35

are more attracted to the idea of bisexual chic than to other men. They are sexual with both genders because it's a cool or trendy thing to do, not because they are especially attracted to both sexes. There are those who really can't make up their minds what they want. And there are those men and women who've transcended labels and don't care what you call them. Obviously, there are a lot of possibilities packed into the word *bisexuality*.

Also see: AC/DC, anima and animus, poppers, switch-hitter, yin and yang

biting

It may not look sexy as a word on a page, but many a couple find themselves biting each other for sexual pleasure. The idea is not to inflict pain (unless you're both into that) but to exploit the

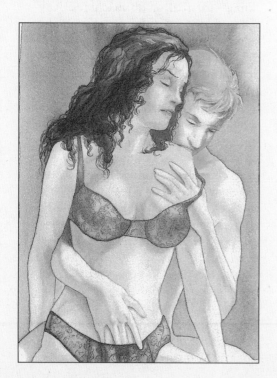

way that sexual arousal raises the pain threshold. True, there are body parts that most people would never want teeth to touch under any circumstances (a certain one of yours no doubt springs to mind). But otherwise, the bite-worthy targets are limited only by the surface areas of both bodies. The intensity can progress from rubbing teeth against skin to eager nibbling to something like a real bite—not a skin-tearing clamper but one that's firmer than you may have predicted in calmer moments.

Just make sure that anything more than a light nip follows smoothly from whatever came just before it. You have to *know* she'll like it before you do it. One way to be sure is if she says, "Bite me." Otherwise, start off with gentler oral play and gradually up the ante, measuring her responses along the way. If those responses are ambiguous, occasionally ask her if she likes what you're doing. If she doesn't say yes, take it as no.

Also see: breath, hickey, kiss, licking, mouth, oral sex, outdoors, rough sex

bladder infection

See: cystitis

blind date

When your first date is a blind date, the advice for any first date applies, only more so. Why? For at least a couple of reasons.

First off, a lot of blind dates are setups by well-intentioned mutual friends. That means you both know that you're expected to hit it off. You also have a kind of permission to jump into bed right after dessert. As a result, your night out together turns into a performance. You try to please your friends instead of yourselves and each other. That's a recipe for disappointment. Avoid it by concentrating on getting acquainted and having a good time in the process. Period. Sure, sex with a virtual stranger on the first date can be thrilling, but making it a goal introduces the possibility of "failure" into what should be a profitable evening of mutual discovery.

If you arranged your own blind date through a personal ad, the whole thing can feel like a job interview. You're tempted to try to come off as the person you think she wants you to be. That implies a pass/fail grading system, which is the opposite of a good time. Don't go there. Just be yourself. Let her know right off that you don't expect immediate evidence of a perfect match.

Then there's the little matter of what exactly you do during this date with a stranger. Careful here. This is where anxiety and eagerness to impress lead to mistakes of excess. Err on the side of conservatism. Choose a restaurant in your or her neighborhood instead of driving 35 miles for some exotic fare that you read about in a newspaper article. Save the experimental theater or underground punk band for when you know each other better. Let the focus be having fun and learning about each other.

Oh, that sigh of relief you hear is coming from her. And it sounds a lot like yours.

Also see: first date, meeting women

blow job
See: fellatio

body fitness

Do yourself a favor: If you're not exercising regularly, start. If you are working out, jack it up a notch. Men in an exercise study told researchers that their sex was more frequent, their performances were more reliable, their orgasms were more satisfying. In the long run, keeping fit through exercise lowers your risk of impotence. In the short run, it lifts your libido. The reasons that fitness may accomplish all these good things include elevated self-esteem, better bloodflow, increased endurance, stronger muscles for moving the right thing the right way during sex, and simply more energy. Any way you look at it, the connection between a fit body and a fun sex life is clear.

Your best bet is cardiovascular exercise. That means some kind of endurance training, such as jogging, running, bicycling, swimming, rowing, or cross-country skiing—for real or on machines. Anything that gets your heart pumping steadily beyond its resting rate will do the trick. Start slow, and work your way up to 30 minutes of moderate exertion at least three times a week.

In addition to gaining endurance, you should pump up your muscles. A basic strength-training routine will also power up your sex life if you stick with it. Any gym or health club should have someone to get you started on a user-friendly program. Or check out an easy-to-follow beginners' weight-training book, such as *The Men's Health Guide to Peak Conditioning.* Pay special attention to your midsection; the muscles there are directly involved in most of the thrusting action. And make sure you strengthen your shoulders and arms with daily pushups and other upper-body exercises. Look at it this way: Would you rather focus on pleasuring her or on not collapsing on top of her?

Also see: abs, aging, athletic sex, back, beefcake, body odor as an attractant, body shapes, disability—overcoming, erection difficulties, exercise, heart conditions, impotence, injuries, Kegel exercises, male body, medications, menopause—yours, muscles, stress, supplements, urologist, weight loss

body image

Most women and plenty of men are unhappy with their bodies. Women are most likely to complain that they're overweight, their breasts are too small or too large, they look old, their thighs are too heavy, and they've suffered the ravages of pregnancy and childbirth, such as stretch marks and cesarean scars. Guys' top-five physical concerns are that their penises are too small, they're losing their hair, they look old, they have beer bellies, and they're too short.

You both need to reclaim your bodies from unrealistic expectations. The fact is, each of you is harder on yourself than you are on each other. When you slide your hand up her leg, you're thinking about the silkiness of her skin and where you're going to touch her next, not about whether she has cellulite or varicose veins—right? Well, when she smothers your face and head with kisses, she's not noticing whether your hairline is receding. She's probably more concerned with what your hand is doing.

Those erotic sensations—not your appearance—are what you should concentrate on. Tell each other how good you're feeling. Make your delight in each other's bodies so obvious that there's no chance for self-criticism.

Your bodies are there to please you, so let them.

Also see: abs, beauty, beefcake, disability—overcoming, erection—firmer, erogenous zones, implants, makeup, mastectomy, media, mirrors, muscles, self-esteem, sexual attraction, size—ass, size—breasts, size—penis, striptease

body odor as an attractant

Life would be a lot easier if we were the dogs that women claim we are. We'd sniff out our partners and then mount them—and they'd never give us any flack for wanting to do it doggie style. Unfortunately, we can't just smell our way into women's beds. Or can we?

Truth is, our schnozzes may have more to do with which women we date—and dump—than we ever realized. One study found that dislike of a partner's odor is

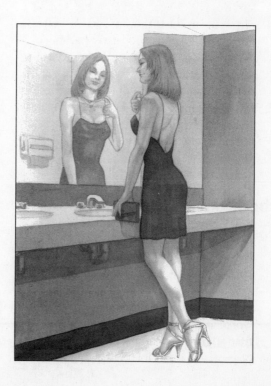

highly predictive that the couple will break up. Okay, that falls into the realm of "duh." But a separate survey showed that 71 percent of men and women rated odor as the *biggest* factor in sexual attraction. Smell turned out to be far more important than looks.

Interestingly, a small Austrian study suggested that the stronger a guy looked, the stronger his stench. Sixteen men wore T-shirts without deodorant for 3 straight days. Then a group of women took a whiff and rated how foul the shirts smelled. The rags with the most offensive odors belonged to the most pumped-up men. According to odor experts, muscular guys have higher testosterone levels, which in turn give them the most powerful odors.

Women's sniffers may be better than ours, thanks to evolution. Experts theorize that because more women than men were needed for the human species to survive, and since women were not as physically robust, they needed a better sense of smell to provide early warning of predators. So the next time she accuses you of ignoring the overflowing trash can or avoiding diaper duty, blame it on your inferior olfactory skills. We'll back you up.

Also see: fragrances, hygiene, muscles, perfume, pheromones, scents, sexy, sweating

body odor—controlling

Think you don't stink? Think again. The unpleasant odor we call funk may not always be apparent to us guys, but it is to the women we love. That's because of their better sense of smell. And while we may welcome the stench that proves we work hard, it can scare off women quicker than a guy who wears polyester someplace where it's visible to the naked eye.

Two glands in our armpits produce the sweat that makes us stink. The ecrine gland pumps out most of our sweat, especially the kind that drenches us when we work out. This sweat in itself hardly smells at all. The odor is actually emitted when bacteria break down the chemicals in the sweat.

The other sweat gland is the apocrine. It becomes active during puberty and produces sweat when we get nervous or sexually aroused. This sweat has a stronger, more distinct odor than that produced when we exercise, and it is also broken down by bacteria.

Here's how to beat B.O.

• Shower daily as well as after workouts and right before a date. Be sure to suds up each time with an antibacterial soap. (We recommend Lever 2000, which won the ladies' vote for best guy soap smell in our independent sniff test.)

• Before you rub on antiperspirant or deodorant, dry your skin thoroughly with a towel. (In case you're wondering—as we were—antiperspirants work by soaking up the moisture on your skin that houses bacteria. Deodorants, on the other hand, cover up B.O. with a pleasant-smelling scent. Deodorants with baking soda do the triple duty of absorbing sweat and odor while also adding a sweet smell to the mix.)

• If you're out to dinner with your date, pass up dishes loaded with garlic or onions. Both have strong odors that are excreted in your sweat for hours afterward. Not to mention the havoc they wreak on your breath.

Now sit back and relax. As sweet as you smell, you're sure to get more than pie for dessert.

Also see: breath, chlamydia, douche, farting, fragrances, hygiene, NSU, perfume, pubic hair, scents, sexy, sweating, vaginal diseases/infections, yeast infection

body oils

Use the ones she keeps atop her dresser or in the bathroom for some slick sex play. Some skin lotions will work. So will massage oils.

Enough of this skin-friendly stuff delivers a tactile turn-on as your slippery hands glide over her even more slippery breasts, buttocks, tummy, and thighs. Couples have even been known to engage in a little sexual oil wrestling, slathering their bodies and then slipping and sliding their way to orgasm. The smart ones throw an old sheet or two over the bed before they grease down.

In this context, all oils are for external use only. They're not to be put inside the vagina or anus, via the penis or otherwise. That means they won't work as lubricants for intercourse, though they look like they will. See our entry on *lubricants* for specifics on the products that are appropriate for internal use. And

don't forget that oil-based products destroy condoms in a flash.

Also see: aromatherapy, massage, ointments, sexual aids

body shapes

Women, you may have noticed, are shaped differently from men. They usually store their fat in their hips and thighs, giving most of them something of a pear shape, as opposed to the apple shape we take on from directing excess fat to our bellies.

But women and men share three basic body types, with relevance for fitness-training goals and attracting the other sex. If you're the reedy ectomorph with little body fat, you probably have more of the slow-twitch muscle fibers that excel at aerobic exercise. If you're a stocky endomorph, your fast-twitch fibers will help you with weight training. If you're a mesomorph, you've got it all, baby. You're just right—not stocky or slim.

Since all this applies to women as well, you can pick your poison: The ecto-

Hot Dates June 25, 1910 President Taft signed a bill making it illegal to transport a woman for the purpose of prostitution. In 1913, the U.S. Supreme Court ruled that the law applied to the transport of mistresses as well.

continued from page 30

after conception. **The longest gestation period? Asian elephants need 608 days**, or a little more than 20 months. And to think that some women get cranky when their little bundles are a week late.

LEGAL BRIEFS

Proving once again that hell hath no fury and all that, **an Alabama woman tarred and feathered her ex-husband's fiancée.** A jury found Marita McElwey guilty of second-degree kidnapping after she had her rival's hair forcibly cut, then did the tar and feathering and left the woman at a garbage dump. All this happened on the day McElwey's ex was supposed to marry the victim. The nuptials were postponed for 2 days.

True or Phallus
A gorilla's erection is three times the size of a man's.

BAWDY BALLADS "Rock Steady," *Aretha Franklin*

continued on page 50

morphic Calista Flockhart? The endomorphic Monica Lewinsky? Or the mesomorphic Catherine Zeta-Jones? You probably have your druthers about female body types, but you'll also probably find that those druthers wane in importance as you start noticing other things you like about her.

Also see: abs, beauty, booty, boxers or briefs, legs, muscles, preference, sexual attraction, sexy, size—ass, size—breasts, size—nose, turn-ons, weight loss

bondage and discipline

A version of dominance and submission in which the dominated submits to discipline (such as spanking or light whipping) while bound. Like all erotic power play, bondage and discipline (B&D) is sexual, consensual, and controlled by agreed-upon limits and a safeword that will stop the action at any time.

What's the attraction? Well, you already have an idea if, to your mutual delight, you've ever held your partner down during sex and really let her have it. Or if she's ever returned the favor. Using constraints to immobilize one partner merely magnifies the potential satisfaction of such an erotic power exchange. And the punishment part? Psychosexual exploration aside, it simply exploits a phenomenon that even the most conservative couples might have noticed—namely, that your threshold for pain is much higher when you're aroused. What the tied-up-and-turned-on B&D player mostly feels (and wants) is intensity. In other words, what hurts when you're not excited can feel great when you are.

Curious? First, forget the image of dungeon dominatrices torturing a nerdy loser with iron manacles; huge, vicious whips; and heavy, metal chains. Today's discerning B&D enthusiasts often prefer "body-friendly" bondage gear such as "Prisoner of Love" kits, with soft and furry handcuffs and an overall feel that's more pleasant than threatening. A cop-out? Not really. Remember, it's the sexual role-playing that counts, not the hardware. Some B&D beginners even use easily breakable ribbons to tie their hands and feet to the bedposts. For them, it's the illusion that counts.

Also see: chains, dominance and submission, flogging, handcuffs, klismaphilia, leather, paddle, playacting, power, safeword, spanking, whips

booty

It's pretty easy to see how a word meaning "rich rewards" turned into sexual slang. A *booty call* can refer to, say, a late-night rendezvous. These days when you're talking about plain old *booty*, you're often referring to a woman's derriere—in an unmistakably suggestive way. But there are lots of other slang choices with which you can complete the sentence "Shake your. . . ." A small sampling: caboose, fanny, rump, butt, arse, stern, tail, hind end, bum, ass, prat, breech, posterior, bottom, backside, behind, rear, seat, gluteal region, keester, culo, buns.

Also see: body shapes, rear entry, size—ass

boredom

Even assuming that you've overcome that primitive urge to mate with all things female, the fact remains that a comfortable romantic routine is dangerously close to a dull romantic routine. The next thing you know, you're caught up in a sexual

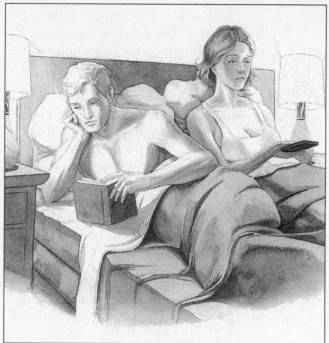

about it. Tell her you'd like to try some new things in bed. (Depending on your partner, you may want to say this casually, without any special inflection or leer, so she doesn't get visions involving cattle prods and hockey masks.) If you're lucky, the talk itself may stir things up a bit.

Oh, and take a look at the rest of your life. Have you fallen into dull routines at work? In your hobbies? In everything? Boring people tend to have boring sex lives. If you crank up the excitement level in all areas of your life, it'll be a lot easier to do it with sex as well.

Also see: depression, fantasies, fatigue, games, marriage, midlife crisis, monotony, rituals, routines, sexual aids, travel as an aphrodisiac, variety

lethargy that taxes your relationship and might even lead to erectile problems.

But that doesn't mean that *monogamy* is just a synonym for *monotony*. First, contrary to Hollywood conceits (and locker room bravado), you're not the only guy in the world who isn't getting laid hourly. Second, you're in charge of your own degree of sexual ennui, for the solution is simple variation—no, not of partners, but of activity with the partner you've chosen. There's an endless supply of shifts and audibles available for your play-calling: new positions, different times of day, other rooms, switched roles. And those are just the basics. Start getting into fantasies, games, clothes, and toys, and the possibilities soar. And we haven't even mentioned Jell-O or duct tape yet.

But you have to go for it. Most couples don't bother. And guess what? That's why they're bored. So talk to her

boss's wife

Forget the stereotype of the plump, overly mascara'd matron stuffed into a garish cocktail dress. These days, your boss's old lady might just be your own age—or younger. And if she decides to come on to you at the company picnic, she just might do it in cutoffs and a halter top. What you have before you in that case is an excellent opportunity to lose your job and reputation—what's left of it, anyway.

There's no upside to this one. Nada. You can't even be flattered, since her motives likely have more to do with power and manipulation than with your intellect or steely buns. And of course, to take her up on her flirtation is to commit professional and social suicide. Trust us on this one, you don't want to even *appear* interested.

Okay, you know all this. But hey, there she is, looking fine and pouring it on pretty heavy. What's a guy supposed to do? Be rude to the boss's wife?

On the contrary, you're supposed to be exceedingly *polite* to the boss's wife. Exaggerated courtesy is your best defense. It tells her, unmistakably but nicely, that you're not interested. It can't be misinterpreted by onlookers. And it's the surest way to diffuse any suggestive comment she may make. Avoid being alone with her, of course. But when you can't, wear her down with your Eddie Haskell act.

What if you're the one doing the lusting? Do we really need to tell you what to do—or what not to do—here? There are lots of shaky reasons to have sex: risk, bragging rights, competition, power, manipulation. Boffing the boss's wife would be all those rolled into one. Immediately seek some other powerfully placed babe to distract you. She may be equally challenging, but at least her husband can't fire you.

Also see: flirtation, job loss, lust, power, trophy wife

boxers or briefs

Ah, the ongoing battle of the bulge. Some guys like the support that briefs give the family jewels. Others prefer to air out their stuff and let it hang, which is what boxers do. Tightie-whities can show off a taut midsection, while undershorts flatter the flabby and sunken-bunned.

Though variety is supposed to be the spice of life, we bet it's conspicuously absent from your top dresser drawer. So, for a day or two, go wild and try a pair of the undies you haven't been using. Test-wear the boxer-brief hybrid as well. Then decide whether you still want to stick with your old standby.

Ask the woman in your life which style of skivvies she prefers to see you in. Even if her answer differs from your preference, be glad she's interested in the subject and the area it covers. Then, respect her druthers. That's not to say you should switch. But don't dismiss the matter as trivial or none of her business. Part of good sex is finding out what matters to your partner.

Besides comfort and sex appeal, another issue some men consider is sperm count. Your testicles hang away from your body because a lower temperature is more conducive to sperm production. So the usual advice is to avoid tight-fitting, temperature-increasing briefs if you want to be fertile. But the scientific research on that is inconclusive. Your drawers will probably be a factor only if you already have fertility problems. And if you think briefs will work as birth control, we have some oceanfront property in Arizona that would be just perfect for you and your growing family.

Also see: body shapes, cross-dressing, dressing for bed, dressing you to look sexy, dry hump, fig leaf, hung, hygiene, lingerie, sperm count, striptease, underwear, undressing

bras

A sadistic killjoy's evil invention, serving no purpose but to separate us from two of life's most exquisite gifts. Still, women are attached to their bras in more ways than one. Or even two. (Who could blame them?) So treat a brassiere with as much respect as you do its contents. It matters to her.

De-bra her with reverence. Don't yank or pull or otherwise rush to get it the hell out of the way. Remove the garment as if unwrapping a priceless treasure, which is exactly what you're doing. Prolong the thrill as the twin marvels of her flesh slowly present themselves for your viewing and fondling pleasure.

All this, of course, is dependent upon getting those famously uncooperative bra hooks apart. Give yourself to the count of 10 to get the little buggers unfastened. Any longer and you're merely fumbling. If you run out of time, look her in the eye and tell her how wonderful it would be if she would do the honors herself. She should be delighted to oblige; if she's not, you didn't have much going in the first place. Realize, too, that many bras nowadays unclasp in the front—a helpful little technological advance that enables us to see what we're doing while we're doing it.

As you may have noticed, there are bras and there are bras. If you're dying to see her in a nice little black lace job, by all means pursue the matter. But do not—repeat, do not—buy one for her as a gift. For a woman, form and function matter at least as much as aesthetics. Bras have to be tried on. And, as mentioned, a woman relates to her bra on a deeply personal level; buying one is something she just has to do herself.

Instead, just happen to come across your choice in a catalog or store display in her presence. Tell her you think she'd look great (or "marvelous" or "sexy," but *never* "better") in that one. Repeat this process until she gets the hint.

Also see: cross-dressing, dressing her to look sexy, feel up, lingerie, size—breasts, underwear, undressing

breaking up

No matter how smart a move it is, ending a relationship hurts. Where an actual divorce is concerned, no matter how quick and amicable and faultless, it's going to be hell for a while. You're going to feel sorry for yourself. When someone about whom you cared (or at least were used to having around) is no longer there, a dose of self-pity is well-earned. You're *supposed* to mope.

What you're not supposed to do is wallow in it for a year. You can recognize wallowing by its dramatic element: It's when you, love's victim, project your sad circumstances into a tragedy of Shakespearean proportions and then play it out endlessly. Seek the comfort of friends and relatives, but don't drag them into supporting roles in your melodrama. Doing so is a useless self-indulgence that distracts you from genuine grieving, while forcing them to check caller ID whenever the phone rings.

Instead, evaluate your relationship for future reference. What went wrong? What part of it was your fault? Did the two of you do everything you could do to make it work? Was it ill-advised from the beginning? More important, reflect on what's really going on with you right now, beyond the heartbreak. The key question: What have you actually lost? A sex partner? A friend? Prestige? The dream of being truly understood by another person? The comfort of a familiar relationship? The answers may not be as wholesome as you'd hoped. But some honest reckoning here will help put the situation in perspective and get you moving forward.

Also see: divorce—avoiding, divorce—issues that lead to, heartache, past partners—dealing with, past partners—longing for, past partners—running into, remarriage, single—suddenly

breast cancer

It hits one in eight American women and is the second-leading cause of cancer deaths among them, after lung cancer. As if that weren't tragic enough, the disease can scar a woman's self-image (or a man's image of her) and then, in turn, the couple's intimacy and sex life. This is true even if she doesn't undergo a mastectomy (breast removal) or lumpectomy (removal of the tumor and a bit of surrounding tissue).

The support and stress reduction provided by an active love life can actually speed her recovery, so if your partner develops breast cancer, her own emotional vulnerability and fears come first, of course. But you may find that you have some issues, too. In fact, it's the man who often shies away from sex after his wife is diagnosed with breast cancer, mostly out of fear and guilt. For example, a man might feel (irrationally) that he somehow caused the cancer by spending too much time fondling her breasts. He may feel guilty about having placed so much emphasis on the beauty of her breasts through the years. Or he may simply fear that he'll hurt her just by engaging in sex.

Then there's the whole mortality thing. Cancer reminds us that death someday will separate us from each other; with that specter suddenly planted in our brains, we sometimes begin shunning intimacy as a defense mechanism.

Another common trap to avoid is the fallacy that working together to maintain your sex life is inappropriate in the face of a life-threatening disease. On the contrary, the two of you *must* talk about sex

after breast cancer. You must ask her doctors specifically about the sexual ramifications of her condition and its treatment. Most of all, you must assure her of her continued desirability.

Also see: hysterectomy, implants, mastectomy

breast enlargement

Cosmetic breast surgery is so popular these days that it's possible the woman in your life has herself perused the plastic surgeon directories a time or two. Five times more breast augmentations and lifts were performed in 1999 than in 1992: In the boob job business, it's an era of boom *and* bust. And no wonder: Most women like the results, the marketing is aggressive, and there's a prevailing expectation among modern women (and, increasingly, men) that they should be able to control what their bodies look like.

What your lady should keep in mind is that breast augmentation is serious surgery. It's not something she should rush into because everybody else is doing it. It's also not the only choice. As a lot of balding men learn, simply accepting a perceived physical imperfection is as effective a way of dealing with it as artificially altering it. It's certainly cheaper.

Your job is not to push her in one direction or the other; it's to understand the intensity the subject holds for her. The potential for emotional pain in a woman's perception of her own breasts is quite real, and an ultra-sensitive topic. You're not going to change her body image with logic. If she does opt for the knife, you should be Mr. Positive all the way. Afterward, don't even think about offering such thoughtful observations as "Hmm . . . they feel a little like Nerf balls." No matter how well-intentioned your comments (or how good-natured your jokes), they're apt to fall flat, as it were. Whatever she asks, your answer is: "You look great." That's actually not a bad piece of advice in general. And it's probably the truth.

Also see: arousal, beauty, body image, breast sensitivity, hypnosis and breast enlargement, implants, media, size—breasts, third-degree cleavage

breastfeeding

It's what those things are really for, after all. If your offspring is being nursed at your mate's bosom, that by no means precludes sexual breast play for you. It does raise some issues that every couple reacts to differently.

She may feel that the baby's suckling is more than enough breast contact, thank you. Don't take it personally. She just may not consider her lumpy, udder-like mammaries to be very sexy. In all honesty, you might not either. This deals you the double duty of reassuring her of her overall desirability while honoring any DON'T TOUCH signs. Talking your way through these temporary sexual detours will definitely pay dividends.

On the other hand, your woman may be so enraptured by her ability to nourish another human being that she welcomes sexual celebration of her noble breasts. The bigger, fuller proportions of her bust could be an arousing change for both of you. If that's the case, you may have already discovered that there's a pretty good chance of milk seeping out when the two of you fool around, especially at orgasm (hers, that is). It's just part of the adventures of parenthood.

One last important piece of advice:

Though breastfeeding does reduce the likelihood of another pregnancy, it's not a form of birth control. Ignore that fact, and she could very well be breastfeeding another brand-new baby 9 months from now.

Also see: bras, breast pain, breast sensitivity, fatigue, kids, lubrication, Madonna/whore complex, mastectomy, mating, nipples, pituitary gland, postpartum depression, size—breasts, topless, witch's milk

breast fondling

It's good to know that one of our favorite teenage pastimes—getting to second base—still scores high on surveys of sexy things folks like. (Uh . . . duh.) In an Internet poll, two-thirds of respondents said that they are sexually aroused by breast fondling (nipples in particular), and two-thirds of *those* people have reached orgasm that way. It would be a shame if your woman were part of the remaining third, who were ho-hum about this most enjoyable of activities, simply because she didn't like the way *you* do it.

There's no one "correct" way to fondle a breast. Some women like it feathery, others quite the opposite; also, women, much like valet parking lots, reserve the right to change their policies without notice.

The female breast is a smooth, soft, alive thing. There's nothing like it in the rest of the universe. Pay homage with your hands. Resist the temptation to clutch a breast or two before the first kiss is over. Nobody likes to be grabbed, especially by surprise. Caress the surrounding area first. Create a little anticipation. It's most pleasurable for both of you (and both of them) to start gently, even if the arousal level is high. Then, once you're in hilly terrain, think beyond rubbing and squeezing. Vary the stroke, increase the intensity gradually, move to the nipples later rather than sooner, and above all, pay attention to her responses. If she seems to be cringing or pulling away, that's a pretty good clue that she's not loving what you're doing. As always, encourage her to let you know what does feel good.

Also see: arousal, bras, size—breasts, topless

breast pain

Those twin mounds of wondrous flesh don't always feel as good from the inside as they do from the outside. Many women go through some kind of breast discomfort—anything from a little tenderness to honest-to-God pain—in the middle of their menstrual cycles and again just before their periods. Your partner may not want to be touched anywhere near the chest on those days. Even a hug can hurt. Your job is to respect that and try to make her—not yourself—feel better. For extra credit, keep track of her menstrual cycle so you know when she's likely to be sore. That saves her the trouble of rebuffing your probing mitts. It's all part of the superior lover's philosophy, which is: Give priority to how your actions feel to her, rather than to you.

If you do get too grabby at the wrong time, here's a way to make up for your faux pas. Have her lie down on her back, blouseless and braless. Fold about ¼ cup of freshly grated ginger into each of two towels, and then soak them with hot (not scalding) water. Place them gently over her breasts and have her leave them

there for 10 to 20 minutes. The ginger's anti-inflammatory effect should reduce the pain and swelling. Even if it doesn't, she'll be so knocked out by your gesture that she'll feel better anyway.

Also see: arousal, breastfeeding, cramps—menstrual, foreplay, PMS

breast reduction

Female breast reductions are considered reconstructive, rather than cosmetic, surgery. The idea is usually to free the poor women of the physical drawbacks—such as the back, neck, and shoulder pain—that go with hauling around those oversize boulders. Male breast reduction surgery, though, is considered cosmetic. Apparently, the approximately 10,000 men who undergo it each year simply prefer not to wear the bra in the family.

Also see: breast enlargement, size—breasts, third-degree cleavage

breasts

Mammary glands that produce and deliver nourishment to newborns. That's one definition. Here's another: proof that God loves us.

Why do we adore *them* so? Because they're beautiful—exquisite hanging sculptures of soft flesh in varying shapes, sizes, and hues. Because they're unique—nothing on our own bodies (or in the universe, for that matter) feels quite like a female breast. Because they're the essence of femininity—at least in our society. Because they're erogenous—contact with them can create a two-way charge of excitement. And because of the intrigue factor: Most of the time, they're at least partially hidden and taboo to touch.

Having said this, we remind you that a woman's breasts are fundamentally different to her than they are to you. Men get so much pleasure out of female bosoms that we sometimes forget that they're attached to a whole person. The most accomplished breast men are sensitive to each woman's feelings about her own breasts. Is she proud of them? Ashamed? Indifferent? Turned on by their erotic potential? Uncomfortable with the attention they get? Gather this kind of intelligence, along with the more specific information you need about how (or whether) she likes them touched. Not only is this a more considerate approach but it also deepens the pleasure and intimacy of breast play for both of you.

Also see: beauty, communication, eye contact, feel up, foreplay, implants, nipples, ogling, size—breasts, topless

gernails-on-the-blackboard experience. So you can't assume your new partner will be pleased by the same breast play that drove your last lover gaga.

Hence the challenge: How do you measure the sensitivity potential of two breasts you've just met? The answer is that you can't, at least not from a distance. Breast size is no indicator of sensitivity. Neither is the breast owner's personality. You just have to feel your way around until you grasp the truth.

Also see: arousal, foreplay, nipple clamps

breast sucking

By you, that is. Of her nipples and any more of the breast that might fit in your mouth. Like any breast play, it's a huge turn-on for some women and a distraction, at best, for others. Keep in mind

breast sensitivity

Female breasts pack so much highly sensitive tissue and so many nerve endings that they seem to tingle with potential, even when there's nothing going on. When there *is* something going on—arousal or orgasm, for example—the way they change their shape and color is a beautiful reminder of their pleasure potential for all concerned.

What's not always obvious, though, is how radically their sensitivity varies from one woman to another. Jessica's pair might be much more arousable than Heather's. And Shasta might love her breast responsiveness, while to Carol it's more of a fin-

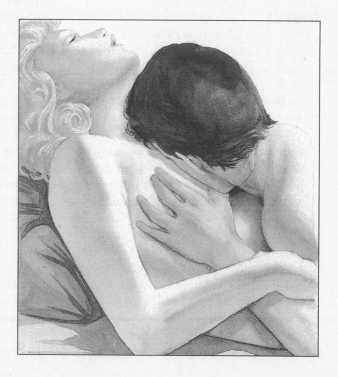

that not all women have even had the experience (and even if your partner has, having it with you is a whole new deal). So don't assume that it's heaven for her. And never forget that you're running your mouth over what can be a highly sensitive part of the female anatomy. Start with soft licks on the breast itself, moving to the nipples gradually and shifting to gentle sucking only when you sense that she's ready and willing. That can be tricky with a new partner since moans and groans are sometimes unleashed for their own sake and don't always mean that she's rhapsodizing over anything in particular. For the clearest signals, you'll find that the English language works beautifully. So stop sucking for a moment and talk to her.

Also see: communication, biting, licking, mouth, nipples

breath

Sexwise, bad breath is a silent killer. You don't know you have it, and she's not likely to clue you in. What she will do, though, is find excuses to keep her distance, possibly as far away as her own apartment.

Women are really and truly turned off by poor oral hygiene. And they're more sensitive to bad odors than we are. Complicating things is the fact that dating itself is dangerous to your breath. Dry mouth—such as that which results from all that talking you do—invites bad breath. So does the alcohol the two of you share. And on a dinner date, you eat but you don't brush.

The best defense here is a good offense. Make it a habit to brush your teeth often. And brush your tongue. That's where odor-causing bacteria gather.

Better yet, get a tongue scraper at a pharmacy. Or even use a spoon. When you're out with her, drink plenty of water. Carry around breath fresheners with chlorophyll. At the end of a meal, munch on that sprig of parsley that you always used to ignore. It's full of chlorophyll, so it will deodorize your mouth as well as mask the food odor. And there's no law against taking your toothbrush with you. It might even come in handy if you end up at her place for the night.

Most important, know your breath status. A good friend can let you know whether it smells okay. But bear in mind that he's not going to tell you unless you ask.

Also see: alcohol, biting, body odor—controlling, hygiene, kiss, licking

brothels/bordellos

They're both quaint old words, as though whorehouses were still gabled Victorian mansions run by fat and kindly madams who lead sing-alongs at the player piano. Today's on-site prostitution facilities are more likely to be massage parlors or nightclubs offering extra services. The legal ones, however—that is, the dozens of "ranches" in Nevada—proudly and openly call themselves brothels. If you find yourself bored enough in Reno or Vegas to consider giving one a try, plan on driving a little; brothels are only allowed in the smaller Nevada counties. Also, be prepared to negotiate directly with the girl of your choice (rather than pay an established house price), and be very specific about what you want. If what you want is unprotected intercourse, forget it: Condoms are required apparel. The licensed brothel sex workers (what the rest of us call hookers) are tested for HIV before they can start, and they get weekly exams for sexually transmitted diseases. The advantage of a legal Nevada brothel, in short, is that you're reasonably assured of avoiding an infection or a raid.

Even with everything safe and legal, we'd recommend thinking about at least two things while you're on your way to the Bunny Ranch.

First, brothel sex is a business transaction, which only further emphasizes the irksome notion that sex is something women have and men want. You'll get much bigger dividends out of putting that same time, energy, and cash into creating situations where you and another unpaid person can be sexual together.

Second, men often go to prostitutes to try things without fear of failure or rejection. It's a sensible-sounding notion that rests, alas, on subordinate myths: that in the eyes of their wives or girl-friends, men are somehow supposed to already be experts at everything sexual; and that exploring new horizons with your steady squeeze is out of the question. In truth, both men and women have to learn *everything* about sex. (It's the one curriculum that never ends. And actually, we like it that way.) Once you accept that, you'll find that fun-spirited, stress-free trial and error with your woman—the one at home—can make for a more rewarding education than any impersonal professional lesson.

And once the two of you master an open, lighthearted, comfortable way of talking about sex, everything's on the table. She may not go for every far-out thing you think of, but the two of you will still be able to experiment with more sexual variations than you'll ever have the time or money to find out about in Nevada.

Also see: escort service, john, money, prostitution, safe sex, STDs

C

cars

A century ago, your ancestors tied their horses to secluded trees and got busy in their buggies. Amish folks probably keep this tradition alive and well today. Since about the start of the 20th century, the rest of us have turned to automobiles when we've felt the need to take our show on the road. By the 1920s, car makers were designing fold-down seats to give lovers beds to romp on. In the '30s, drive-in theaters came along, giving amorous young people a convenient alibi for the evening. The '50s witnessed the debut of the roving sex-mobile known as the van.

Cars offer the opportunity to literally take sex to new places, thereby adding excitement and variety to a relationship. They allow partners to have sex in public places—more privately. In a 1999 survey, 14 percent of men and 1 percent of women admitted they'd been the re-cipients of sexual favors while driving (which suggests that the 1 percent of women got around). Six percent of men and 2 percent of women said that, while actually driving the car, they'd performed sex acts on passengers. We're sure the folks at Allstate were just thrilled by this news.

Our advice: Put the car in park before you shift yourself into overdrive. Maybe it's not quite as exhilarating, but it's a whole lot less dangerous.

Also see: feel up, hickey, lubricants, quickies, risky sex, road erection, road head

casting couch

The office furniture upon which would-be starlets offered their sexual favors to powerful film producers or directors in exchange for getting cast in movie roles.

The venue may not always have been the sofa, and the aspiring newcomer may not always have been female, but sex-for-screen-time trades were especially common during the 1930s and '40s in Hollywood. And today? Well, power in today's film industry is more diffuse, harassment laws are more prevalent, and feminism is more effective. So the practice may now be less common than in the past. But sex is still often considered a negotiable commodity, and until that changes, the casting couch will live on—and not just in Tinseltown.

Also see: beauty, beefcake, movies, power, prostitution, sex symbols

celibacy

Strictly speaking, it's the chaste, unmarried life, such as a monk vows to uphold. But since *unmarried* and *chaste* are far from synonymous in the real world, you usually hear *celibacy* used as a synonym for abstinence.

Also see: abstinence, sex—lack of, virginity—hers

cervical cap

A relatively new birth control option in the United States, it's a small, thimble-shaped, rubber device that fits over the cervix and stays put via suction. Covering the cervix keeps sperm from reaching the fallopian tubes and, possibly, an egg. The cervical cap works much like a diaphragm, but it's smaller and simpler. And it can be kept in place longer—up to 48 hours—without risking complications such as toxic shock syndrome. Like a diaphragm, it must be specially fitted by a physician because cervices vary in size.

And a woman will need to be refitted after weight changes of more than 10 pounds, full or partial-term pregnancy, or abdominal surgery. Its effectiveness—80 percent, with typical use, roughly the same as a diaphragm's—depends on using it along with spermicidal jelly.

Also see: contraception, diaphragm, nonoxynol-9, sponge

cervix

The opening to the uterus. It is through this bulblike portal at the back of the vagina that sperm attempt to pass on their eggward journey. The cervix pulls itself up and back as the vagina opens up during intercourse, allowing it to dodge your thrusting penis. If you do hit it, that's pretty much the end of the line since the cervix isn't very flexible. Repeated cervix ramming by a lengthy member is probably going to be uncomfortable for at least one of you, although (as in so many other sexual maneuvers) there's a blurred line between pain and pleasure. Some people suggest that the cervix has its own set of responsive nerve endings that are the source of the intense orgasms that seem to originate deep within her body.

Also see: diaphragm, hung, hysterectomy, Pap test, pregnancy, size—vagina, sponge, sympto-thermal method, tampon, uterus, uterus—tipped, vagina

chains

Along with whips, they're the very symbol of sadomasochistic bondage play, and they exude a certain dungeon aesthetic that some folks find appealing. But there must be 50 ways to immobilize your lover, and chains are low on the list. They're unwieldy, not to mention cold, hard, and uncomfortable. Most folks who get tied up in sex prefer more body-friendly ways of going about it, such as furry belts or knotted soft fabrics. And as a flagellation tool, strong chains are definitely a no-no. Too dangerous. If you want the chain symbolism, a necklace or a purse chain should suffice. The point of bondage is erotic power play and heightened intensity, not cut wrists or a damaged tailbone. Use a heavy attitude, not heavy equipment.

Also see: bondage and discipline, dominance and submission, kinky, safeword

chakras

Literally translated from the Hindi, *chakras* means "wheels of spinning energy." They are energy centers distributed in more or less a straight line, from the first chakra at the base of your spine, through your genital area (the second chakra) and solar plexus (the third), and on up through your heart (fourth), throat (fifth), and brow (sixth), to your crown (seventh). What makes this concept relevant to your Western sex life is that, according to Eastern philosophy, you have the capacity to experience orgasm in any of these seven chakras.

Now that's an attention grabber if there ever was one. But don't expect such migrating orgasms tonight. You'll need to dedicate some time first to learning about the tantric and Taoist approaches to sex. Simply put, each of the seven chakras is said to play a vital role in your physical and psychological functioning. A fair simplification is that the three lower chakras have a larger physiological component, while the four higher chakras are more obviously related to your psychological makeup. There are many good books available on this subject. Try David Pond's *Chakras for Beginners,* or search www.amazon.com or www.sacredcenters.com for other books and videotapes on chakras and tantra.

Committed followers believe that paying attention to your chakras can help you experience a more complete orgasm. They recommend that as you're making love (or masturbating), you might try to let the sexual energy flow out to the first, third, and fourth chakras. Relax your breathing, inhale through your nose, and exhale through your mouth. Squeeze your pubococcygeus (PC) muscles on the exhale. This, according to the doctrine, will pump energy throughout your entire body. Focus on one chakra at a time, moving on only when you "feel" the heat in that area. The idea is to prolong the act not by stifling sexual sensations but by giving them more room to flower. Ideally, at a certain point you'll have a full-body orgasm. And when you do come, you'll feel the pleasure from the base of your spine to your heart.

Well, okay, maybe not. Mostly, you're going to feel it in your johnson. At least for now. But an all-encompassing climax is something to work toward, at least if you believe Sting, Woody Harrelson, Richard Gere, and other tantric devotees.

Also see: orgasm, religion, spiritual sex, tantra, yogi

chlamydia

Probably the most common sexually transmitted bacterial disease that most people have never heard of. In women, untreated chlamydia can lead to pelvic inflammatory disease, chronic pelvic pain, and ectopic pregnancy. It can cause infertility in both women and men. Antibiotics knock it out quickly, but you won't seek treatment if you don't know you have it, and about 85 percent of women and 40 percent of men with chlamydia notice no symptoms. If symptoms do show up, they'll probably include mild pain when you urinate and a slight discharge from your penis. If you notice any of these problems, immediately have them checked out, and tell your partner (we hope you'd have sense enough to do both of these without our telling you to). If your lover complains of pain during intercourse or if you notice that her vagina is producing unusual discharge or an unpleasant odor, she may be infected.

Also see: ectopic pregancy, infertility, pelvic inflammatory disease, safe sex, STDs

chromosomes

When you shoot those millions of sperm cells within the body of your beloved at the climax of intercourse, you also determine the sex of anyone conceived due to your moment of ecstasy. Why does this depend on you and not her? It's all in the chromosomes, rod-shaped structures in your cells that contain your all-determining genes.

Most people have 46 chromosomes, arranged in pairs (though people with Down syndrome have an extra one). All but one of those 23 pairs are matching copies of the same chromosome. The 23rd pair are the sex chromosomes, and they play by their own rules. In men, they're not identical; we call one X and the other Y. In women, they *are* identical—both are Xs. Unlike other cells, your sperm cell and her egg cell each carry only half of the 46 chromosomes, one from each pair. So her egg has one of her two Xs, no matter what, while each of

Hot Dates **1913** Each night, thousands of young people filled the dance halls in Chicago, prompting the Illinois Senate Vice Committee to hold hearings on what it called the largest menace to the chastity of women.

continued from page 35

Answer:
False. The reverse is true. The average man sports about 6 inches, while a gorilla measures a measly 2. Yet another reason to pity King Kong?

Seemed like a Good Idea at the Time. . .
As recently as 1940, at least one medical textbook included instructions on how to cauterize the clitorises of women who were frequent masturbators. Surgeons performed the procedure on mental patients and criminals.

Foreign Affairs
The *Kama Sutra* suggests this solution for lengthening your penis: Before sex, rub it with warm water, then smear on honey and ginger. **Note: Do not try this near beehives.**

In Extremis
Now this was truly the odd couple. In South Wales in 1972, an ambitious **male dachshund reportedly snuck up on a sleeping female Great Dane** and had his way with her. Doggoned if their tryst didn't produce 13 "Great Dachshunds" with short legs, big heads, and raised ears.

BAWDY BALLADS "I Want Your Sex," *George Michael*

continued on page 57

your sperm cells contains either one X or one Y. If the sperm that fertilizes the egg has an X, the resulting XX pair creates a female. If it has a Y, the resulting XY pair creates a male. You're a man because a sperm with a Y chromosome got to your mom's egg first.

Actually, your Y chromosome didn't directly provide your manly features. Rather, it kicked off a chain of events that resulted, at about week 8 of your fetal existence, in the male hormone testosterone pumping through your sexless embryonic body. Testosterone then guided your development in a manward direction. The Y chromosome made the decision, but testosterone did the work.

Also see: anima and animus, androgyny, genetics, hermaphrodite, hormones, mating, micropenis, testosterone, transvestism, yin and yang, zygote

circumcision

More than 60 percent of American men have already had their penises' foreskins surgically removed, usually shortly after birth. Let's put this in perspective: Worldwide, more than 80 percent of males are *not* circumcised.

Many American males, especially Jews, have it done for religious reasons. There are health factors too; circumcised men run a lower risk of contracting sexually transmitted diseases. Hygiene convenience also comes into it since a man with his foreskin intact needs to roll it back to clean under it daily and after intercourse. But mainly, there's the momentum of custom—the father's been clipped, so the son tends to be as well. Also, since circumcision is the norm in America, aesthetic preference mostly runs that way.

That momentum has been slowing down a bit, and we may be starting to follow in the footsteps of our brothers from abroad. These days, the medical establishment doesn't unanimously encourage circumcision as a routine procedure, so parents often make their own decision. That decision might be influenced by a small but vocal save-the-foreskin movement that's criticizing infant circumcision as unnecessary, risky, painful, and abusive. What's more, the activists claim that circumcised adult men are mutilated, deprived of sensitive skin that's rightfully theirs, and performing sexually at a disadvantage. Some even go so far as to advocate re-creating your foreskin.

Our advice regarding your newborn son is to proceed as you surely would have anyway: You and the boy's mother should inform yourselves, talk to the doctors involved, discuss the pros and cons with each other, and then make the decision you both think is best. As for your own foreskin status, don't worry about it. If you're circumcised, do you really feel "mutilated"? Do you know anybody who does? Didn't think so. Moreover, there's zero evidence that the presence or absence of a foreskin has any effect on performance or pleasure. In general, women don't care which kind of penis you have, and those who do are split down the middle, since it's purely a matter of taste. Finally, we think the whole idea of a foreskin-reconstruction procedure is batty. There may be legitimate concerns about infant circumcision, but you're an adult. And, hey, you have enough things to think about without unsolicited criticism of your perfectly fine penis.

Also see: foreskin, frenulum, glans, penile cancer, phimosis, prepuce, smegma

C

clitoral orgasm

A female orgasm triggered by stimulation of the clitoris. For the majority of women, it's the most available kind of orgasm. Put simply, most (not all) American women seldom climax from vaginal stimulation alone; they need direct stimulation of their clitorises.

Problem is, you don't often hear it put that simply. Some claim that the clitoral variety is the only true female orgasm; a century ago, the prevailing belief was that only vaginal orgasms were "mature" and "correct." Some women report a marked difference in feeling and intensity between the two; others report none. Some who are capable of both prefer vaginal orgasms, others clitoral, and still others like them equally.

Obviously, there's a lot of subjectivity here. What's true for everybody, though, is that the nerves that supply the clitoris also supply the vagina—and the G-spot, for that matter. So we're in a sense talking about different routes to the same destination.

Also see: afterplay, breastfeeding, breast fondling, cervix, cramps—menstrual, cunnilingus, disability—hers, faking orgasm, female ejaculation, get off, Janus Report, manual stimulation, nipples, oral sex, pee—her—during orgasm, uterus, Venus butterfly, vibrator, virginity—hers

clitoris

This supersensitive nub of flesh above the vaginal opening exists for one reason

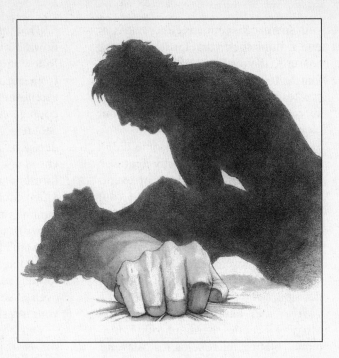

and one reason only: to get her off. It (not the vagina itself) is where her most intense sexual pleasure comes from. That makes the clitoris the answer to every man's prayer: a magic button for pleasing a woman.

So why isn't it pushed more? Lots of reasons, the most curious being that intercourse only sometimes gives the clitoris direct stimulation. You may curse this as a flaw of evolution. But you'll be happier if you take it as a cue to engage in sex play that will indeed include the clitoris, such as using your (or her) fingers or your tongue or a sex toy. This you can do before, during, after, or instead of intercourse. (Quick tip: You may have some difficulty using your tongue during intercourse.)

There's another reason for clit neglect: Like a properly prepared martini, a good clitoris is hard to find. It's not very big. It's seldom where you think it should be.

And even though arousal leads to engorgement of the clitoris—a kind of female erection—the organ has a counterproductive habit of retracting into its surrounding hood of flesh exactly when her stimulation is peaking. Many a finger or tongue has withdrawn in confusion at this point, so tantalizingly close to paradise—not a pleasing development for her. And then the hidden treasure is hard to relocate.

There are two good solutions. One is communication. *She* knows where everything is, and she probably also knows when and how she wants you to touch her. All she has to do is tell you . . . or show you. The latter, for the record, can be an incredibly sexy experience in its own right.

Meanwhile, all *you* have to do is ask. Clitoral attention provides a fine opportunity to refute the charge that men won't ask for directions. Or see for yourself: On your next trip downtown for cunnilingus, leave a light on and check things out. Every vulva has its own beauty, and here's your chance to explore this one. One part of you or another will be spending a lot of quality time here. Why not know the terrain?

Also see: cunnilingus, dildo, French tickler, glans, licking, missionary position, nymphomania, prepuce, pudenda, sixty-nine (69), standing positions, vagina, vulva

clumsiness

The cure for sexual clumsiness comes down to being patient. (Lots of practice may help, but you were going to try that anyway.) Take it easy. Go slow. The klutz is grabby on a date, rushing to start sex, rushing to finish it. The smooth operator, on the other hand, makes no move before its time. When, and only when, two body parts have announced clearly that they're ready for each other—be they hands, lips, genitals, or any combination thereof—contact will almost surely happen without awkward complications.

Once you slow down, it's easier to pay attention—an equally important clumsiness preventer. Key in on what's going on with her at any given moment—at dinner, in the car, in bed. Read her signals. Act accordingly. It's when you insist on blindly imposing some preconceived game plan that a sexual session turns into a Keystone Cops routine.

Just as important, pay attention to how things feel for you. Are you actually aroused? Do you want more touching or desire more stimulation? Being more conscious of what's actually happening makes you more graceful.

Also, be yourself. Striking a sexual pose to impress her (or to boost your own confidence?) means being constantly "on" instead of relaxed. And guys who aren't relaxed get clumsy. In fact, banish the whole idea of performance from your lovemaking. Remember, your partner is just that: a partner, not a spectator. You're not performing *for* her; you're working *with* her.

When clumsiness happens, it's often a team effort, so laugh about it together. Sex is supposed to be fun, after all.

Also see: anticipatory anxiety, first time with a lover, laughter, performance anxiety, relaxation, self-esteem, sexual etiquette, shyness, spectatoring, techniques

cocaine

The euphoric effect it creates by stimulating the brain's pleasure centers is

C

probably responsible for its once rampant reputation as a sex drug, because people who feel good also feel more sexual. However, any sexual benefits are dependent upon the anesthetic being taken only in occasional small doses—discipline rare among coke users, as Robert Downey Jr., Darryl Strawberry, and myriad other fallen idols can amply testify. (Yeah, we know, you can handle it better than those guys. Sure you can.) Larger doses, steady use, and crack smoking impair sexual function, often to the point of impotence. Also, people who do a lot of cocaine don't connect well with others, which obviously discourages sexual union. Finally, a low or lost libido is common among heavy users, meaning that cocaine is ultimately the exact opposite of a sex drug.

Also see: aphrodisiac, drugs

cock ring

It's just what it sounds like. But a cock ring (also known as a penis ring or constriction device) is for play, not for show. Essentially, it acts as a mild tourniquet that slows bloodflow out of your penis. Since erections are all about blood, this has led to some exaggerated ideas about what a cock ring can accomplish. It will not help you get an erection. It will, however, help many men hang on to their erections before ejaculation, and the extra blood down there can give you a wider erection—benefits that your woman may really appreciate. Some men also find that a cock ring encourages their half-ons to firm up into full-ons.

A cock ring's surest and highest use, however, is as a sensation enhancer. When you fit the ring against the body

wall—that is, behind your testicles—some unusual and often pleasurable feelings announce themselves during arousal. This is also the preferred position for firmness. How, you ask, can a ring get behind your testicles? Well, one made of an elastic material will stretch enough to let the balls poke through, one by one. But your safest bet is a removable and adjustable cock ring that uses Velcro, snaps, or a bolo tie to open and close. Such a ring is usually made of soft leather or latex. Never use a solid metal ring that slips straight on like a wedding band. That's how emergency room docs get the stuck–cock-ring stories they swap over coffee.

More safety tips: Never try to make your own cock ring using makeshift devices such as rubber bands or string. Adjust the ring so it's not so tight at full erection that you lose all sensation; if you can't adjust it, don't use it. Never keep it on for more than a half-hour—20 minutes your first few times. Left in place too long, it can cause irreversible damage to the soft tissues of your penis. This should go without saying, but we have to mention it: If you feel pain, see bruising, or experience numbness or a loss of sensation, remove the ring. Ditch cock rings altogether if you have a blood-clotting disorder, diabetes, or vascular or nerve disease, or if you regularly use anticoagulants, aspirin, or any other blood-thinning medication.

Advanced cock ringmasters can enjoy some little extras. The most popular are the "clit bump" and other similar attachments designed for her pleasure. You can also get a setup to hang a small, compatible vibrator on your ring to get things buzzing. Is it any wonder that American technological ingenuity is admired the world over?

Also see: erection—firmer, French tickler, injuries, orgasm—delayed, ointments, penis pump, priapism, sexual aids

coitus

No need to add this one to your everyday vocabulary; it's a medical and scientific term usually referring to pro-creative sex.

come

A handy alternative verb for those who consider "I'm about to ejaculate!" to be too scholarly an utterance for such a pleasurable imminent event. *To come* actually substitutes for *to have an orgasm* or *to climax* and is therefore a suitable addition to both the male and female sexual vocabularies.

By the way, *come* is not really a gutter word these days; it's regularly used in

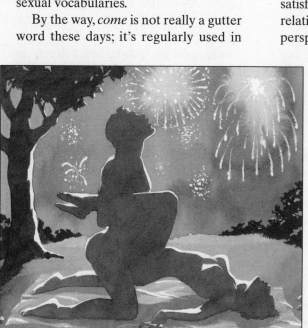

C

any frankly sexual context—such as a sexologist's advice ("Don't worry about coming too fast") or a couple's intimate conversation ("It felt wonderful when you came").

Also see: cum, ejaculation, get off, orgasm

commitment

A word unknown to men. So we're told, anyway.

For the record, commitment can be anything from going steady to an official vow of till death do ye part. But it's always a clear decision that the relationship—however you define it—is a priority, that there's a "we" along with the "I," and that you both want it that way.

Commitment is a good thing; most of us truly need the companionship and the attachment (not to mention the sexual satisfaction) that comes with a committed relationship. So why do guys mumble and perspire and find a reason to leave the state for a few days when the reality of it draws nigh? Truth is, there are so many powerful reasons for our aversion to commitment that it's a miracle any of us ever get hitched.

Those who explain everything in evolutionary terms point out that male humans are genetically wired to spread seed. Then there's psychology. Boys, unlike girls, face the difficult developmental task of giving up their early identification with their mothers. There's maturity. Younger adults who are just becoming fully aware of the shortcomings of human relationships often understandably postpone serious attachments. There's timing. Some guys really aren't ready yet for that strange and scary journey through the tunnel of committed love. And there's popular culture, with the nonstop media message that the single life is where all the fun is.

But the most powerful reason of all is social conditioning. Even in these supposedly enlightened times, we're told from the time we toddle that we should enjoy our "freedom" while we can because, one day, some woman is going to "get" us and take it all away. Then, we're vilified for heeding that same warning. Go figure. So it's not all your fault that you fear commitment, good buddy.

By telling you that, we have now empowered you to break the cycle. Before you do, though, get straight just what it is you're committing to. Sexual exclusivity is what usually comes to mind, but the sticking point may well be something else—like having children or retooling your social life or controlling your money. Both of you will feel better if you resolve these issues. It may not be the most romantic conversation you'll ever have. And that's good. Be as unromantic as you have to be to take care of this stuff. Then you can be romantic for the rest of your lives.

Also see: affairs, companionship, desertion, discretion, infatuation, intimacy, jealousy, lust, marriage, monogamy, rituals, wild women, workaholism, young men/older women, zipless sex

communication

This word pops up a lot in relation to sex. In fact, you'll see many permutations of it throughout this book. So much of our advice boils down to "Ask her . . ." or "Tell her . . ." that you may get sick and tired of hearing the message. It's necessary for us to keep repeating it, though, because so many couples avoid talking to each other about sex. And if you and your mate are among those who maintain a vow of silence about it, you're missing out.

Communication is simply the ability to comfortably exchange information with your partner about one another's thoughts, feelings, desires, problems, and anything else that matters to you as a couple. The word comes from the same Latin root as *common*. And what you're doing when you talk to each other freely and openly is cultivating the common ground you've chosen to occupy. It comes down to intimacy. Good sex is more than just rubbing genitals. Its meaning—and much of its pleasure—comes from connecting deeply with another person. By definition, that kind of human connection requires communication.

The problem is that for a lot of guys, communication just doesn't seem to come naturally. And truth be told, women don't do much better. We tell ourselves that because we're already sexually intimate with somebody, overt communication isn't necessary. Our thoughts should be obvious, shouldn't they?

Disabuse yourself of that notion. Your thoughts are not obvious. Whatever good things come out of an ongoing relationship, mind reading isn't one of them. Let the words flow freely, and you create intimacy and better sex. Bottle them up, and misinterpretations abound, resentments fester, hostilities multiply, problems grow. All of that bad stuff gets played out in the bedroom sooner or later.

You'll be relieved to learn that communication doesn't require frequent, heavy-duty encounter sessions. What you want are lines of communication that are always open, not scheduled conferences. Share your feelings and listen to hers even when the issue is relatively minor. Once you can deal with a debate about the best way to squeeze the toothpaste tube, you can work your way up to more sensitive issues. Yes, sometimes the two of you will indeed need to sit down and have a serious discussion. But ongoing communication will help you avoid those tense dialogues that feel like emergency meetings of the Security Council. When one of you utters the dreaded words *We need to talk*, it's a dead giveaway that you should have been talking a lot more all along.

When it is necessary to have a heart-to-heart, tackle just one issue at a time. If you get into a litany of complaints, you're not so much communicating as having it out. And stay upbeat: No matter how much you're bugged by something, bring it up with a positive attitude—especially if it's something in the bedroom that's bothering you.

Let's face it, sex is a loaded topic. She may interpret a simple request as criti-cism. You may take an innocent suggestion as a full-bore attack on your manhood. Either one of you may feel that you're risking rejection just by bringing up the subject.

Or you might worry that conversations about sex will kill the spontaneity and spoil the fun. It usually doesn't work that way. Sex holds more mystery and wonder than you could ever talk to death. Good-natured exchanges about what gets each of you turned on or off make both of you more receptive—not less—to an endless supply of delights and surprises.

Let her know what you like, and find out what she likes. Try to frame suggestions for change in terms of something she already does that pleases you. For example, if you'd like her to be more physical during intercourse, start by telling her how good her body feels when she moves. From there, it's easy to let her know that more movement would feel even better.

And go ahead and talk during the heat of action. Pillow talk not only reveals what you like but also deepens the intimacy level. Just don't voice complaints during the fireworks or the after-

Hot Dates 1915 Projectionists toured the country with a film called *A Free Ride*. Directed by A. Wise Guy and shot by Will B. Hard, it was the first known stag film to hit America's screens.

LEGAL BRIEFS

She'll leave the light on for you: Police in Florida said a woman driving nude on Interstate 95 turned on the light inside her car to give passing truckers a better view. Truckers spread the word about the woman via CB radio and jockeyed for a better look at her. Police arrested her and **charged her with being a traffic hazard**. She also was charged with drunken driving and possession of marijuana.

Seemed like a Good Idea at the Time...

For nearly 2 decades, famed topless dancer Carol Doda made her en-

True or Phallus?

A penis reaches its full size by the time a man turns 21.

BAWDY BALLADS "I Want a Little Sugar in My Bowl," *Nina Simone*

continued on page 62

glow (although you should mention the changes you'd like when the mood allows). "That feels wonderful" is good in-sex communication. "I hate it when you do that" isn't.

On that same note: Lighten up. Nowhere is it written that sex has to be a solemn topic. A playful attitude makes communication a lot easier and a lot more fun. And once the words start flowing, you'll find out something else: that talking about sex can itself be a turn-on.

Despite that, don't communicate everything. Sharing personal sexual information invigorates your sex life together, but filter the flow for the sake of her feelings. You don't really need to tell her that her lovemaking style reminds you of some former lover or how you sometimes fantasize about making it with your shapely next-door neighbor. Keep the focus on the pleasure you share together.

Also see: arguing; begging; cybersex; discretion; divorce—avoiding; divorce—issues that lead to; Don't ask, don't tell; Internet dating; laughter; making up; past partners—talking about; phone sex; secrets; sex therapy; sweet talk; talking dirty; teasing; whispering

communication—nonverbal

Most people call this body language, which is fine, but keep in mind that there are ways to communicate nonverbally that aren't done with the body per se. For example, a sigh says a lot. So do certain actions, such as when you clean up the bedroom before she comes home. And so can the *lack* of an expected action, such as your decision not to respond to her come-hither pose.

There are at least three important areas of your sex life where nonverbal communication matters a lot. One is during courtship, especially those charged moments when the two of you first notice each other. At that point, what you say is less important than how you say it. And neither matters as much as your actions—such as the timing of your smile, the position of your body, the subtleness of your touch.

Another crucial area is the daily life of your relationship, where domestic bliss is helped along by your ability to decode your partner's signals and understand her unspoken feelings. Time is the best teacher here; couples tend to develop an intricate unspoken language over the years.

And the third is during sex itself, where almost everything is communicated nonverbally, often in impressive detail. The lingua franca of the bedroom consists of moans, groans, motions, and touches. A guided hand or a well-timed "Mmmmm" communicates a lot.

But the best piece of advice about nonverbal communication is this: Don't depend on it 100 percent. By its very nature, body language is imprecise and open to interpretation—and misinterpretation. If confusion is the only other alternative, it's better to resort to plain English.

Also see: courtship, eye contact, flirtation, grunting, kiss, meeting women, moaning, signals, smiling, winking

companionship

It may sound like the very opposite of hot sex, but it's part of the package if you're planning to live on this planet for more than a few years. *Companionship* means a caring and trusting friendship with your sexual partner. It means really knowing her and letting her really know you. You want to cultivate that kind of companionship with your sexmate so that the sex in your relationship keeps getting better instead of burning itself out.

Reaping the rewards of companionship usually requires giving up two alternatives. One is the torrid sexual attraction of a new romance. The other is having lots of different sexual partners, which many men and women desire. The first is inevitable since the heat of new sex cools quickly on its own. But why would any right-thinking guy give up the renewable thrill of playing the field for a monogamous companion? Because, deny it as we may, many men eventually prefer a sexual partner who's a lifelong friend. Yeah, you may already have a best friend, and you may already have a sexual partner. But combine the two in one companion and you've created the kind of self-perpetuating intimacy that's a prerequisite for a comfortable yet ever-improving sex life.

Also see: commitment, communication, death of a partner, desertion, escort service, eye contact, financial difficulties, intimacy, soul mate

compulsive behavior

It's what's going on with people who are repeatedly driven to engage in a sexual activity that they get nothing out of—no pleasure, no escape, no nothing. Any sexual activity that you can't help but continue despite the harm it's causing is probably an example of compulsive behavior. It might, for example, be masturbation that makes you constantly late for work, or rough anal stimulation that causes chronic pain. Another might be

the constant and inappropriate use of sex to avoid handling life problems.

Compulsive, let us emphasize, does not simply mean "frequent." You can masturbate six times a day without there necessarily being anything compulsive about it. A robust appetite for sex doesn't automatically qualify as compulsive behavior. What does qualify is when you can't stop your behavior without extreme psychological discomfort. Also—along with a lack of actual pleasure from the activity—frustration, shame, and guilt are quite common.

The gamut of sexual compulsivity ranges from people who function normally in their day-to-day lives to those who are simply out of control. If you are obsessed with unwanted, intrusive sexual thoughts or behaviors that cause trouble in other areas of your life, talk to a therapist who is comfortable and experienced with this disorder. Some therapists prescribe medication such as Prozac or lithium.

Also see: fantasies, fetish, paraphilias, perversions, sex addiction, sex therapy

condom

It's like Kodak film: It captures that special moment. By trapping your ejaculated semen and preventing skin-to-skin genital contact during intercourse, this superthin, penis-hugging sheath does double duty, preventing pregnancy as well as the spread of sexually transmitted diseases. Condoms are cheap, readily available, socially acceptable, portable, and disposable, which is probably why they've been around in one form or another since at least 1000 B.C. These days, they're also dependable as hell, with a 97 percent effectiveness rate at preventing pregnancy, as long as you use

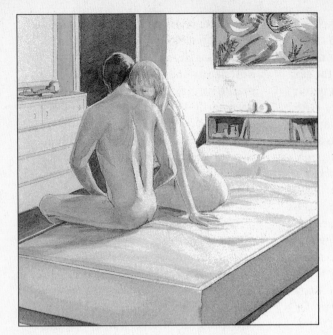

ally during intercourse to make sure the rubber is still in place. And always hold the condom securely around the base of your penis as you withdraw after ejaculation, to keep the little bugger from sliding off.

Even infrequent rubber users shouldn't have much trouble mastering those safety suggestions. Still, lots of men (and women) consider condoms a nuisance. The whole process seems like an unwelcome interruption. And covering up body parts during sex—especially *that* body part—hardly seems to be in the spirit of uninhibited pleasure.

But there are cures for these complaints. First of all, remind yourself that using a condom is not as big a nuisance as unwanted pregnancy or HIV. So don't curse your condom as a distraction; appreciate it as an instrument of hale-and-hearty, worry-free sex. Then, stop taking mood-killing, willy-wilting condom time-outs. Instead, incorporate the sheathing into the sexual flow. Put the condom on slowly and sensually, in plain sight. Or let her do the honors.

Finally, think of condoms as everyday sex toys. Experiment with sizes, colors, and the little sensuous extras like bumps and ribbing. There's no shortage of options. Like everything else about sex, condoms should be fun.

Also see: anal sex, body oils, contraception, Cowper's glands, diaphragm, dildo, femoral intercourse, French tickler, IUD, K-Y jelly, lubricants, morning-after pill, nonoxynol-9, ointments, Pap test, period, Pill—the, premature ejaculation, prophylactic, rectum, role reversal, rubber, safe sex, STDs, suppositories

them right and they haven't expired. Expiration dates are printed right on the packets; make sure yours are not out of date. As a rule of thumb, latex condoms have a shelf life of 3 to 5 years. But prolonged exposure to sunlight, high temperatures, or mineral or vegetable oils can speed their deterioration.

Let's review the basics: For the best protection against STDs, use a less porous (and much more common) latex condom rather than the lambskin variety. Put the condom on before your penis makes any contact with her vagina or anus. To maximize sensation, first daub the inside of the tip with a drop of a water-based lubricant such as Probe, Astroglide, or K-Y jelly. Also leave a little slack at the tip so your semen has someplace to go. Condoms with reservoir tips have slack built in, but either way you should squeeze the air out after you've rolled the condom on a little bit. Then finish the rolling. Reach down occasion-

condom—polyurethane

On the evolutionary scale of condoms, the polyurethane variety was supposed to be the best thing since ribs for her pleasure. Upon their late-1994 debut, we were told they were the ultimate for safe sex and pregnancy prevention. London International Group, the maker of the first such condom, the Avanti, even promised greater sensitivity because these synthetic sheaths were half as thick as those made of latex.

As is usually the case in such instances, the truth is neither here nor there.

The polyurethane prophylactic does have its upside. Some men—and women—do cite a greater sensitivity and comfort. Plus, unlike latex condoms, the polyurethane version is odorless and can be used with oil-based lubricants. Polyurethane also is a welcome alternative for the 1 to 6 percent of the general population (5 to 10 percent of health-care workers) who are allergic to latex.

Alas, its disadvantages may deflate some of your enthusiasm. Many brave volunteer couples have plunged into condom research in the name of science, and the resulting studies appear to show that polyurethane sheaths break and slip off at a much higher rate than latex ones. In a series of small studies by the California Family Health Council in the early 1990s, the Avanti condoms broke an average of 9.5 percent of the time, compared to a 1.5 percent average failure rate for latex condoms. A later study by the council showed similar results: Breakage rates during intercourse or withdrawal were 7.2 percent for the polyurethane condoms versus just 1.1 percent for latex.

Also see: lubricants, prophylactic, rubber, safe sex, STDs

contraception

Talk about taking things for granted: Technological advancement has given us contraception that's safe, easy, available, and effective. So what do we do? We complain. About the cost. About threats to spontaneity. About the few remaining risks. About the general hassle of it all.

The truth is, contraception—the prevention of unwanted pregnancy using birth control devices or agents—has changed the way we think of sex. For the better.

Modern contraceptives work in lots of ways. *Barrier methods*—such as the diaphragm, the cervical cap, the female condom, and the sponge—are temporarily placed inside the vagina to block sperm from reaching an egg. (The male condom, of course, keeps the sperm out of the vagina in the first place.) *Spermicides* are substances that actually kill sperm once they're in the vagina, and they're typically used to supplement other methods. *Hormonal birth control* prevents ovulation so there's simply no egg to impregnate; the Pill is by far the most popular, but there are also longer-lasting implants and shots as well as the morning-after pill.

You can find information throughout this book on the major methods. Which one is best is up to you and your mate. But we can tell you two things, the first of which you've probably heard before: The responsibility for birth control is not hers, or yours, but shared—just as the consequences of an unwanted pregnancy are shared. In practice, that means you should be just as unwilling to participate in unprotected intercourse as she is. Our second piece of advice may sound radical: Consider contraception a part of sex, not a sidetrack from it. Think of the

C

birth control (and safe sex) conversation with a new partner not as an anti-romantic obligation but rather as a thrilling prelude to pleasure. After all, talk is a turn-on, and what could be a sexier topic than arranging to have great, carefree sex with each other? The same holds for applying a birth control device—your condom or her diaphragm, for example. Don't approach it as an imposition. Make it a mutual rite of pleasure. Foreplay, if you will.

Also see: abstinence, beds, boxers or briefs, cervical cap, condom, diaphragm, douche, dry hump, erection difficulties, femoral intercourse, first time with a lover, IUD, kids, male pill, morning-after pill, nonoxynol-9, Norplant, oral contraceptive, Pap test, Pill—the, religion, rhythm method, safe sex, sexual revolution, sponge, sympto-thermal method, tubal ligation, vasectomy

costumes

They're proven purveyors of sexual pizzazz. You want to look hot for each other anyway; erotic costuming merely takes

that idea to a higher level. Even if just one of you dons over-the-top garb—say she slips into a G-string and pasties with a feather boa and high heels—you both feel the heat. Turn it up further by getting into the spirit of the thing yourself, perhaps using the Chippendales dancers as role models. But don't limit yourselves to our two admittedly clichéd suggestions. Choose whatever the two of you consider turn-on costumes. At the very least, you'll have some laughs.

Spicier still is using costumes to up the ante during sexual role-playing. For instance, if it's going to be one of those nights where she takes total control to "do" you, starting things off with her in a nurse's getup and you with an arm in a sling will fuel the fantasy by adding a touch of authenticity. The potential pairings are limited only by your imagination—and the movies and television programs you've seen. Cop and speeder? Princess and serf? Cocktail waitress and customer? *I Dream of Jeannie? Mork & Mindy? Death Slaves from the Planet Zoron?* Okay, we're kidding about that last one. But whatever you come up with,

Hot Dates **1915** The U.S. Supreme Court ruled that film was not protected by the First Amendment: It was "a business, pure and simple." Thirty-seven years later, in 1952, the highest court overturned that ruling.

continued from page 57

Answer:
False. Sorry, but by age 17 it's as big as it will get.

trance at San Francisco's Condor strip club on **a trick piano that descended from the ceiling to the stage**. You'd think that would be a really cool place to have sex.

You'd be wrong.

While assistant bar manager James Ferrozzo and nude dancer Teresa Hill made beautiful music to-

gether, something triggered the switch that raised the piano from stage to ceiling—thereby crushing Ferrozzo to death and trapping the naked Hill beneath him until a janitor reopened the club the next morning.

Police said Hill was so drunk she didn't remember climbing on top

BAWDY BALLADS "Guido the Killer Pimp," *Tangerine Dream*

continued on page 73

it's a good idea to test-drive the costume fantasy by playing it out in your mind when you have some private time. See if it really does anything for you before you bring it up with her.

Finding the costumes is the easy part. Overcoming embarrassment to actually wear them is harder. Try simply blurting out that you're turned on by the idea of her dressing up as a cheerleader, admitting out loud that you're a bit embarrassed about it and afraid she might consider the idea ridiculous. She may respond that she does indeed consider it ridiculous—but she'd love it if *you* dressed that way. Now you're getting somewhere. However she responds, the idea is on the table, which means that half the battle is won.

Helpful hint: Look for a context that helps the project flow. The obvious choice is Halloween night, when putting on a costume isn't just easy, it's darn near obligatory. From there, it's a simple matter of moving your little costume party into the bedroom.

Also see: cross-dressing, fantasies, games

couch

The living room couch is right up there with the kitchen table and the shower as an alternative site for sex. We get told a lot these days that we have to take the action out of the bedroom. Break the routine. Spice things up. And it's good advice. To quarantine sex to one small room robs you of your potential as a sexual being. There's a great big universe out there, and it's full of places in which to get it on. One of those places is the couch, where it's easy and natural to turn your attention away from a *Sanford and Son* rerun and focus it on that desirable being sitting next to you. It's also great for spontaneity. It's nice to just sort of flow into the act of lovemaking while you're messing around on the sofa, instead of having to risk breaking the spell (and giving everybody a chance to rethink things?) by getting up and adjourning to the bedroom. So by all means, go for it.

But . . . in the real world—the place where real people have real sex with real bodies—the couch is a damn awkward venue for actual intercourse. The seating area is not big enough, the arms and coffee tables get in the way, and you have to worry about kicking over lamps or those glass-framed pictures of the kids. So don't let the advice industry convince you that you're a boring couple if at some point you move the action off the couch and onto a bed.

This is not to say that you *can't* get down on the davenport. In fact, a couch is a great piece of furniture for oral sex since one of you can sit back while the other kneels on the floor and goes to work. But if you do go for full sofa sex, here are two suggestions: Lay a blanket or sheet between the fabric and your bodily fluids. And try a seated rear-entry position—you sit on the couch, she sits on your lap facing away from you—for a better fit with the natural contours of the furniture. More important, you both get a view of the television.

Also see: athletic sex, boredom, casting couch, rear entry, variety

courtship

Go ahead and sniff at its prissy connotations, but courtship is a powerful, evolution-hardened strategy that moves two people from total strangerhood to sexual intimacy. That's a pretty amazing piece of business, when you think about it.

Our friends in the animal world sometimes turn courtship into a dance. So do we, in our complex, drawn-out, yet often unself-conscious way. Men and women court each other with signals—a series of subtle cues and responses that depend (like any dance) on timing, rhythm, and lots of nonverbal communication.

All of the steps in this dance have one thing in common: sensuality. Whether you realize it or not, just about anything you do to woo your woman has to do with sound, taste, motion, beauty, touch. That's why the oldest courting tools—music, dining, dancing, flowers, the kiss on the hand—are still the best. Use them.

Further, courtship plays itself out in stages. It doesn't matter if they take place over a few hours in a nightclub or a few years under the watchful eyes of old-school parents; the stages stay the same.

1. Mutual eye contact gets the ball rolling. Without it, nothing's likely to happen. But once it's made, it demands a response, which usually means . . .

2. An approach. If she approaches you, great. If not, the fact that she made eye contact is your invitation to break the ice.

3. Once you're near her, don't just stand there. Talk. Forget everything you've seen in the movies. Successful courtship talk has more to do with tone than with content, the best tone being sweet and musical, almost singsong. If that sounds very unlike James Bond's sophisticated banter, well, it is. Courtship

conversation isn't about suave. It's about making her feel good and warm and safe and sexy. Impress her with your deep knowledge of particle theory some other time. Right now, compliment her hair.

4. Then move on to the next step, the turn. If things are progressing smoothly, the two of you will keep shifting your positions until you're facing each other straight on.

5. When you're aligned, touch. Believe it or not, she usually initiates it, often with a slight, fleeting brush of your arm while making some unrelated comment. Don't be fooled by the subtlety. This is a probe, and you must respond in kind. Touch back with equal restraint.

6. Moving in synchrony is what you'll find yourselves doing now. You lift your glass, she lifts hers. You somehow reach toward each other simultaneously. You sway in rhythm together. Suddenly, dancing seems like a very good idea.

7. Caressing—touching with a purpose—comes next. This is where the initiative usually shifts from mostly hers to mostly yours. It's as if she were telling you, "Okay, I've done my part; now you take it from here." It's a mixed blessing since going too fast or too slow is equally likely to kill the deal. By now, though, you should have a pretty good idea of her pace and preferences.

8. Touching progresses to kissing. Though the initiative is yours, she must make it clear that she wants to be kissed. Women are usually pretty good at that, so once the encouragement is there, go for it. A woman who signals for a kiss and doesn't get it is not a happy camper.

9. Sooner or later comes the whole enchilada. But at the threshold of intercourse (the first time, anyway), it's wise to supplement all those signals with more overt communication—for consent, for safer sex, for a friendly sense of relaxation.

Incidentally, if you're wondering why you should bother with all this rigmarole in a case where you're both ready to jump straight to the last stage, consider: Courtship itself is a turn-on. Each stage holds out the promise of more to come. Anticipation is continuously stoked and never quite quenched. Even after consummation, a sort of continuous feedback loop of desire has been created, making the two of you eager to start the whole process all over again, right from stage one. That's why courtship should never end, even after decades of marriage.

Also see: boredom, communication—nonverbal, dating, eye contact, flirtation, meeting women, one-night stand, pickup lines, seduction, signals, sweet talk, unwanted advances

Cowper's glands

Two pea-size glands below the prostate that provide prelubrication assistance by secreting a few drops of clear fluid through the urethra when you get aroused. Those drops often contain some sperm, which is one reason why any unprotected penetration—even without ejaculation—is a pregnancy risk. So put on a condom before you put your pecker anywhere near her vagina. The name of the gland, by the way, comes from its discoverer, the late-17th-century English surgeon and anatomist William Cowper (pronounced "Cooper"). He'll forever be a part of you.

Also see: arousal, condom, lubrication

crabs

They're really lice. But when they infest your pubic area, they certainly make you feel crabby. That's because they also make you feel intense itching as they feed on your blood and lay their tiny white eggs, or nits, in your pubic hair.

The tiny lice can live outside a host for up to 2 days, which means that they can be spread by simple contact, not just by sexual intercourse. So you and your sex partner don't have to suspect each other of infidelity if the little buggers show up.

Also see: pubic lice, scratching, STDs

cramps—leg

Screaming at orgasm is great—if you're screaming in ecstasy.

Unfortunately, pain sometimes strikes at the most inopportune times, thanks to excruciating leg-muscle cramps. It so happens that a lot of the triggers that cause charley horses happen naturally during sex, including muscle overexertion, decreased bloodflow to the muscle (perhaps from sustaining a certain position), overflexing the muscle while thrusting, and dehydration. (When sex is imminent, you don't normally say things like "Wait, honey, I have to get a glass of water first.")

Don't even think about soldiering your way through the pain. Stop what you're doing and stretch the cramped muscle by contracting its antagonist. That is, if the cramp is in the back of your calf, contract the muscle in the front of your calf by pointing your big toe toward your forehead and pulling your toes up with your hands. Then, massage the cramped muscle—or have her do it for you, assuming she hasn't bolted from the bed at the sound of your bloodcurdling shrieks. A hot bath will get both of you feeling relaxed and ready to pick up where you left off.

There are a few things you can do to avoid the cramp in the first place. That water we talked about? Make a point of drinking it throughout the day. A good rule of thumb is to multiply your body weight in pounds by 0.7 (thus a 200-pound man needs 64 ounces, or eight 8-ounce glasses, every day). And take advantage of her inevitable disappearance into the bathroom to sneak in a cramp-discouraging runner's stretch: Stand a few steps in front of a wall with one leg forward and bent at the knee. Reach out to the wall with both hands at chest level, and lean into it without lifting your heels. Feel the stretch in your back leg and hold it for 20 seconds. Then switch legs and repeat. We guarantee you'll be done before she finishes doing whatever women do in there.

cramps—menstrual

She's likely to get them at "that time of the month." And you, being the helpful, empathic guy you are, can actually do her some good. That's because some women report that orgasm helps alleviate the cramping, bloating, and other discomforts of their periods. So offer to do some sexual healing; it's something she herself might not ordinarily think of in her cranky state.

Your woman may respond in one of two ways to your notions of having sex at that particular time. She may be delighted at your interest. Or she may run at you with an ice pick. (In which case, you shouldn't force the issue. You only

brought it up for her benefit, remember?) Either way, you'll take her mind off her abdomen for a while.

The downside? If she goes along with the idea but her cramps return later, you may have to do it all over again. Poor guy.

Also see: breast pain, PMS, tampon

cross-dressing

Wear women's clothes, and you're cross-dressing. Those usually called cross-dressers, however, tend to be relatively low-key in their sartorial habits—unlike, say, drag queens.

Sporting an evening gown at a Halloween party may be cross-dressing in the generic sense, but true cross-dressers are in it for the long haul. And there are a lot more of them than you might think. Poke around certain big-city clothing stores and you'll find a decent supply of king-size hosiery and extra-extra-extra-large dresses—way too big for even most big, beautiful women. Guess who's snatching up the merchandise?

How to accommodate cross-dressing in a sexual relationship? Do you tell a prospective partner? Hide it from your wife and risk being found out at the worst possible moment, as in the hilarious scene from Woody Allen's *Everything You Always Wanted to Know about Sex (But Were Afraid to Ask)*? There are no pat answers. Some women won't get it, no matter what. Others, if they know you as an all-around swell guy with more to offer than a pretty dress, will be happy to make things work.

One rule always applies, though: Don't raid her wardrobe for secret tryons. You'll stretch her things—one of the surest ways to tick off a female. If you're going to dress like a woman, be a man about it. Buy your own clothes!

Also see: arousal, drag, fetish, homophobia, homosexuality, paraphilias, transvestism

cum

A slang term for what Monica Lewinsky had on her dress. (That's semen, for those of you who spent the late 1990s on another planet.) *Cum* is the noun form of the euphemism *to come*, meaning "to reach orgasm." (We bet your high school English teacher never gave you that grammar lesson.)

Also see: come, ejaculation, get off, gusher, semen, wet spot

cunnilingus

Now here's a medical term for oral sex that really sounds like what's going on. As you probably know, it's the sexual stimulating of her genital area (labia, clitoris, and vaginal opening) with your lips and tongue.

The secret here is to enjoy it. Don't do it "for" her. Don't "give" it like a gift. Go down on your partner in the spirit of mutual pleasure. Get into the sensate experience of cunnilingus instead of just trying to bring her off. Make yourself comfortable and settle in for a good time. Look for ways (like music, scents, positions) to heighten the pleasure—*your* pleasure. Sound selfish? On the contrary, you'll be a more enthusiastic and generous oral lover. You'll be less likely to get impatient about just how long you have to do this before she's had enough. And you'll find

it easier to get creative—to explore, experiment, and stumble upon new ways to please her. When you're having fun, it's easier for her to have fun.

Then again, maybe you just don't like the idea of getting your face down there and going at it. Give it a chance. Give it a few chances. It's worth the effort since a lot of women are crazy about cunnilingus and since it gives you a fine opportunity to pleasure your partner without needing an erection. But look, if it remains clear that this thing isn't for you, don't do it. Just be forewarned that for some women your disinclination in this area is a deal breaker.

Also see: beard burn, clitoral orgasm, clitoris, eat, fellatio, give head, Janus Report, licking, marathon, oral sex, pregnancy, tongue, vaginal injuries, yeast infection

cybersex

Name your technological advance—movable type, the camera, the telephone, the automobile—and we humans will find a way to use it for sex.

The computer is no exception. With the Internet, you've got a fast and far-flung personal ad service. You've got a cheap and easy porn-viewing machine, with more selection and interactive possibilities than any X-rated video store could dream of. But when people talk about cybersex, they usually mean the online sex chats that two people at opposite ends of the globe can engage in to get each other off. Toll-free, no less.

It's like two-way phone sex, but with a keyboard. You'd think the typing requirement would leave you at least one hand short of the number needed for communication *and* pleasure. Think again. Folks seem to manage just fine. When you move from a group chat to a private one with your chosen date, the two of you are free to type messages back and forth, building to whatever sexual crescendo you choose. The appeal is safe sexual interaction with total anonymity and no other human being actually present.

Here's a FAQ for you. (That's a frequently asked question, in cyberparlance.) How do you know that the person on the other end is really what she says she is and not what *he* isn't saying *he* is? You don't. Lots of tricks have been suggested to trip up gender frauds—for example, asking your cyberpartner's panty hose size—but the truth is, there's really no way to know for sure. Many stay off the Net for just that reason. Others find it an additional turn-on.

If you do choose to pursue Net nookie, ideally, you want to do it to practice the social skills and nurture the courage you need for real-life interaction with the opposite sex. Going online as a *substitute* for developing those skills is almost certainly a bad idea. Another bad idea is doing it at the expense of quality time spent with your real-life partner. And if you're married, don't kid yourself:

Engaging in cybersex on the sly may very well constitute a form of infidelity in your wife's eyes.

Nonsense, you say? Then why are you doing it on the sly, bubba?

Also see: arousal, dial-a-porn, extramarital sex, Internet dating, phone sex, pornography, videos

cystitis

A bladder infection—usually hers, not yours—marked by frequent and painful urination. There's no one cause. But, like other urinary tract infections, it can come from usually well-behaved intestinal bacteria that migrate and multiply after the urethra becomes irritated due to sexual intercourse. Hence the moniker *honeymoon cystitis*, as women are more at risk when they resume intercourse after a layoff or dramatically turn up the frequency. It's a good idea for your partner to urinate immediately after intercourse to flush out bacteria.

What can you do? Use plenty of lubrication to help prevent the friction that chafes the urethra and can cause cystitis. And show plenty of patience to help her get through the antibiotic cycle if she does get it.

Also see: pee—painful, urethritis, urinary problems

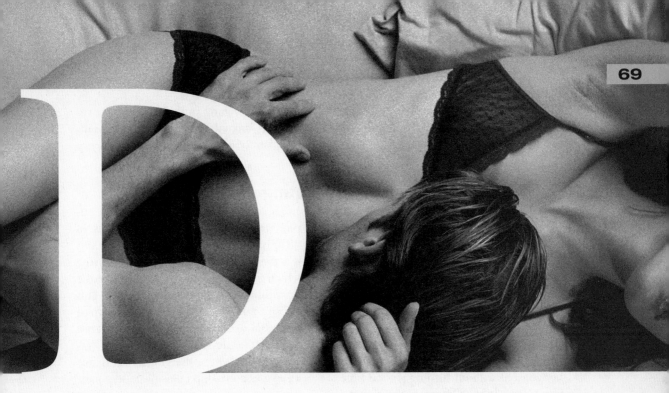

danger

It's a turn-on. Or at least it can be, especially if you fall into that category of human beings whom psychologists describe as risk takers. These are the guys who need a dose of danger to get excited about anything, be it a business venture, weekend sports, or a roll in the hay. For them, danger is an aphrodisiac.

That's not as extreme as it sounds. Fear excites your body in much the same way that sex does—by getting your heart beating harder, your lungs breathing faster, and your muscles tensing tighter.

Take a look at a roller coaster full of screaming 20-year-olds. Is it really so surprising that some people actually experience sexual arousal when they're scared?

Also see: bars, boss's wife, emotions, injuries, risky sex, safe sex, STDs

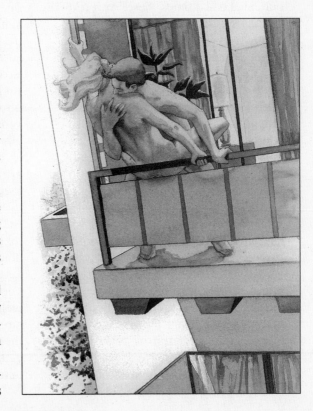

D

date rape

Date rape is forced sex. It is rape. Period. That alone should convince anybody to refrain from it. The confusion occurs because of the *date* part of date rape. It means that the victim and perpetrator have some kind of social relationship (hence the alternative term, *acquaintance rape*). It also means that the force used may come not from weapons or brute strength but from coercion, intimidation, or simply getting her intoxicated. The damage of a date rape can be just as devastating as that of a stranger's attack, but the broken boundaries aren't as clear.

Where does seduction end and coercion begin? And how can you be sure of her consent without turning a good time into a deposition? Common questions of our enlightened times, these. As it turns out, the surest way to deal with them is totally consistent with the best sex: Never pressure a woman for it. If she says no to intercourse or to any sexual touching along the way, back off. Don't interpret it. Don't try to figure out a way around it. Just back off. The world isn't going to end. You may lose a sexual "opportunity," but this is the adult, manly, legal way to go.

Pressure and good sex don't go together anyway. The best sex results from two willing and eager people who have already talked about it and anticipated it, and who are relaxed enough with each other to concentrate on mutual pleasure. You don't get there by pushing, and amid today's litigious climate, you don't want to take a chance by assuming that her protests are insincere. Let the activists and academics argue about whether no always means no. The kind of consent you're waiting for is "*Oh* yes!"

Also see: gang rape, lust, no, rape, rejection—sexual, seduction, sex offenders, Spanish fly, unwanted advances, violence

dating

In some circles, it's a contemporary euphemism for "having sex with," as in "Biff is dating Buffy." More traditionally, it's the series of social outings during which a man and a woman explore the possibility of a sexual relationship. If it doesn't take place against a backdrop of potential sex—however remote—it's not dating. It's ride-sharing.

Dating is where the human sex dance known as courtship takes place, at a pace less breakneck than at singles bars. Early on, much of the dance is nonverbal. While the two of you exchange comments on the movie you just saw, a silent conversation about where things stand sexually might be going on at the same time. Pay attention to it. For example, does she lean in toward you and touch your arm when she tells you that she really enjoyed the show?

Those are cues that might signal growing sexual interest. Encourage them. Respond to them. But don't press the issue. The number-one rule of dating is: Do not be pushy about sex. Breaking that rule is not just unseemly, it's self-defeating. Dating allows the two of you to enjoy yourselves together, get to know each other, and sooner or later feel comfortable enough to act on your mutual attraction. You can't do any of that when you're too preoccupied with getting laid to pay attention to her as a person. And she can't do it while she's busy defending herself from your heavy artillery.

Also see: courtship, first date, first time with a lover, Internet dating, match-making services, mating, personal ads, pickup lines, rejection—romantic, singles scene

death of a partner

It's a tragedy for anybody, but it's especially tough for men, many of whom have traditionally relied on their women for emotional support, friendship, and companionship as well as the more practical household stuff. And a lot of us make mistakes that discourage recovery. One of those mistakes is self-recrimination. "If only I'd done this or that . . ." is a typical reaction that's neither realistic nor helpful.

Another error is jumping into a new sexual relationship prematurely. Better to finish your grieving first. And better to do some existential reflection. The men who recover best from the deaths of their lovers are the ones who seriously explore the meaning of it all. Sample questions: What did our relationship mean to me? Where does her loss put me? What do I have of value to offer the world? The best recoverers also contemplate, rather than dodge, the larger questions about life and the universe that naturally announce themselves at this time. Such reflection is difficult, time-consuming, uncomfortable—and absolutely necessary. It requires a high level of focused consciousness at a time when it may be more tempting to sleep-walk through the pain. But it's the only way to truly get on with your life.

Also see: breaking up, breast cancer, companionship, heartache, necrophilia, past partners—longing for, single—suddenly, young men/older women

depression

This is right up there with anxiety at the top of the list of psychological disorders that can screw up your sex life. Depression can describe a mere bout with the blues or a serious clinical condition characterized by sadness, retarded motor functions, feelings of inadequacy, and even thoughts of suicide. There's a sex connection at both ends of that range, with different people affected in different ways. Some men actually become more sexually active when they're depressed, probably because it's the one and only thing they're comfortable doing that involves other people. However, depressed men are more apt to suffer from low libidos, not high ones. Many experience erection problems.

Depression, with its feelings of lifelessness, helplessness, and isolation, is by no means rare. Take note of any ongoing feelings of boredom with your sex life. They could, of course, be no more than the logical consequence of a static pattern of routine sex. If that's the case, vary the pattern and break out of the routine. But complaints of sexual boredom also set off red flags with sex therapists; they're sometimes a sign of depression.

Getting more exercise, eating less sugar, and increasing your social interaction with friends can all be helpful in battling depression. If these strategies don't help, you should see a doctor.

One thing to keep in mind if you seek treatment for depression is that some common antidepressant medications—

D

such as those, like Prozac, that inhibit the uptake of the neurotransmitter serotonin—can cause problems with sex drive, erection, or orgasm and ejaculation. So, even if the condition itself doesn't shrink your libido or your penis, the pills might. If your medication seems to be hurting your sex life, ask your doctor to experiment with dosages or prescribe something else.

Also see: boredom, emotions, empty-nest syndrome, heartache, job loss, menopause—hers, midlife crisis, PMS, postpartum depression, Prozac, sex—lack of, single—suddenly

desertion

We're not necessarily talking about the door-slamming, I'm-leaving-forever-and-taking-the-TV-with-me kind. It can be a thousand little rejections that happen any day, any minute, without either of you really intending them. Say she mumbles, "I'm listening. . . " but keeps sorting through the mail while you're talking about vacation ideas. To the rest of the world, that's just impolite; to you, it's worse. You're attached to this woman and she to you. You're each part of who the other is. When one of you operates according to that attachment and the other doesn't, it feels like desertion. And it's not a good feeling.

For these occasional moments, take a simple approach. Ask her when would be a better time to talk. (In all likelihood, she'll be happy that you actually *want* to talk, so she'll focus her full attention on you.) If her distraction has been going on long-term, try to find out if there's an underlying issue. Problems at work, with family, with your relationship? Be prepared for a long-term answer.

What if you're the one who's feeling distant? Remember, everything is magnified in the bedroom, where expectations of intimacy are highest. That's why you hear so much talk about being "in the moment" when it comes to sex. If she's particularly tuned in to you while making love and you come off as mechanical or distracted, she feels abandoned.

There are two wrong ways to deal with this. One is to do your damnedest to be present and connected all day, every day, and every time you have sex—permanently non-abandoning, so to speak. No human being could pull that off. The other is to master the motions of connectedness, throwing in some eye contact here and some stock phrases there. Forget it. You're not fooling anybody.

Do this instead: Tell her when and why you're feeling disconnected. Make clear that it's temporary. That way, you air it out and defuse it at the same time. If sex is at issue, consider words to this effect: "I love making love with you, but I'm kind of preoccupied right now. If we do it now, I may not be as into it as I'd like to be. But if that's okay with you, let's go for it." She may be horny enough to want to plunge ahead anyway. And you know what? You may not mind.

Also see: commitment, companionship, toys

desperate

It's what you never want to be. If you feel starved for sexual gratification, you're going to start acting a little bit too pushy around women, a little bit too sexually aggressive, a little bit . . . well, desperate. That won't get you anywhere except further along the cycle of desperation. Next thing you know, you'll be looking for love in all the wrong places. Against your better judgment, you'll hook up with somebody who can offer only her own sexual or emotional desperation. The blind lead the blind.

The way out of this mess is not a better sex-seeking strategy but an overhaul of your thoughts on the nature of human sexuality. Lose the notion that sex is a scarce commodity. Focus more on really getting to know different women than on getting laid this very night. If sex is in the cards, it'll be more likely to happen when a woman feels relaxed and comfortable with you. Should you make her feel desired? You bet. Just don't make her feel like prey or like you're working against some kind of clock.

Strategy summary: If you want a steady flow of sex, don't try to force it. Create the conditions for it.

Also see: begging, courtship, dating, masher, matchmaking services, meeting women, personal ads, pity sex, rejection—sexual, seduction

DHEA

No matter how stellar our sex lives may be, we're always looking for ways to make them better. This goal, noble though it seems, makes us vulnerable to pills and potions promising better sex in a bottle. One such gimmick is DHEA, short for dehydroepiandrosterone, which is purported to throw both our sex drives and our sex lives into high gear by boosting testosterone levels.

Male virility depends largely on testosterone levels, and DHEA levels indirectly affect them. DHEA is a precursor hormone, or hormonal middleman, that is produced by your adrenal glands and then converted into testosterone. Your natural supply of DHEA peaks at age 25 and declines steadily thereafter. Proponents of DHEA say replenishing the waning supply is a key to maintaining virility as well as youth.

Nice theory. Trouble is, in practice, there is *no* evidence that taking DHEA supplements can boost sex drive, potency,

Hot Dates | **1916** Birth control advocate Margaret Sanger opened the nation's first birth control clinic in Brooklyn. It was open only 10 days before the vice squad shut it down and arrested Sanger.

continued from page 62

of the piano or Ferrozzo climbing on top of her.

Foreign Affairs

In some parts of Africa, it's believed that half a man is twice the man. **Those who want to have large families have one testicle removed and burned** as an offering to the fertility god. This is supposed to make the men more potent. What, then, is the sound of one gland slapping?

In Extremis

The most married person in the world is not Mickey Rooney or Larry King but Mongkut of Siam (now Thailand), the real-life prototype for *The King and I.* Mongkut had 9,000 wives and concubines.

Legal Briefs

A doctor and his wife, en route from Munich, Germany, to San Diego, were arrested during an intermediate stop

True or Phallus?

In the early 1980s, the toy surprise in some boxes of Cracker Jacks was a tiny pamphlet with photos of nude men and women titled "Erotic Sexual Positions from around the World."

BAWDY BALLADS | "Let's Spend the Night Together," *the Rolling Stones*

continued on page 78

or staying power—or even raise testosterone levels at all. The recommended dose is too small to make a difference in a healthy man's already-high natural testosterone levels. And the amount needed to provide measurable testosterone uptick would actually prove toxic.

Indeed, even smaller amounts of DHEA have been shown to lower HDL (the "good" cholesterol), thus increasing your risk for heart disease. The hormone can also make existing prostate cancer proliferate faster. And because high testosterone levels speed production of red blood cells, supplementing with DHEA may even thicken your blood and raise your risk of having a stroke.

Our take? Skip the middleman. If you suffer from low sex drive, ask your doctor to test your testosterone levels. Testosterone supplementation is available by prescription.

Also see: hormones, testosterone replacement therapy

dial-a-porn

The commercial version of phone sex. What you get in exchange for a bloated phone bill is sometimes no more than a semi-explicit recorded message. But you can also engage in live conversation with a woman you'll never meet. Or you can join a party line of several strangers participating in a fantasy-filled verbal free-for-all. Since dial-a-porn first took off in the 1980s, the government has attempted (often successfully) to "regulate" it—that is, suppress and censor it. Despite that, and despite stiff competition from Internet porn, the calls keep, well, coming.

Dial-a-porn does offer anonymous fantasy fulfillment, a free hand (two if you use speakerphone), and a kind of

safe sex that might not even qualify as cheating, depending on the rules of your relationship. On the other hand, it can be ungodly expensive since most services charge by the minute and train their agents (that's what the hired humans attached to the voices are actually called) to stall for time. FCC regulations also limit what agents are allowed to say, which in some cases means coded conversations that are more silly than stimulating. ("I bet you'd like to give me the shaft. . . . ") Besides, the whole idea of talking sexy with an "agent" isn't our idea of a good time. All things considered, an eager and loquacious real-life wife or girlfriend is a better—and cheaper—partner for phone sex.

Also see: compulsive behavior, cybersex, moaning, phone sex, pornography, talking dirty, voice

diaphragm

It's the oldest and most popular of the female barrier birth control methods (the kind that literally block sperm from getting to an egg). A diaphragm is essentially a saucer-shaped rubber cup that gets coated with spermicide and then placed over the cervix, at the back of the vagina. The barrier, then, is both physical and chemical. Diaphragms are cost-effective since one can last for 2 years. And they work; if used correctly with no mishaps, the effectiveness rate is 94 percent. (In the real, fumble-fingered world, that rate is more like 80 percent.)

If your sex partner inserts a diaphragm, you're excused from condom use—at least for birth control purposes. What you can do, though, is participate in what might be called the diaphragm lifestyle. For example, the diaphragm must be put in place no more than 2 hours before intercourse. In spontaneous encounters, that probably means an intermission for diaphragm insertion just when things are getting hot. And on those fortunate occasions when you're ready to go back for seconds, a spermicide reload is necessary first. These pauses in the action may seem like good times to run to the fridge for a beer. But it's better to stay with her, and maybe even help. At the very least, hand her things. Try to make it a sexy ritual instead of an unwelcome interruption.

Afterward, be aware that she has the responsibility of taking care of what is, after all, a piece of medical equipment. A diaphragm must be washed after each use, dusted with cornstarch, inspected occasionally for tiny holes, stored in a special case, refitted if she gains or loses weight (including after pregnancy), and packed when the two of you go away for the weekend. A little recognition of her efforts would no doubt be appreciated.

Also see: cervical cap, contraception, nonoxynol-9, sponge, STDs, toxic shock syndrome

dildo

What's the difference between a dildo and a vibrator? A penetrating question. In general, they're both phallic-shaped sex toys. And from a woman's point of view, both have the advantage of never getting tired, never losing the mood, and never watching baseball on television. But the joys of vibration are best applied externally, exciting the pleasure-packed nerve endings of the vulva, clitoris, anal opening, or penis head. The nonvibrating dildo, on the other hand (or even on the same hand), is like Roger Clemens—it

likes to work inside and is most effective when it keeps moving in and out.

This brings up another question on your mind: "Why would she want a fake penis in her vagina if she can have mine?" Well, she's better qualified to answer that than we are. Ask her. You'll probably find that it has nothing to do with your penis size or your performance, nor with any problem in your sex life together. A dildo, like any sex toy, isn't for "fixing" one or both partners. It's for enhancing sexual pleasure. So don't think of it as just her thing; think of it as a toy for two. She can play with it in your presence, while you watch or participate (by, for example, orally pleasuring her). Alternatively, you can do the inserting, leaving her hands and mouth free for reciprocal favors. And if you've both learned to like anal stimulation, two more orifices become eligible receivers. In that case, she can use a special harness to mount the dildo on her pelvis so she can experience doggie-style intercourse from what is usually your point of view, as the two of you engage in some serious role reversal. The possibilities, as they say, are endless.

An added bonus: A dildo is a good safe-sex option. Just make sure you wash it thoroughly or put a condom on it before transferring it from the anus to the vagina or mouth. And always use a lubricant for anal insertion.

If you're intrigued, start by shopping together online, via mail order, or at one of the modern, nonsleazy sex shops where you can actually see what will be getting into you—and the options abound. A veritable cottage industry of dildo designers has come up with numbers that look like dolphins, mythical figures, hands or feet, or simply abstract forms that are pleasing to the eye. Some

D

day, the Museum of Modern Art may offer a retrospective on Non-Penile Representation at the Dawn of the Dildo Revolution: Form and Function. Meanwhile, you and your lady can choose between a dildo that looks just like an erect penis and one that doesn't.

Check the material. Silicone-based dildos are much better than the predominant mystery-rubber kind. They're easier to clean (you can pop them in the dishwasher—top rack only), and they last longer. Size, though, is your main concern. Too big will be uncomfortable, especially if it's going up an anal canal. Too small might be disappointing, especially if it's going into a vagina. How do you know what size is just right? After all, test-inserting a dildo is impossible online, and it's frowned upon at the sex-shop display shelves.

You can try using the finger-comparison test, but by far, the most accurate solution is produce. Finish laughing, then go on down to the supermarket, select zucchini and cucumbers in lots of sizes, go home, wash them, insert them one by one (using a condom and, if you're testing them for anal use, a water-based lubricant), pick her favorite (and yours, if applicable), and then measure its circumference. You now have a size guideline, without having done anything that folks haven't done for thousands of years. And you'll both be smiling during the salad course tonight.

Also see: anal plug, phallic, role reversal, sexual aids, Venus butterfly

disability—hers

Getting up enough nerve to ask a woman out on a date is tough enough even when the woman doesn't have a physical disability. If she does, that raises another whole set of issues. Do you mention the disability or ignore it? Help her open a heavy door or let her do it herself?

Your best bet when charting these murky waters is to remember that, though she's really no different emotionally or intellectually than any other woman, there may well be some sensitivity hurdles you need to put behind you before the two of you can relate to one another as just a man and a woman.

If she uses a wheelchair, sit down so you're at eye level when talking to her. She gets around with crutches? Go ahead and ask her how she came to need them. It's better to ask than to skip the topic altogether. (Do that, and you risk sending her the message that it makes you feel uncomfortable or, worse, embarrassed.) Just don't make every conversation about those crutches. Her disability is only one small aspect of who she is; make it a small aspect of your relationship as well.

Realize also that she may be reluctant to share her whole life story until she gets to know you better. And for the record, there are plenty of nondisabled people who feel the exact same way.

If she seems to need help, say, getting up from a chair, don't rush to her aid without first asking if she would like some assistance. Women with disabilities don't want to be viewed as weak victims who need to be rescued. The things she's able to do for herself give her dignity and independence, and you don't want to take those away from her.

When it comes to working up a sweat between the sheets, the key—as in any intimate relationship—is communication. Be especially sensitive to her body language. She may be reluctant to tell you if something is uncomfortable for her, so as not to hurt your feelings or make you feel incompetent. Keep in mind that certain positions may be painful or just plain impossible. That doesn't mean the sex has to be stale. Some couples coping with disabilities say they've overcome challenges in the bedroom simply by being more creative. And, hey, coital creativity is your middle name, right?

Depending on the nature of her disability, she may have trouble reaching orgasm. If that's the case, focus on what feels good for her, and for you, rather than on the pursuit of orgasm. The fact that the big O may be elusive at first does not mean it's a lost cause. In fact, half of all people with the most serious disabilities—spinal cord injuries—report having orgasms, and most folks who don't reach orgasm still report being sexually satisfied.

disability—overcoming

The only guys who aren't one accident away from a disability are those who've already had that accident.

For the differently abled, the unfortunate stereotype of the asexual "cripple" is just one more challenge to meet. In most cases, physical handicaps don't suppress the libido. Even those whose nervous systems are so damaged that erection and orgasm are out of the picture can still express their affection and passion in satisfying ways. It's simply a matter of taking the advice we give all our readers: Expand the boundaries of sex by redefining sexuality more broadly.

Also see: back, body image, heart conditions, injuries, sickness

discretion

Generally, it's considered polite, respectful, and mature to be discreet about your sexual relationships and behaviors—meaning that what you and your partner do privately should remain private. An obvious exception would be confidential discussions with a qualified relationships counselor, psychotherapist, clergy person, or medical provider.

Sure, you're not going to keep quiet about your hot one-nighter with that woman you'll never see again. She's going to tell her own friends about it, just like you'll tell yours.

But it's a different story if you're in a steady relationship. If your friends have met your woman, blabbing about how good she is in bed only guarantees that they'll start imagining what she looks like naked and spread-eagled—just in case they don't do that already. (Do you really want to make her the subject of laughter and derision?) And God help you if your buddies are dumb enough to let her catch them snickering about her (or if she hears it third-hand from a girlfriend who's seeing one of them). If she finds out that you've violated her confidence, you're likely to lose her trust and cause her embarrassment and other difficulties. Then you won't have to worry about keeping mum about those romantic little interludes, because there won't be romantic little interludes anymore.

Believe us, you don't want her talking to the girls about you, either. In a good relationship, a woman most likely considers your sex life to be the most sacred of intimacies. If she lets other women in on your personal secrets, it may mean that she's unhappy with the way things are going and she's seeking sympathy and advice.

Also see: best friend's wife; commitment; communication; Don't ask, don't tell; fantasies; intimacy; jealousy; past partners—talking about; secrets

divorce—avoiding

One long-shot strategy for avoiding a divorce is to ask for one. Spouses have been known to react in utter disbelief, having been going along their merry ways without a clue that anything was wrong. That right there reveals at least two defects in your relationship that you can try to fix: a woeful lack of communication and an assumption that a good marriage takes care of itself. The shock of hearing the question can stun a complacent spouse into working on problems like these and may actually help save the marriage.

Another strategy, surprisingly, is to argue more. If you're avoiding verbal spats, you're probably avoiding whatever problems are behind them. You're also behaving as though you can't resolve conflicts together. If you want your marriage to survive, turn that around. Now.

There are some factors that may statistically work against a marriage's success: marrying young, being a child of divorced parents, and going in with unrealistic expectations. But once you exchange vows, it's your marriage to win or lose. Dedication and communication are your best defenses against failure. And if a crisis arises, more dedication and communication—as well as professional counseling—are better alternatives than prematurely throwing in the towel. True, avoiding divorce isn't always smart; some marriages are better off dissolved. But settling for divorce simply to avoid the hard work of keeping a marriage alive is a mistake, and it's disrespectful to both your mate and yourself.

Divorce is a topic around which industries have sprung up, so we can't possibly answer all of your questions here. Suffice it to say that if you think your marriage is in peril, there are any number of books, marriage counselors,

Hot Dates 1918 to 1925 A Massachusetts doctor wrote a series of sex manuals that recommended positions other than the typical missionary position and advised delaying orgasm to allow one's partner to catch up.

continued from page 73

Answer:
True. The snack's distributor blamed the gaffe on a prankster.

after a 13-year-old girl and her mother, who'd been seated nearby on the flight, told airline personnel that **the couple had appeared to be having sex**. Also arrested were two unrelated male passengers who threw food and drinks at flight attendants attempting to intervene in the couple's frolicking.

The wife, by the way, was a lawyer and part-time judge.

Seemed like a Good Idea at the Time. . .
An Ohio woman survived 4 days one January wedged in the front seat of a car with **the decomposing corpse of her boyfriend**

BAWDY BALLADS "Love to Love You Baby," *Donna Summer*

continued on page 89

psychotherapists, support groups, and wise old relatives who may have useful advice for you.

Also see: arguing, breaking up, communication, marriage, matchmaking services, remarriage, trust—rebuilding

divorce—coping with

See: breaking up, past partners—dealing with, single—suddenly

divorce—issues that lead to

One of them is sex. If you consider it the center of your relationship, a partner who will never share your erotic vision can be frustrating at best and unresolvable at worst. (This leaves aside the question of whether sex *should* be the center of your relationship, but that's another story.) Sex in a marriage is like your penis itself: It becomes that much more important to you when it's not working right.

Of course, problematic sex is less of an issue for some than for others. This is true of just about any factor in a marriage— money, property, power, child rearing. There's no rating system that applies equally to all. But there are two situations that clearly stand out: substance abuse and violence. If there's active, destructive alcoholism or drug abuse in a union, that relationship is in jeopardy. If there's physical violence, it should definitely end.

There's also one overriding issue that you can use to assess all the others: whether or not the two of you truly like each other. Not love each other. Like each other. All spouses inevitably have problems. Spouses who genuinely like each other can work together to over-

come them. If you like your wife as a person, it's easier to feel that it's worth working on whatever specific issues are threatening your marriage. If you don't, there may not be much point in making the effort.

Also see: adultery, affairs, arguing, communication, frigidity, Madonna/whore complex, marriage, marriage—open

doggie style

Zoologically accurate slang for intercourse wherein you enter her vagina from behind. Variations abound, of course, but the most doglike rear-entry position has the two of you on your knees.

One drawback here is the nomenclature. *Rear entry* sounds coldly mechanical. *Doggie style* sounds like a fashion rag for the canine set. Solution: Give it your own name. *Rump bump, over the moon, that thing I really like*—just get creative; it's all good.

Also see: animals, exercise, G-spot, rear entry, standing positions

dominance and submission

It's not what it looks like. Yes, it's sex play where one partner submits to being dominated by the other. Yes, it usually involves exaggerated fantasy role-playing about, say, a kidnapper torturing a hostage. Yes, somebody may be tied up in the process. And yes, there may be a little high-intensity physicality that looks like pain (though it shouldn't necessarily feel like it). But true dominance and submission is not one partner getting off at the expense of the other; it's always consensual. It's always planned out. It's always under control.

D

The more accurate term for it is *erotic power play*. Think about your usual lovemaking. Don't the two of you constantly manipulate control and surrender in subtle ways just before and during sex? Erotic power play simply eliminates the subtlety and highlights the opportunities.

The hard part is conquering your shyness and bringing up the idea in the first place. One way is to talk after conventional sex about any obvious power play incident that cropped up. Example: In the throes of passion, she gritted her teeth and threatened to do such and such to you until you begged for mercy. If that intrigued you, tell her how much you liked it and that you'd enjoy taking it further. Then talk things out together.

If it's a go, you have some planning to do. Deciding who'll be the "top" (dominator) and who the "bottom" is only the beginning. You also need to agree on roles, which can be as generic as mistress and slave, or more creative, like the librarian and the linebacker. Then sketch out what you'll actually do, both during sex and leading up to it. That may sound overly scripted, but unless you negotiate compatible roles that you both see as a turn-on, you're not going to have a good time of it. It's hard to wing your way through such unfamiliar sexual territory. Most important, you need to agree on a safeword that will stop the action if one of you becomes uncomfortable.

Of course, there are cautions to heed when considering this kind of activity. Some people may be uncomfortable with rough play because it reminds them of something bad that happened in their pasts. They include women or men who have been raped, people who have childhood histories of physical or sexual abuse, and others who have been exposed to much violence in their lives. For those who haven't completely dealt with those experiences, being on the receiving end of anything that even resembles physical trauma can lead to flashbacks and freak-outs. At the very least, it is not going to make for a superlative erotic adventure.

Also see: bondage and discipline, chains, flogging, games, handcuffs, klismaphilia, leather, paddle, playacting, power, rough sex, Sade—Marquis de, safeword, spanking, whips, wrestling

Don't ask, don't tell

The phrase has come to describe a compromise policy concerning homosexuals in the U.S. military: "We won't ask you if you're gay if you don't do or say anything to make us think you are." But *Don't ask, don't tell* is also the way a lot of U.S. marriages work: "I won't tell you if I'm fooling around, and I won't ask you if you are. But if you are, just make sure I don't find out about it." Sound familiar?

Well, you won't get any value judgments here. The problem, though, is that this is usually an unspoken, de facto arrangement. In other words, the couple has a don't-ask-don't-tell policy about its don't-ask-don't-tell policy. That may be a comfortable way of dealing with (or, rather, not dealing with) the specter of infidelity. But it creates a barrier to communication and intimacy. Hard as it is, it's generally more desirable for couples to put these cards on the table.

Also see: affairs, homosexuality, outing

douche

Flushing out the inside of the vagina with a jet of water or cleansing liquid is a centuries-old hygiene practice. But if your partner is among the 40 million American women who douche regularly, she's wasting her time.

The very idea of a hygienic douche implies that there's something foul about the vagina. The truth is, it's a self-cleaning organ. A regular bath or shower gets the area plenty clean. Now, if you're uncomfortable with the natural smell and taste of your partner's healthy vagina, that's an issue. But it's not one she can simply wash away.

On the other hand, a persistent foul odor from the vagina could indicate an infection. If that's the case, the woman needs a medical exam, not a douche. In fact, douching often makes things worse—or even causes vaginal problems in the first place—because prepared douching products contain chemicals that upset the balance of the vagina's natural pH and healthful bacteria. The result is often an increase in yeast and bacterial infections.

Douching also has a long, unsuccessful history as a birth control strategy. If your partner uses it as your sole means of contraception, start thinking of names for the baby.

Also see: hygiene, klismaphilia, Pap test, pelvic inflammatory disease, suppositories, vaginal moisture, yeast infection

douche bag

It holds whatever vaginal cleansing solution a woman uses to douche. It's fitted with a hose and valve so she can hang it shoulder-high as she sits back in a tub, inserts the hose in her vagina, and opens the valve to jet the liquid—usually a mix of vinegar and water—into action. When she feels full, she closes the valve, removes the hose, and lets the fluid flush out.

With such a use, *douche bag* is also an irresistible term of insult in the Howard Stern name-calling tradition. We'd hazard a guess that, these days, there are more men who've been called douche bags than women who've ever used the apparatus. Store-bought douches come with disposable nozzles, which most of the women who douche use instead.

Also see: bidet

drag

At its simplest, *dressing in drag* is trendier slang for the generic term *cross-dressing*—that is, wearing clothes of the opposite gender. But in practice, drag usually points to some specific homosexual, transvestite behavior. It might mean donning certain fantasy garments for arousal purposes. It might mean dressing up for a drag party. It might describe the sartorial statement of a female impersonator, also known as (you'll love this) a gender illusionist. If you want to fine-tune your lingo, think of drag as more theatrical or over the top than cross-dressing. Drag usually implies gayness; cross-dressing usually doesn't. Cross-dressers tend to look like the housewife down the street. Drag aspires to Mae West.

Also see: costumes, cross-dressing, gender bender, homosexuality, transvestism

D

drag queen

He's a gay man who not only dresses up in stereotypically female garb but also plays the role to its outrageous max in a melodramatic manner. The effect is intentionally comic and often laced with biting wit.

Is there a lesbian equivalent? You bet. And she's called a—ta da—drag king.

Also see: femme

dreams

Most of us dream about sex, whether we know it or not. Some sex dreams are disguised beneath symbolism, while others—like the ones where we're sporting donkey dongs and chasing after Pamela Anderson—are a bit more direct.

These times of racy REM sleep feature such unmistakable signs of arousal as erections and vaginal lubrication. Many people even experience orgasms in their sleep. Eighty percent of men report having had wet dreams, especially in their late teenage years and early 20s. Forty percent of women, usually those in their 40s, admit to having awoken in the middle of orgasms at least once in their lifetimes.

People who frequently daydream about sex don't dream about it as much during sleep as do those who spend few daylight hours fantasizing. Sex dreams and nocturnal orgasms also seem to be a safety valve—an outlet for sexual frustration—for people who don't have sex partners.

We also tend to dream bisexually. Indeed, regardless of your sexual orientation, you've probably had homosexual dreams. And you may dream of sex acts that you'd never commit while awake.

Not to worry if you've had dreams like these. Sex therapists tell us that dreams are okay no matter the subject. Since they're often symbolic, there's no point in taking them too seriously.

According to Sigmund Freud's studies, men often have the Oedipus dream, in which they engage in sexual activity with their mothers, usually symbolically. Freud also surmised that long objects such as poles and sticks are common phallic symbols in dreams. Meanwhile, dreams of boxes, cupboards, and empty rooms symbolize vaginas. If you dream of ascending stairs, opening a locked door, or entering a narrow space, you could be dreaming of intercourse.

We'd tell you more, but we're ready for our nap now.

Also see: fantasies, Freud, heterosexuality, hypnosis and performance enhancement, lover, sexual thoughts, succubus, wet dream

dressing for bed

When it comes to sex, we men are more visually oriented than women, so we're interested in what she's wearing just before she's wearing nothing. Women, well aware of this, do a pretty good job of dressing seductively for our bedroom benefit. But even the best of them can start preferring convenience to sexiness once she thinks that it doesn't matter to you anymore.

So here's a brilliant suggestion: Let her know that it matters.

Compliments, not complaints, get the job done. When she does slither into bed sporting something slinky and fetching, tell her how much you like her in it. Then tell her again. Use magazines or movies to give her ideas for future bedroom garb. (You do this, incidentally, by telling your woman how hot *she* would look in whatever diaphanous negligee is on display, not by pointing out how hot the model looks. But you knew that.)

Use some discretion before you go out and buy her outrageously sexy lingerie. Women have varying levels of comfort with their bodies. Yours may be mortified at the very thought of slipping into such a thing and may then resent you for "forcing" it on her. Gauge her feelings by toying aloud with the idea in her presence. Take the pressure off by approaching the whole idea of lingerie as good clean fun—which is about all these highly impractical garments are good for.

A good way to encourage comely attire in the bedroom is to take the lead yourself. Here, you'll need cues from her, since the only three things all women agree on when it comes to men's bedwear is that it shouldn't (a) stink, (b) be covered in transmission fluid, and (c) be awash in vestiges of your last sexual encounter, with someone else. Use the old magazine trick to draw out her opinions. Wear something that makes you feel sexy, and see what she thinks. Or just flat-out ask her what she'd like to see you in. Don't succumb to anything that makes you feel ridiculous. Do keep an open mind. It's the bedroom, after all.

The main thing is to keep sexiness on the agenda. Slack off for too long, and you'll both sink into the Dreaded, Sex-Stifling Swamp of Sweatpants.

While we're giving the *S* words a workout, here's one last suggestion: socks. Have a clean pair handy and put them on her at some appropriate point—especially if she's a new partner away from her dresser drawers. It's an im-mutable fact of life that women's feet are always cold. Your warming gesture shows thoughtfulness, while saving her the inconvenience of re-socking herself and the embarrassment of asking to borrow some.

Also see: costumes, lingerie, playacting, striptease, underwear, undressing

dressing her to look sexy

Your basic task here is to stay the hell out of the way. That means two things, mostly.

One is that you should lose whatever residual 1950s qualms you have about your woman looking like a million bucks in front of other guys. If you have a good relationship, you know that her sexiness ultimately is for you. If you don't, you have more serious issues to deal with than her attire. Two is to remember that she, not you, knows her idea of a sexy getup. Most women are only too happy to consider their guys' sartorial preferences, but no matter how hot you think an outfit is, it's a loser if it doesn't turn her on. If she feels out of place in her clothes—in particular, if she feels uncomfortable with the way a certain garment highlights her self-perceived "flaws"—she won't feel sexy. Just remember to tell her that she looks great no matter what she's wearing. A garb's sexiness starts with the erotic effect it has on *her,* not on you.

Also see: arousal, beauty, jealousy, lace, latex, lingerie, leather, makeup

dressing you to look sexy

Women have the edge when it comes to fetching fashions. They can look hot

D

simply by wearing less and showing more. That's probably not going to work for you.

What *will* work is dressing to show self-confidence and the implied power and means that go with it. When you want to dress to kill, put on what makes you feel like a studly world-beater. If it's a power suit that does the trick, so be it. If it's jeans and a flannel shirt, more power to you. This is a highly individual thing having to do with the image *you* feel most comfortable presenting.

That's not to say that anything goes. Here are a few of the things that don't go.

• There is nothing less sexy to women than a dirty human being in even dirtier clothes. So even if casual bohemian is your chosen idiom, bump it up a notch when you're seeing her in a datelike setting. We say this several times in this book, but it never stops being true: The implied message—"You're special"—is a tremendous turn-on for her.

• Never dress noticeably younger than you are, no matter how sexy it makes you feel. You're not fooling anyone. What you're telling her is that you're not confident enough about who you really are.

• Beware, too, of worrying too much about hiding your flaws. Reasonable adjustments, such as fits that de-emphasize flab, are fine. Less fine are lift shoes and baldness-covering hats, which betray, again, a lack of confidence. Besides, you can't hide forever. Are you planning to wear shoes to the beach? To leave your hat on during sex?

• Don't overadvertise. It's enough to choose clothing that's cut to reveal your taut glutes or bulging biceps. Lose the fishnet tank top, though, unless your quarry is some pre-legal 'N Sync groupie (in which case you should think twice anyway).

• Finally, the best fashion advice has nothing to do with clothes: Get in better shape; all your clothes will suddenly look sexier. Women, of course, appreciate a good male body. More important, they respond to what it says about you: that you care enough to work at looking good, for them and for yourself.

Also see: boxers or briefs, crossdressing, latex, leather, power, self-esteem, sexy, slick, striptease, underwear, undressing

drugs

Most recreational drugs are sex-impairing, dangerous, or both. At best, they reduce arousal and the intensity of orgasms. At worst, they can make you temporarily impotent. That's a pretty strong argument against undermining the healthy pleasures of sex with the unhealthy risks of getting high.

To have the best possible sex, it's wise to avoid even legal recreational drugs. You may not think that nicotine and alcohol have much in common with heroin or amphetamines, but they're all drugs and they all can be detrimental to sex. In the long term, nicotine can damage the veins responsible for your hard-ons, leaving you impotent. Having one too many beers can leave you limp that very night, not to mention the havoc that heavy drinking can cause over time.

Just as significant as the physical effects of drugs are the mental consequences. A stoned or buzzed sex partner can't be a focused, present, in-the-moment lover. Drugs cause the intimacy and subtle communication that intensify sex to go up in smoke (or take a powder). When you're being controlled by a controlled substance, your body goes through the motions, but your head is somewhere else. If she took the drug, too, the two of you may be having sex at the same time, but you're not really making love together. And if one of you isn't under the influence, that person may feel alone, abandoned, or superfluous. None of this is conducive to satisfying sex.

Also see: AIDS, alcohol, cocaine, divorce—issues that lead to, infertility, LSD, marijuana, medications, poppers, rape, rave, smoking, Spanish fly, steroids, yohimbine

dry hump

To rub your clothed genitals against another's clothed genitals or clothed thigh or any other part of her clothed body. It can be a fully clad simulation of intercourse or a brief dress rehearsal. Just remember that the word *dry* can be misleading: Hump enthusiastically enough, and one or both of you are going to have moist underwear, if not an embarrassingly visible wet spot to deal with. Still, with one caveat, dry humping is as safe a sex act as you're likely to experience and a recommended way for you and the one you love to pass time in an otherwise unoccupied elevator.

Now for the caveat: What starts out as underwear-to-underwear humping may unintentionally end up bringing skin directly in contact with skin, or fluid directly in contact with fluid. In such cases, you aren't dry humping; you're having sex. And you may well be exposing yourself to all the incidentals—such as pregnancy and disease—that go with it.

Also see: abstinence, femoral intercourse, hump, safe sex

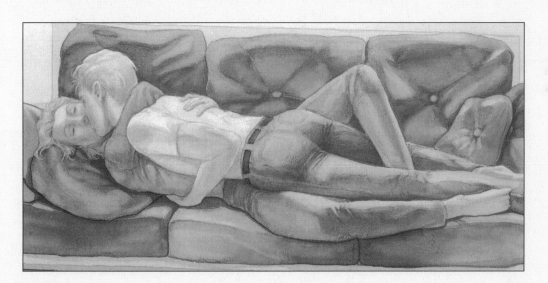

eat

For our purposes, of course, we're talking about slang for cunnilingus—oral stimulation of the female genitals. Used this way, *eat* and *eat out* are both a bit on the crude side and don't exactly provoke the most pleasant image of this mutually pleasurable sex option. So it's a good bet that if she invites you out to eat tonight, she has dining in mind—at least at the beginning of the evening.

Also see: cunnilingus, oral sex, sixty-nine (69)

ectopic pregnancy

Occasionally—1 to 5 percent of the time—a successfully fertilized egg implants itself outside its proper place in the uterus. The resulting ectopic pregnancy cannot produce a viable fetus. Also called a tubal pregnancy (since the fallopian tube is the usual site of implan-

tation), it's a dangerous and potentially fatal condition requiring surgery.

Most women can conceive normally after treatment and are encouraged to resume sexual relations as soon as they want to. A key thing for both of you to know is that a major risk factor for ectopic pregnancy is pelvic inflammatory disease, which in turn is usually caused by untreated sexually transmitted diseases such as gonorrhea or chlamydia. So pay attention to STD prevention, and have any infection treated right away.

Also see: chlamydia, fallopian tubes, gonorrhea, pelvic inflammatory disease, STDs, tubal ligation, zygote

ejaculation

The projection of about a teaspoonful of sperm-containing semen from your penis is so associated with orgasm that we usually consider them the same thing. Technically, they're not, since you can theoretically have an orgasm without ejaculating. Don't count on that though.

What you can count on is that once you reach what's known as ejaculatory inevitability, nothing in the world is going to stop the semen from coming. What you feel at this stage is the fluids from several glands gathering in the urethra, the tube that the semen rushes through to get out. Then, the urethra and penile muscles contract, the bladder opening closes (so that no urine gets into the mix), and the seminal fluid has no choice but to spurt out the opening of your penis. That, sir, is ejaculation. So do yourself a favor: Once you hit ejaculatory inevitability, don't try to hold back. That just ruins a good time. If you want to delay ejaculation, learn to recognize the feelings that come before you come.

Not being able to ejaculate is another matter. Physical causes might include prostate troubles, diabetes, neurovascular problems, medications, even cancer. If you can come while masturbating but not during intercourse, the cause is probably psychological. See a sex therapist. And there's another offbeat condition, retrograde ejaculation, that results in nothing coming out when you ejaculate. Instead, the semen shoots backward into the bladder because the valve that's supposed to prevent that very thing has been damaged. While this doesn't necessarily ruin the pleasure, it makes it hard to father children. The most important advice about ejaculatory problems? If there's any pain, see a doctor. Orgasm may not always make the Earth move, but it should never hurt.

Also see: aging, come, depression, fellatio, female ejaculation, gusher, orgasm, pee after sex, premature ejaculation, prostate, retrograde ejaculation, semen, sloppy sex, urethra, urologist, wet dream, wet spot, zinc

Electra complex

The female equivalent of the Oedipus complex, it has to do with a girl's erotic attraction to her father. This is the stuff of psychoanalytic theory, so don't take it literally. But don't ignore it, either, because it has relevance for any guy with a steady sexual partner.

Know that the little girl lives on inside the grown woman. You can expect her, at times, to relate to you as if you were her father. Let her. As long as it doesn't dominate your relationship (and she doesn't hate her father), no harm is done. Besides, there are going to be times when you won't mind being the little boy.

Also see: Freud, *Lolita,* male body, trophy wife, young men/older women, young women/older men

emotions

Your body's sexual arousal is all about stimuli, physical responses, electrochemistry. But all that hard science can be easily overridden by those fuzzy things we call emotions. What happens to your glorious erection when you hear your partner's paroled boyfriend knocking on the door? You know what happens. Fear is that powerful. So are other negative emotions such as guilt, worry, and anger. And so especially are the big two, anxiety and depression. Ignore these emotions at your own risk. If they're getting in the way, it's best to resolve them first and *then* make love—

especially if they have something to do with your bedmate.

Of course, on the flip side, you already know the impact that more positive feelings can have on your intimate interludes. We hope you've had the luck to celebrate a raise or new job or some other success by riding (or being ridden) as high as you feel. And when your most predominant positive feelings are love, affection, or caring for the woman you're with, that's sure to make for more satisfying sex.

But don't count on positive emotions to always override physical problems. After his wedding reception, many a newlywed is exceedingly happy—and exceedingly tipsy. Tipsy often wins, and consummation gets put on hold.

Emotions color your experience of sex in subtler ways as well. Your technique might vary with your emotions. You may proceed tentatively because of some lingering pang of guilt. There may be some extra oomph in your thrusts from some leftover anger. Sometimes, you want to be taken care of during sex because you're feeling insecure. Other times, you want to run the show because you're feeling on top of the world. None of this is bad. Indeed, the emotion factor helps provide the variety and expression that mark the best of intimate relationships.

So if emotions affect sex, does sex affect emotions? It sure as hell can make us happy, as that just-laid grin attests. Whatever the cause of that feeling— endorphin release, relaxation, sense of accomplishment—it's fantastic. But the best thing that sex can do for your emotions, if you let it, is liberate them. For a lot of us, the throes of sexual passion are the only times when we find it relatively easy to tap into our emotions and express them. And that feels good.

Hot Dates | **1920** Trojan condoms made their debut. They were marketed for disease prevention—not birth control—and were sold in gas stations, tobacco shops, barbershops, and drugstores.

continued from page 78

straddling her. The couple had indulged in sex, drugs, and alcohol with the engine running while parked in a garage.

Police said the boyfriend apparently died of carbon monoxide poisoning. The woman escaped with just a case of hypothermia.

Foreign Affairs

The popular notion that Eskimos rub noses as a form of intimacy is not quite accurate. In truth, **they place their noses and mouths against** each other's cheeks in order to smell each other.

In Extremis

The testicles of the blue whale are about 2½ feet long and weigh about 110 pounds. No wonder he's blue.

LEGAL BRIEFS

When a Wyoming woman caught two men burglarizing her apartment, did she scream? Dial 911? Nope. She invited one of the culprits to spend the night.

True or Phallus?

The sculptor who created a Pietà statue in a New Jersey church was asked to perform breast-reduction surgery on his artwork after some parishioners complained that the Virgin Mary's bustline was too ample.

BAWDY BALLADS | "Sam—The Hot Dog Man," *Lil Johnson*

continued on page 94

Chalk up another reason to have frequent sex.

Also see: animals, anticipatory anxiety, arguing, danger, depression, fears/phobias, financial difficulties, guilt, heartache, hormones, infatuation, jealousy, love, lust, making up, mood, passion, performance anxiety, relaxation, self-esteem, trust—rebuilding

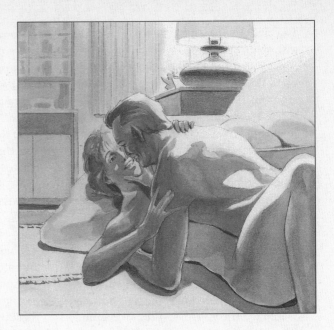

empty-nest syndrome

It refers to that time in life when the kids are grown and gone, leaving the two of you free to bounce around the bedroom like bunnies, the way you did decades ago. Sounds great—and it *can* be great—but they call it a syndrome for a reason. Though there's more time (and space) for sex, there's also less to distract you from relationship and personal issues that can make sex problematic. So if you haven't been communicating as a couple, let the kids' absence inspire you. Get to know each other again—or maybe for the first time. This won't happen automatically. You have to make it happen.

Forget about recapturing the sex of youth. You wouldn't want to even if you could. By now, you've learned that sex can be slower, deeper, more intimate, more enriching. That's a good thing. Stay with it. Explore it further.

Also be aware that an endless second honeymoon may not be your mate's highest priority now. Traditionally, her empty-nest problem has been described as an emotional letdown that comes with the end of her child-rearing mission in life. It's just as likely that what's bothering her is the sudden realization that until now, her life has been lived for others. She just may develop her own agenda, and sex with you may not be at the top of it. Don't resist. Encourage her in her pursuits. Have your own as well. Just stay close.

Do new things together. We're not necessarily talking about sex here. We're talking life. Go to Europe. Start big projects. Volunteer. Save the world. And communicate all the while. Two fulfilling lives don't preclude an active sex life. They nourish one. Bored people often have boring sex.

Also see: aging, depression, intimacy, Madonna/whore complex, menopause—hers, midlife crisis

epididymitis

Didymos is Greek for "twin" or "double." *Epididymis* is the name for the coiled tubing that sits atop, or *epi*, each testicle, providing a site in which sperm mature and await their marching orders.

It's a safe guess that few guys know much about their two epididymides and that fewer care—unless those epididymides get infected and inflamed. If that happens to you, you'll have pain and swelling in your scrotum, tender testicular lumps that are hot to the touch, difficulty urinating, and perhaps a discharge from your penis. Epididymitis is no picnic.

It's a bacterial infection that has many possible causes, including migrating germs from a sexually transmitted disease such as chlamydia or gonorrhea. Antibiotics usually take care of it. While you're waiting, you can try to reduce the discomfort by applying ice compresses, soaking in a hot tub, wearing an athletic supporter, or lying in bed with a pillow under your buttocks to raise your scrotum—always one of our favorite activities anyway.

Also see: chlamydia, gonorrhea

erection

It's what nature gave you instead of a penis bone, which would've been awkward to have around all of the time.

An erection is a reflex. You can't, alas, will one into existence. (Nor can you will one *out* of existence, as many a mortified 13-year-old has discovered during fourth period biology class.) Rather, the brain needs to respond to some kind of sexual stimulation. That stimulation can be physical, as when a curvaceous nymph rubs your genitals. It can be mental, as when you think about a curvaceous nymph rubbing your genitals. It can be aural, as when a curvaceous nymph whispers into your ear that she'd like to rub your genitals. Or it can be visual, as when you watch a curvaceous nymph rub her own genitals. Whatever it is, your brain responds by marshalling your body's heavy hitters—the circulating blood, the autonomic (involuntary) nervous system, and chemicals—to work together to create an erection.

This they do by sending more blood into your penis than is allowed to drain away. There, the blood gathers in special erectile tissue, mostly in spongelike cylinders called the corpora cavernosa and the corpus spongiosum. That accumulation builds up a hydraulic pressure, rendering your penis bigger, stiffer, and ready to rumble.

Also see: arousal, clitoris, hung, impotence, pee after sex, penis, refractory period, road erection, size—penis, stimulation

erection difficulties

The essential thing to know about erection problems is this: The erectile dysfunction that those earnest-looking guys in the Viagra commercials are talking about is not the same thing as those occasional episodes of unwelcome limpness. If it's episodic, it's not erectile dysfunction. Erectile dysfunction (or impotence) is a consistent inability to get or keep an erection satisfactory for sexual intercourse. That has nothing to do with the nearly universal male experience of not getting it up from time to time. Occasional power failures are normal. Repeat, *normal.*

In fact, there are circumstances when you're not *supposed* to get it up. Too much alcohol in your system is one of those circumstances. So is outside stress, such as tomorrow's IRS audit. So is stress from the sexual encounter itself, such as performance anxiety or worrying about birth control. So is anything else that interferes with the complicated electrochemical biology and psychology of erectile function. The reason for the system's failure may not be clear at the time, but you can bet there is one. It's your body's way of telling you that this is not a good time for intercourse. It's not your fault.

That doesn't make it any easier to take, does it? But you can handle it. First, remind yourself that it's an isolated case that says nothing about you as a man. You are not your penis. Resist the male urge to tough it out, as if trying harder would change things. Don't ignore what you're both thinking about; that just makes it seem more important than it need be. Go ahead and let her know you're disappointed—but not humiliated. Keep the mood light. Continue paying attention to her. Then, simply do something else together. Bringing her to orgasm orally or manually are two obvious choices, but they're not the only ones. Do whatever you've been doing that you both enjoyed. Focus on the positive things about being together. You can have intercourse some other time.

By the way, sometimes guys create erection problems when there aren't any. It's natural for erections to come and go during a love session. For example, if you divert your attention by going down on her, your erection may take a recess. Relax and it'll come back. Panic and it may not. Like everything else about sex, erections don't appreciate being rushed.

As for true erectile dysfunction, lots of factors—physical and psychological—can cause it, most of which are more likely as you get older. One thing you can do on your own is try to notice whether you get erections in your sleep. Do you occasionally wake up with a hard-on, even though you can't achieve one for intercourse? Can you get erections under certain circumstances and not others? If so, these are good indications that your plumbing is okay and the problem lies elsewhere. Even so, if you're consistently getting soft-ons, you need to see a doctor. Ongoing erectile problems often indicate a more threatening condition, such as cardiovascular disease. Also, a doctor can uncover some other cause, such as medications or diet. And finally, there are treatments—including Viagra—that can get you up and going again.

Also see: abstinence, aging, anticipatory anxiety, fears/phobias, heart conditions, impotence, injuries, papaverine, performance anxiety, Peyronie's disease, priapism, prostatectomy, sex therapy

erection—firmer

Firmer than what? Maximum hardness for one guy is Jell-O for another. What's more, your own firmness is far from consistent—you'll have nights of steel and nights of rubber. Even during the same sex session, your erectile rigidity is going to vary. So what? She doesn't need a lead pipe to enjoy herself (if she did, she'd just go find one—to hell with you). Nor does your own pleasure depend on maximum stiffness. If it's firm enough to get the job done, it's firm enough.

Put it in perspective: Erection firmness peaks at age 17. So by the time you're 40 or so, you may notice a difference. By 60, you surely will. But steadily softer erections aren't a progression toward impotence. Less rigidity is natural, if it's gradual. If you experience a sudden, drastic reduction in stiffness, you should see a urologist to check for venous leakage or bloodflow problems. Medications or anxiety could also be the culprit. But in most cases, it's just a question of aging.

Still, if you're hell-bent on being, well, unbent . . . Lots of guys insist that a cock ring will upgrade a half-staff to a full mast. Viagra supposedly does nothing for men who don't medically need it, but that doesn't stop guys from telling researchers that "recreational" Viagra use emboldens their erections. The only stiffness strategy we really recommend is to pay more attention to your overall arousal than to your penis. Heightened excitement often means a firmer erection. And even if it doesn't, you'll be less likely to care.

Also see: alcohol, arousal, cock ring, French tickler, priapism, road head

ment with every square inch of both bodies and see which can give or receive pleasure. You'll find areas that work for both of you. You'll also find plenty of spots that turn on one and not the other. You may discover exquisite joy in a foot rub that only tickles her. She, in turn, may squeal with delight at a light lick at the back of her neck. And once you're fully aroused, other parts of your body that were ignorable a few minutes earlier can suddenly surprise you with their capacity for sexual pleasure—if you give them a chance. That chance will never come if you confine the action to the traditional erogenous zones. Don't limit. Explore.

Also see: booty, breasts, clitoris, frenulum, glans, G-spot, labia majora and minora, legs, lips, male body, mons pubis, mouth, nipples, penis, perineum, prepuce, pudenda, rectum, scrotum, skin, stimulation, toes, tongue, touch

erogenous zones

Formally, those areas of the body that produce the most sexual excitement or libidinal gratification when stimulated. Traditionally, that means the genitals, breasts, buttocks, anus, and mouth. If formal and traditional sex is what you want, that's all you need to know. But if you'd prefer a rich and varied sex life that's more satisfying to you and your partner, throw out the whole notion of erogenous zones. Think of the entire human body as one giant sexual-pleasure center.

That's not just the sexually correct thing to say. It's a view you can use. Instead of privileging a few body parts, experi-

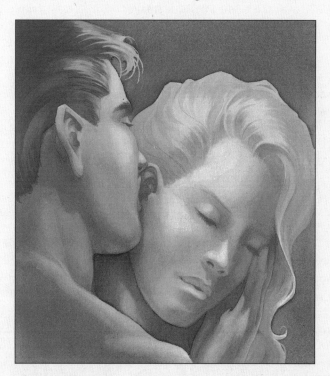

erotica

"Sexually oriented material." As definitions go, that's awfully general. Still, try pinning it down any tighter, and you're going to get nothing but arguments. Why? Because people don't just have different opinions about what is and isn't erotica. They actually *experience* the same material differently.

And that may be the key thing to know. Whatever the work in question—an erotic painting, a nude photo, some turn-on text, an explicit video—there's going to be more than one reaction to it. It's not just that some will find it arousing and some won't. It's also that some may consider it liberating, others downright dehumanizing. There are also basic gender differences: Women often compare themselves to and identify with the females in erotic images, while guys just content themselves with drooling over the women in those images.

Sex involves so many complicated emotions that it's crucial to consider the possibility of conflicting reactions if you'd like to enjoy erotica with your wife or girlfriend. Find out about her past experiences with erotic material. What does she like? Dislike? Then pay close attention to her responses during the screening or reading or viewing.

If your individual reactions are way out of whack, it's not going to work. Try something else.

Also see: erotic literature, pornography, voyeurism

erotic films

In one sense, *The Bridges of Madison County* fits in this category—at least for some women—since it deals with erotic attraction. But it's safe to say that when most of us talk about erotic films, we're thinking not so much Eastwood and Streep as Holmes and Lovelace.

Once cheap, grainy, and clandestine, glossy erotic films are now common cable fare and just a credit card swipe away at decent hotels. Not to mince words, they're all about showing people having sex—either in explicit, penetrating detail (hard-core) or with implied

Hot Dates Circa 1923 Courting forever changed as chaperoned meetings gave way to modern dates and etiquette books became the new moral guardian.

continued from page 89

Answer:
True. And the sculptor reluctantly agreed to the alteration. Good thing Michelangelo's David wasn't nearby.

Later, the woman discovered that she was missing $260. The guy who stayed denied taking the dough, saying **his accomplice must have pocketed it**.

Seemed like a Good Idea at the Time. . .
In Los Angeles, a woman perched on a bridge railing during an apparent lovers' quarrel tried to avert her beau's kiss and **fell 50 feet to her death**. Her companion reached out to save her, with similarly tragic results. Moral: If she hollers, let her go.

Foreign Affairs
The Malay people of Malaysia believe that **babies are conceived in men's brains**. It's thought that, after the

BAWDY BALLADS "Baby Come and Get It," *Pointer Sisters*

continued on page 103

but unmistakable simulation (soft-core).

Actually, porn is evolving somewhat of late, now that women are exerting their influence behind the camera as well as under the male actors. As a rule, male-produced porn intentionally keeps the environment on the explicitly sexual side and the dramatic development next to nil to divorce the action from everyday life. But the new "women's erotica" surrounds the sex with more-believable dialogue, real human relationships, and unfolding dramatic development—like, perhaps, a doomed affair between a middle-age photographer and a bored farmer's wife.

All this makes erotic films more appealing to some women, smoothing the way for you and your partner to have a rousing time watching sexy videos together. That doesn't mean X-rated movie dates are right for all couples. You should discuss it beforehand; no surprises. And you must accept it if her response is not what you'd hoped. Don't try to coerce her into getting used to it; this isn't hockey or country music.

If you're going to introduce X-rated videos into your mutual bedroom, forget about doing it as "education." Sure, you might pick up some ideas from a porn flick, but for the most part, what those ladies and gentleman are doing—or appear to be doing thanks to editorial enhancement—is not realistic. By no means should you consider them role models. If you want education, turn to one of the fine instructional sex videos on the market. Watch erotic films for entertainment.

Porn does offer one valuable lesson, though. Good erotic videos are graphic demonstrations of how women and men can be happy, relaxed, and unashamed as they truly enjoy sex. Sad to say, that's an eye-opener for a lot of people.

Also see: lesbian, movies, pornography, size—penis, third-degree cleavage, videos, X-rated

erotic literature

Believe it or not, there was a time on this Earth when the most stimulating fare required you to read—and not just the label of an X-rated videocassette. But even in an era as saturated with accessible visual erotica as ours, erotic literature is far from dead. It can be raunchy, as in *Penthouse* "Forum Letters." It can pretend to be something else, as in popular romance novels. It can be sophisticated, as in books from the irresistibly named Kensington Ladies' Erotica Society. Whatever the case, it's everywhere.

There are real advantages to erotic literature. One is the detail. The written word can describe a lot more than a camera could ever show. This may float your boat a little higher. And printed porn takes you inside the heads of the protagonists. That makes it easier for you to explore what kinds of characters, situations, and actions you're more likely to respond to sexually. This is information you can take back to the real world and use.

You don't have to read alone. Reciting turn-on prose aloud to each other is a good way to introduce erotica into your sexual relationship. You're more in control than when you watch a video, and you're more aware of each other. If you both enjoy your little story hour, run with it. Take roles, each reading the dialogue of a character. Change the roles. Act out the scenes. Improvise.

Also see: erotica; *Joy of Sex, The*; *Kama Sutra*; *Lolita*; *Penthouse*; *Playboy*;

Playgirl; pornography; Sade—Marquis de; zipless sex

escort service

Essentially, a prostitution agency.

Escort services charge more than street hookers do—elite call girls make up to $2,500 per night. Still, some guys consider them the preferred route to a paid lay. Here are a few of the reasons why.

• You get more for your money: Escorts charge by the night, not by the trick.

• You're less likely to get busted. (You didn't think the high cost made escort services legal, did you?) It's easier for cops to spot solicitation on the street than to know what's going on behind closed doors. We're not saying the local precinct won't stage a sting at the neighborhood escort service. It just doesn't happen as often. In fact, top-end escort agencies are quite discreet (Heidi Fleiss notwithstanding). Most don't advertise, and they shirk the IRS via overseas bank accounts and by headquartering outside U.S. jurisdiction.

• Hiring an escort is nearly effortless. A guy arranges for "companionship" by flipping through the Yellow Pages to the "Escort Service—Personal" listing and making a phone call (hence the synonym *call girl*). Higher-class escort services are harder to find—they rely on word of mouth.

• Escorts will visit a client anywhere he wants, even in the comfort of his own home. What's more, elite call girls provide more than a once-and-done sex act: They spend whole nights with clients and are often the eye candy adorning company executives and other wealthy professionals during vacations, business trips, and parties. And when a client finds an escort he likes, he can arrange to be a regular.

Think the converse of this scenario—getting paid to pleasure women—sounds like *your* dream job? Think on this: Physically speaking, a woman can have sex with any guy, any time. With the help of a good lubricant, her equipment always works. Not so for a man. And if a guy can't get stiff, he may wind up, well, stiffed.

Also see: brothels/bordellos, gigolo, john, money, prostitution, trick

estrogen

You don't know women if you don't know estrogen, the principal female sex hormone. More accurately, it's a *class* of hormones from the steroid family that includes estradiol, estrone, and estriol. Estrogen is what makes a woman a woman, starting in early fetushood, when it's instrumental in shaping her vagina, uterus, and ovaries. Later, estrogen is responsible for the mood swings, breast development, and rounding hips of budding female pubescence. Higher-than-usual estrogen levels contribute to various discomforts (for both of you) just before her period. And estrogen manipulation is why birth control pills work.

Most important for her (and therefore your) sex life is a woman's estrogen-driven tendency to seek closeness and nurturing contact as part and parcel of being sexually turned on. We testosterone-powered men aren't opposed to the intimacy thing, but we tend to think that . . . well . . . it doesn't need to be overdone. What we have here is a chemical conflict between the sexes. Accommodating it is the ongoing challenge of a sexual relationship.

Her estrogen production drops drastically with menopause around age 51. From a feminist point of view, there's a certain advantage in this, since her chemically mandated "caretaker" urge is now better able to yield to more self-assertive goals. But sexually, the estrogen decrease can cause some problems, such as drying and thinning vaginal walls, painful intercourse, and lowered libido. What's more, the higher incidence of female cardiovascular disease after age 50 points out the heart-protecting qualities of estrogen. Other postmenopausal problems show that estrogen also protects bones and aids memory. For those reasons, many women in their 50s and beyond replenish their estrogen supply through estrogen replacement therapy, also known as hormone replacement therapy (HRT). There's controversy about that, though, with strong feelings on both sides. The pro-HRT camp sees it as a quality-of-life advantage since today's postmenopausal women can expect to live several more sexually active decades. Opponents see HRT as unnatural and an unnecessary breast and uterine cancer risk since estrogen, amongst all its other qualities, can have a cancer-promoting effect. The overall significance of that effect is is part of the controversy.

Estrogen, by the way, influences your own sexuality as well. Just as women manufacture a tad of testosterone to fuel their sex drives, men produce a little estrogen from their testes. And as your testosterone levels dip a bit in later years, your estrogen is freer to encourage the more "feminine" virtues of nurturing and harmonizing. The new chemical balance can give you a best-of-both-worlds sexual persona, and it's one reason why older men enjoy a reputation as better lovers.

Also see: hormones, menopause—hers, morning-after pill, ovaries, Pill—the, pituitary gland, PMS, vaginal moisture

eunuch

A man who's been castrated, meaning his testicles (not his penis) have been removed. Historically, the dirty deed was done on purpose to keep the soprano supply plentiful and, earlier, to create a class of harem guardians and chamberlains for Asian and Roman emperors. (The word *eunuch*, in fact, comes from the Greek for "guardian of the bed.") Today, it's usually accident victims or surgery survivors who find themselves two nuts short of an Almond Joy.

You can win bar bets by knowing that many eunuchs do have the ability to get it up. Those who've had both or, usually, one testicle removed because of testicular cancer are given testosterone patches or injections if they need them to help things move onward and upward. Guys who are gelded due to prostate cancer, however, don't get the extra testosterone, since the entire purpose of their operations was to stem the flow of the tumor-feeding male hormone at its sources. But patch or no, the testosterone loss caused by castration doesn't necessarily prohibit arousal.

Also see: pederast, testicular trauma, testosterone replacement therapy

excitement

In sexology lingo, it's the first of four phases of the body's sexual response. A lot goes on. Blood rushes to your

E

penis. It gets erect. Your testicles move up in your scrotum. Your penile opening enlarges. Your breathing and heart rates increase. Your muscles get tenser. Your nipples may firm up. In women, the excitement phase brings lubrication of the vagina and a swelling of its tissues with blood. Men tend to move from the excitement phase through the other three (plateau, orgasm, and resolution) much faster than women do.

Also see: arousal, foreplay, premature ejaculation

exercise

During sex, that is. And why not? Physical fitness improves your sex life. That's a given. And sex itself is a fitness-promoting aerobic workout, as long as you're vigorous about it and not too eager to get it over with. All that's missing for the full-package sex workout is some muscle building. Conveniently for you, an eager crew of can-do sex therapists and physical trainers got together to design some flagrante-delicto exercises that get you fit as well as off. No, you don't have to take any barbells into bed with you. You just need her co-operation.

The bent-over row works your upper back, with your beloved supplying the weight. As she lies facedown on the floor, hold both ends of a towel that runs under her belly. Stand over her with your knees bent and your back straight. Using the towel, slowly lift her toward you (she lets the tops of her feet rest on the floor) and penetrate her from behind. Her body makes a 45-degree angle with the floor, and she supports herself with her hands just above her knees. Move her up and

down with the towel, controlling things so you stay inside her. Let her down very slowly when you're through or too tired to continue. Don't try this if you have lower-back problems. And just as in the gym, it's bad form to let your weight crash to the floor.

In ab-solutely doggie style, you concentrate on your abs. While on your knees, enter her from behind as she lies facedown with her head and shoulders flat on the floor, her legs bent at the knees, and her butt as high as she can get it in the air behind her. Do standard rear-entry thrusting, but concentrate on your abdominal muscles, making sure that they (and not your legs) do the work. You can help to isolate your abs by trying to lift her up with each thrust, rather than bearing downward into her. You get extra credit if you actually lift her.

The prurient press is the pushup routine of your teenage fantasy. With her pelvis supported by a pillow or two, enter your prone, faceup partner while keeping your body horizontal. Your sole support should come from your hands flat on the bed or floor below her shoulders. Bend your arms to lower yourself deep into her, and then raise yourself, pushup style, until you're as high as you can get without losing penetration.

Got it? Now get down and give us 50!

Also see: abs, athletic sex, beefcake, body fitness, depression, Kegel exercises, muscles, rug burn, sickness, sperm count, sweating, weight loss

exhaustion

You're probably not as exhausted after sex as you think you are. Sure, you're breathing hard. And, sure, you're in no condition to jump right up and mount the stationary bicycle—especially after one of those nonstop thrusting marathons or particularly athletic sessions. But that tired feeling mostly reflects the great release of physical and emotional tension that comes with ejaculation. Call it the exhaustion of satisfaction. And enjoy it as one of the perks of good sex.

Tempting as it may be to ride this calm wave to sleep, try quietly sharing this sexual epilogue with your partner, who'll be feeling the same afterglow if she climaxed. You may find that the "exhaustion" soon passes and that you're ready for a little afterplay. Or stationary biking. Or you may enjoy the intimacy of actually *sleeping* together.

Also see: afterglow, afterplay, athletic sex, fatigue, refractory period

exhibitionism

Who's an exhibitionist? You are.

This is not to say that you're a flasher, an aggressor who exposes his genitals to shock an unwilling victim. But you are an exhibitionist nonetheless. Somewhere inside, every guy wants his sexuality noticed, displayed, admired.

That's why a new partner's expression of awe when she first lays eyes on your manhood is about the most gratifying response you can hope for. That's why the idea of 50,000 people wildly cheering a center-field demonstration of your sexual prowess at Yankee Stadium is a pleasing fantasy.

If it were up to biology alone, there'd be a long line of potential performers in the Yankee Stadium outfield. Of course, to function as a society, we have to cool it. So the word *exhibitionism* is usually interpreted as antisocial behavior, of

which an all-too-real example is the compulsive who exposes himself inappropriately, offensively, and illegally.

Still, exhibitionism—tempered by discretion—can be a rich source of sexual pleasure. Your steady sexual partner should be a safe and willing audience (and may be a bit of an exhibitionist herself). Start by complimenting each other more. Create an unabashed atmosphere that nurtures each other's exhibitionist tendencies. Strip for her—and do it like you mean it. (She'll love it.) At dinner, give her an unexpected glimpse of what your clothes usually cover. Forget to wear your underwear on a Sunday outing, and let her know it. Have a conversation about upcoming sex, loudly enough that others might hear. Some couples push the envelope, arranging to be watched while making love. Others put a doll in the room and pretend.

Just be careful around strangers. They may have a stricter interpretation of the aforementioned "antisocial" behavior than you do. And realize that attitudes about sexual displays, like many of today's conventions, aren't always guy-friendly. One wise wag put it this way: If a man watches a woman undress, he's a voyeur. If a woman watches a man undress, he's an exhibitionist.

Also see: compulsive behavior, fantasies, masher, mirrors, outdoors, paraphilias, perversions, public places, risky sex, sex offenders, sex therapy, striptease, swinging, third-degree cleavage, topless, undressing, voyeurism

extramarital sex

Sex outside marriage. Usually, *extramarital* refers to a married person being sexual with somebody who is not his or her spouse. Two single people enjoying sexual relations are engaging in *premarital* or *nonmarital* sex.

Also see: affairs, cybersex, marriage—open, ménage à trois, promiscuity, swinging, variety

eye contact

An awesome turn-on, and one that many men underrate. The sexual power of eye contact is so immediate that some cultures forbid it. (Or did you think the veil was a fashion statement?) The rest of us use eye contact to attract partners for sex, please them during sex, and keep them around for more sex. Not for nothing are the eyes sometimes referred to as the most erotic part of the body.

If a stranger tickles your sexual fancy, making eye contact is your first assignment. The reason is simple: Eye contact cannot be ignored. She may avert her gaze. She may give you the finger. But then again, she may smile. If she does, *something* has started. It's up to you to figure out what it is . . . starting by responding to that response. Similarly, a lack of eye contact tells plenty and is a useful step in the mating dance. Many a poor schmo could have saved himself hours of striking out if he'd bothered to notice that she never even looked at him when he approached.

Maintaining eye contact during intercourse is the special privilege of the human species. Take advantage of it. A woman wants to know that you're "present" during sex—that is, making love to *her* rather than just getting your rocks off. Looking into her eyes says it all.

And keep making eye contact regularly with your partner when you're together in nonsexual situations. It reinforces the attachment—that here-for-each-other companionship—that's at the heart of any long-term relationship.

Also see: communication—nonverbal, companionship, courtship, flirtation, lovemaking, missionary position, signals, size—eyes, wandering eye, winking

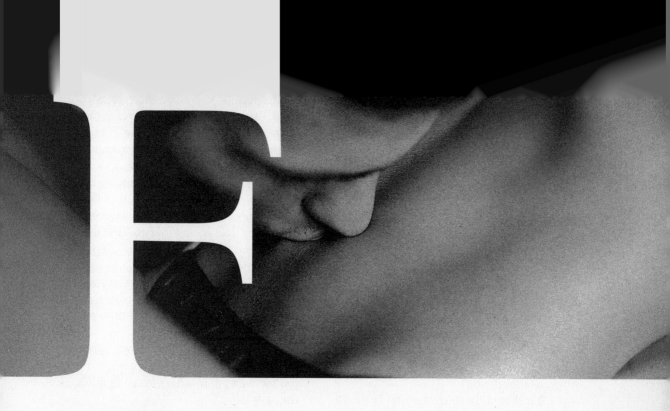

faking orgasm

The running gag is that if fewer men faked foreplay, fewer women would fake orgasm. As things stand, lots of women sometimes fake it, and some fake it often. Why might *your* woman do this? To please you. To let you know that she's having a good time. To reassure you that you're a good lover. What better proof of all those things than a smoking climax? And if it's not happening for real, a false crescendo of moans and cries will do the trick. No harm done, right?

Maybe. Even well-intentioned deception isn't exactly a desired ingredient in a sexual relationship. It's certainly not going to help real orgasms happen. And there may be some performance anxiety going on—*her* anxiety about being sufficiently responsive to you. Eventually, faked orgasms may be the only ones she'll have. While you're in the room, anyway.

You don't have to suspect that your partner is faking orgasms to help her not need to. First, destroy the justification for

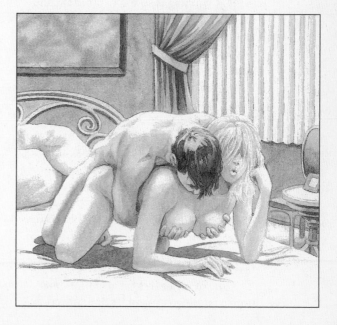

fraud by finding a way to let her know that your ego doesn't depend on whether you "give" her an orgasm during sex. Sure, you want her to feel good and be satisfied, but the idea that you're a good lover if she comes and a bad one if she doesn't gives you too much credit either way. Getting that important point across is a step toward encouraging more mutual trust about each other's sexual needs. She should feel comfortable letting you know that she hasn't come yet. And you should feel comfortable receiving that information.

Also, take to heart that one-liner about foreplay. Women do need more time for arousal. And they're much more likely to climax during sex if there's generous stimulation.

But that still avoids the real issue. If your woman fakes an orgasm during intercourse to please you, it implies the following: (1) that sex is a challenge, (2) that intercourse is the playing field, (3) that victory comes with her orgasm, and (4) that winning is so important that she may have to rig the results to do it. The fact is, though, that for most women, intercourse is not a feasible route to orgasm. And trying only makes it harder.

Instead, think about re-choreographing your sexual sessions. Play down the idea of orgasm during intercourse. Help her come via oral sex, manual sex, vibrator sex. Encourage her to take things into her own hands and get herself off—with you there. Any of this can happen before intercourse, after intercourse, or instead of intercourse. All those things are just as much "real" sex as intercourse.

They're certainly more real than faked orgasms.

Also see: clitoral orgasm, communication, cunnilingus, manual stimulation

fallopian tubes

Your sperm's Valhalla—their final reward. Each of a woman's two ovaries are connected to her uterus by one of these passages. Upon ovulation, her mature egg moves into the tube attached to the ovary from which it sprung and awaits fertilization. If one of your valiant little vikings completes the long swim through her vagina, cervix, and uterus—and then is lucky enough to pick the egg-occupied tube rather than the other, usually empty one—he gets to fulfill his destiny and dive into the egg. The newly conceived zygote then moves out of the tube and into the uterus.

Also see: cervical cap, ectopic pregnancy, fertility, hysterectomy, ovaries, reproductive system—hers, tubal ligation, zinc, zygote

fantasies

Sex in your head, generally with you as the star. All those hot scenarios and lusty narratives that screen regularly at the triple-X multiplex of your mind spring from the erotic content of your sexuality. They're part of the human side of sex that makes the act more than just a physiological imperative. All you have to do with your fantasies is enjoy them. And never, ever feel guilty about them—not even when you fantasize about doing things that are probably immoral and definitely illegal in most states.

You are not in complete control of your fantasies' scripts. Thus, fantasizing about something does not necessarily mean you really want to do it. This is true even of fantasies about a real-life female whom you know you shouldn't be thinking about that way. Part of the beauty of fantasy is that it allows a harmless release of erotic feelings that are there whether you think they should be or not.

This brings us to a question that may be troubling for you (and for your partner, in particular): Should you feel guilty for fantasizing about one woman while making love with another? No, not at all. This is actually one of the most common uses of fantasy. Remember, fantasy's chief function is to heighten arousal. So don't think of it as betrayal; think of it as a tool for improving sex with your regular partner. Besides, who's to say she's not doing the same thing? (We know, she couldn't possibly think of anyone but you. Just humor us here.)

Should you and your partner verbally share your fantasies? There are a lot of upsides to doing so. Sharing deepens intimacy. It suggests new avenues of mutual sexual pleasure. Talking about fantasies can be a turn-on in its own right. For some couples, it may be the only way that certain subjects—say, anal sex—ever come up.

Just be careful. She may have no desire to hear your fantasies; in fact, the very idea of your having them may bother her. Even if she's game, there are some fantasies better left unshared—for instance, personally touchy subjects like your appreciation of her younger, slimmer sister. And even as open-minded as you may think you are, once you actually start hearing about what she'd like to do to Sven the tennis instructor, you may not find her fantasies so charming. You may, in fact, be unable to get the images out of your head. Before you open this can of worms, make sure neither one of you is going to go shrieking away from the dirty, little wrigglers. Potentially contentious fantasies should be among those you keep in your private stock so you can continue to take advantage of no-fault, no-consequences, secret sexual fantasies.

Oh, and about the above-mentioned illegalities and other unusual fantasies: Sex therapists assure us that the *occasional* idle thought is nothing to worry about. Seek a therapy consult if your fantasies routinely involve violent, destruc-

Hot Dates | 1927 Actress Mae West spent 8 days in jail for her performance in the boisterous play *Sex*.

continued from page 94

cranial conception, an expectant father experiences 40 days of the same sorts of food cravings that will plague his wife later. Then, the baby supposedly travels from dad's head to his liver, said to be the center of emotions. After the chip off the ol' blockhead has acquired the father's rationality and emotions, it journeys to his penis, finally picking up the usual route to the mother's womb.

In Extremis

A boar produces about 85 trillion sperm during ejaculation; a horse between 4 trillion and 13 trillion. A man produces a paltry 40 million to 600 million.

True or Phallus

An earthworm has both a penis and a vagina.

BAWDY BALLADS | "Steamy Windows," *Tina Turner*

continued on page 110

tive, or socially unacceptable behavior and if they have cropped up suddenly, are intense enough to distract you from everyday activities, or recur a number of times over a period of days. We're not saying these are signs of trouble . . . necessarily. But only a therapist can help you be sure.

Also see: best friend's wife, bestiality, boredom, compulsive behavior, costumes, dreams, exhibitionism, games, gang bang, gang rape, heterosexuality, homosexuality, incest, microphilia, necrophilia, paraphilias, pedophilia, perversions, phone sex, playacting, rape, risky sex, rough sex, sex symbols, sex therapy, sexual thoughts, taboos, underage, violence, voyeurism, wife's best friend, zoophilia

farting

Look, inadvertently letting one go in the midst of passionate sex can happen, though for most of us who aren't Belushi's Bluto, it shouldn't happen that often. You'll be pleased to know that despite the widely held belief that we guys consider audible gas-passing to be a legitimate mode of self-expression, she's as likely to have dealt it as you are. Either way, it's embarrassing.

But it's also understandable. Sex, after all, is about a physical letting go. Ceding control is part of the magic, and it often results in involuntary activity that would be thought gross in other circumstances. Like drooling. Or moaning. Farting is no different. It just smells worse.

If you're the guilty party, go ahead and clear the air by expressing your embarrassment. But also stress the positive, letting her know that you're so engrossed in making love with her that you lost control.

And if she's clearly embarrassed at having done it herself, reassure her that you're enjoying the lovemaking, and tell her that you like the way she lets herself go.

Then open a window.

Also see: body odor—controlling, laughter, sexual etiquette

fatigue

Every couple has nights when they'd rather just sleep than sleep together. That's okay. But if one or both of you are consistently too pooped to party, don't just accept it. Are you one of those hardworking couples who always puts off sex until midnight and then decides you couldn't be bothered after all? If so, a little schedule tweaking and reprioritizing are clearly in order.

Even when you really are too tired for intercourse, don't rule out all physical contact. Just hugging and touching with no intention of going further keeps you connected and feeling good, tired as you may be.

If sex is just one of many things throughout the day that you feel too tired to do, see a doctor. Constant, debilitating fatigue could be a symptom of an underlying health condition, possibly a serious one.

Sometimes, one partner is not really physically tired but simply tired of less-than-satisfactory sex. Consciously or otherwise, she might be using fatigue as an excuse to avoid dealing with a problem in your sexual relationship. So might you, for that matter. Get the issue out in the open and try to solve it: What you're working toward is the special kind of fatigue that follows a mutually rewarding lovemaking session.

Also see: afternoon delight, appointments, atmosphere, biological clock, boredom, depression, gusher, marriage—lack of sex in, pregnancy, relaxation, sickness, stress, time-saving tips, withholding, workaholism

fears/phobias

Fear doesn't have to be a full-fledged phobia to mess with your sex life. Simple, nonclinical fear can do it. Some fears are healthy; they keep you from doing stupid things. But inappropriate fears—the ones that ignore facts and skew your behavior—get you into trouble instead of out of it. A case in point is what one sexologist calls EFRAIDS: exaggerated fear reaction to AIDS. Instead of enjoying safe sex in any of its available forms, some people simply fear that any sex might kill them.

What's more, sexual fears work so insidiously that they often bring about what we fear most. For example, a major cause of erection difficulties is fear of erection difficulties.

A fear or phobia may have nothing to do with sex and still affect it. A fear of, say, messiness makes it hard for you to enjoy sex. If you're hung up on dirt or germs, your woman may never be clean enough for you. Such problems are compounded by a tendency to load anxiety onto sex. Just as you might say that you're afraid of the dark when what you're really afraid of is vicious nocturnal animals or muggers, you can feel that you're afraid of sex when it's really women or loss of control that you fear.

So, do a personal fear inventory. Try to identify your fears so that you can confront and neutralize any problematic ones. They may not be obvious, but thinking about anything that you find distasteful about sex may point you in the right di-

rection. Also, try teasing your own fears out of problems that you've been attributing to your partner. Do this by asking yourself what the problem might be about if it weren't about her. Say you've always been disappointed because you assume she's not the kind of woman who could understand your sexual fantasies. Try to think of an alternative reason for your discouragement, one without her in the picture. You might come up with this: You're worried that your fantasies are too weird to be acceptable to other people.

Now you can stop wasting your energy blaming her and start thinking more clearly about the issue. Maybe you'll realize that you have nothing to be worried about. There's no reason why anybody's personal fantasies need to be acceptable to other people—they're *personal*. And pinpointing the fear itself puts you in a position to take the necessary steps toward getting over it. Sometimes it can help to talk with your friends or your partner. Other times, the answers may lie in therapy or medication. Either way, identifying the problem means that you're on your way to conquering it.

Also see: AIDS, anticipatory anxiety, danger, depression, emotions, hang-ups, injuries, performance anxiety, sex therapy, sickness

feel up

Though it can refer to manual contact with the vagina, you may recognize this phrasal verb as teen terminology for what a professorial type might refer to as "prolonged fondling of one or both female breasts." Textbook, backseat-of-the-car feeling up requires some dexterity since it's so often done with blouse and brassiere more or less in

F

place. Both the adolescent and the older man feel up their partners for the thrill of it or for *her* benefit or both.

Most men of all ages love touching and squeezing breasts. We join you in the fervent hope that your feeling-up days are far from finished!

Also see: bras, breast fondling, cars, foreplay, implants, labia majora and minora, tickling

fellatio

It's not one thing. It's a lot of things. A few erection-encouraging slurps of your penis's shaft is not the same as prolonged sucking (which is what fellatio meant back in its Latin incarnation). Being taken down deep into her throat is not at all like having your entire genital area lightly nibbled. An energetic, head-bobbing effort to get you to orgasm—or an absurdly ineffectual, literal interpretation of the term *blow job*—is certainly different from a slow-motion tongue bath as extended foreplay. And whether she swallows your ejaculate or executes an 11th-hour retreat to take it elsewhere also affects the experience.

Contrary to the usual assumption (at least among women), not all of us would sell our children for a good session of head. Even some of us who like it have a hard time reaching orgasm through fellatio alone. And we can't make assumptions about women's thoughts on the matter: They're all over the map on this one. Some can't get enough, some tolerate it just to please you, some won't even attempt it. And there's no way to tell in advance where a new lover stands on the issue. If it's important to you to know sooner rather than later, find a way to ask her.

Not all the technique in fellatio is hers. After all, you're the one wielding an engorged appendage in the vicinity of another person's face. You're putting her in a tricky position and—especially if you're on top—a vulnerable one. Nothing wrong with any of that, mind you, but it's easy to get carried away by the throes of pleasure and start shoving or thrusting in a way that's going to gag her, send her running from the room, or provoke her to feel a vague kinship with Lorena Bobbitt. So keep her comfortable. You want both of you to feel good about the diversion.

That's why a good approach to fellatio with a new partner is to let her run the show. Give her a chance to show you what she likes. And give her plenty of warning about your approaching ejaculation so she can discourage it, encourage it, or gulp it down as she sees fit.

Finally, think of fellatio (and cunnilingus) as the sexual equivalent of good pasta—appropriate as both a side dish and a main course. Intercourse is great, but it doesn't have to dominate the menu. If you both like oral sex, try it as a frequent entrée.

Going down, anyone?

Also see: cunnilingus, glory hole, oral sex, prostitution, road head, sodomy, vacuum devices

female ejaculation

There does seem to be such a thing, though what's being ejaculated is something of a mystery. Only some women ejaculate, and only sometimes. The clear or milky liquid they release at orgasm isn't semen, obviously. Experts believe the fluid, which may be part urine, spurts out of two ducts on either side of a woman's urethral opening. It often comes with her second or third orgasm, and some experts believe that it requires G-spot stimulation.

Sorry we can't be more specific about this understudied aspect of female sexuality. But answer us this: Would women be as sexy if there were *nothing* mysterious about them?

Also see: clitoral orgasm, come, ejaculation, G-spot, lubrication, pee—her—during orgasm, sloppy sex, urethra, wet spot, witch's milk

femme

Pronounced and sometimes spelled "fem," this derivation of the French word for "woman" describes a lesbian who projects a clearly feminine appearance. The more extreme version—lots of makeup, high heels, frilly dresses—earns the term *high femme* or *lipstick lesbian*. A femme is the opposite of the more masculine-looking *butch* lesbian.

Don't assume that a feminine/masculine dynamic exists within a same-sex relationship. Outward traits don't necessarily reflect gender roles, hence the saying "Butch in the streets, femme between the sheets." And a femme, high or otherwise, will not necessarily choose a butch lesbian as her partner.

Also see: androgyny, anima and animus, lesbian, yin and yang

femoral intercourse

Or interfemoral coitus. Or interfemoral intercourse. All are fancy names for humping her thighs. And by that, we mean actually inserting your erect penis between her closed upper legs and thrusting away. The sensate possibilities are inviting, you must admit, especially if she assists your efforts with appropriate shifts and well-timed squeezes. And as long as you don't let the action migrate too far north, she's not going to get pregnant. (Though we still recommend a condom for protection against sexually transmitted diseases.) Of course, the penis/thigh action in and of itself doesn't do much for her, orgasmically speaking. But as a low-effort way to please her man—like, maybe after she's been on her feet shopping all day—she may love this variation.

Also see: dry hump

fertility

The physiological ability to reproduce. Your fertility depends on a sufficient number of healthy sperm in your semen. If you've got 'em, you're a fertile fellow.

Note that fertility has nothing to do with erectile capacity. Infertility and impotence are two entirely different problems. You can have consistent monster erections and spew bucketfuls of cum but still be infertile if your sperm are subpar or too few.

After puberty, male fertility is also independent of age. While women stop producing fertile eggs at menopause, most men are potential fathers-to-be well into geezerdom. So if you're enjoying a May-September romance, keep those condoms on the nightstand, right next to your denture glass.

Of course, even if you're pumping out plenty of potent tadpoles, they're all for naught unless your mate is also fertile. A woman's fertility requires that her ovaries produce healthy eggs and that her fallopian tubes are clear so that your sperm can reach those eggs. And, of course, planting your seed requires the two of you to do the deed at the right time in her

F

cycle. That often requires repeat visits to the bedroom, but who's complaining?

Also see: biological clock, boxers or briefs, contraception, infertility, menopause—hers, ovulation, pregnancy, puberty, reproductive system—hers, reproductive system—yours, semen, sperm count, trophy wife, vasectomy reversal, zygote

fetish

You have a fetish if there is an object or body part that you eroticize in a compulsive way. The key word here is *compulsive*. The fetishist has such an unusually strong attraction to something like, say, shoes (or cigars or feet or hair) that the object pretty much becomes a prerequisite for a satisfying sexual experience. So if satin sheets or jiggling midriffs are your favorite turn-ons, don't call them fetishes unless they're a mandatory requirement for a good time.

If you don't already have a fetish, it's unlikely that you'll suddenly develop one: The attachment is usually rooted in childhood or adolescent experiences. So go ahead and enjoy your particular preferences, as long as they are not harmful to you or your partner (and if they are, you should consider therapy). But also enjoy a diversity of turn-ons, which are not available to true fetishists.

Also see: compulsive behavior, preference

fig leaf

Actually, if you check Genesis 3:7, it should be *fig leaves*, plural, not that single leaf-shape thing you sometimes see positioned strategically on sculptures. Adam and Eve sewed them together for loincloths after discovering—with surprise and shame—that they were naked. Thus they begat the fashion industry.

Fig leaves are no longer the fabric of choice, but shame persists. So does a certain sense of vulnerability. Embarrassment aside, men cover up to protect the family jewels from wayward objects, sniffing beasts, and the cold. Combine the physical threat with the typical male concerns about size and visual appeal, and you begin to think the first couple was on to something with those fig leaves.

But though modesty is useful (and recommended) in the street and backcountry, try a little less in the bedroom. If all your sex is happening under the covers with the lights out, you may be letting shame limit your pleasure. Many of the best lovers are comfortable with their own nude bodies. So let it all hang out. Both of you.

Also see: body image, boxers or briefs, guilt, hang-ups, hung, underwear

financial difficulties

They'll bite you in bed as well as in the wallet. Serious money woes—losing your job, looming bankruptcy, lacking health insurance—mean serious worry. And worry is a sworn enemy of sexual desire, not to mention erections.

The thing about money is that it's symbolic. It often reflects a guy's sense of self-worth, especially if he considers himself Mr. Provider. So if you go belly-up financially, you may feel like you're belly-up as a human being. Obviously, the solution is to solve your financial problem. We can't do that for you—at least not in this book—but we can tell you what to do in the meantime to ease the burden on your sex life.

In a serious relationship, your best bet is to share your fiscal woes with your sexual partner. Problem is, money is right up there with sex at the top of the list of subjects that couples are least likely to talk to each other about. And now you have to talk about both at the same time! A tough task, but the alternatives are tougher. To her, anything short of full financial disclosure comes off as controlling and manipulative. So talk now or fight later. Tell her what the problem is, right down to specific numbers. And tell her how it's making you feel. She'll appreciate it. You'll feel like you've taken a load off your shoulders. And the source of any

sexual problems will be out there for both of you to see and deal with. Instead of a secret, you'll have a partner.

Also see: communication, companionship, emotions, job loss, money, power, size—wallet

F

finasteride

When you're finally tired of arguing over whether Miller Lite tastes great or is less filling, you may feel like debating whether finasteride is a baldness antidote or a prostate pill. We'll settle this for you: It's both. Finasteride stops testosterone from converting to dihydrotestosterone (DHT), a hormone that appears to be a key factor in both inherited male-pattern hair loss and prostate enlargement. As a baldness pill, it's prescribed under the name Propecia. As a prostate pill, it's Proscar.

Proscar is one of several treatments for an enlarged prostate. For those men who respond to it—not everybody—it's been shown to shrink the prostate over a period of 6 months to a year. Proscar must be taken indefinitely, or the pesky organ will grow again, bedeviling a guy with symptoms ranging the incredible gamut from frequent urination to . . . difficult urination.

Men whose prostates are only minimally enlarged or whose problems are not related to the organ's size don't seem to be helped by Proscar. And it seems to be effective for other men in only 30 to 40 percent of cases. So it is but one option in treating the condition.

During the drug's testing phase, its manufacturer made an interesting discovery: Some of the study subjects also grew more hair. It was a stroke of plain, dumb luck for the pharmaceutical com-

F

pany, who found two drugs in one, as well as for men fretting over recalcitrant hair follicles.

The only difference between the two pills is that Proscar is five times the dosage of Propecia. The pills cost about the same, so some balding men get prescriptions for Proscar, cut each tablet into five portions, and save a bundle.

Also see: hair, prostate enlargement

first date

Sex on the first date? That's the usual question. But even after it's answered, there's still another one: Will there be a second date? So why not concentrate less on whether you'll be having sex and more on who you will—or won't—be having it with?

If you and she have wildly different reasons for dating, you probably won't be seeing each other for very long, no matter how great her legs are. Since you can't al-ways know her intentions ahead of time, your first date is the time to find out about them.

That means actually steering the conversation at some point toward a little chat about your respective goals—compare agendas, if you will. Maybe one of you is searching for a permanent mate, and the other is in a major play-the-field mode. Maybe one of you is looking to expand your social life, and the other wants to date one person precisely to avoid the crowds. Maybe neither one of you knows what the hell you want. It's worth discussing.

Of course, implicit in this advice is that you know your own dating expectations. For example, if you're bent on an adventurous fling that'll take the two of you from Brazil to Borneo and back, there's little sense in asking out a single mother with two toddlers and a full-time job.

Once you're out on that first date, be yourself, no matter what. Adopting a

Hot Dates 1930 The Motion Picture Production Code was established. It prohibited showing nudity, lustful kissing, rape, biracial relationships, and childbirth. Within a year, ticket sales dropped by 30 million.

continued from page 103

Answer:
True. Earthworms, when they stumble across each other in the dark, have intercourse that lasts 3 to 4 hours. The tiny penis of each finds and enters the tiny vagina of the other.

LEGAL BRIEFS
Your education dollars at work: A San Francisco State University arts major was cited for misdemeanor indecent exposure after he climbed atop a campus building and shaved his pubic hair before 1,000 spectators.

The student said he was completing a homework assignment requiring him to do something in public at which he was unskilled and which **he might look clumsy or ugly** doing. The student called his performance "perfect art, . . . a real public transformation."

A pubic one too.

Seemed like a Good Idea at the Time. . .
Bill Clinton was not the first president to be guilty of sexual peccadilloes. Way back in 1899, French president Francois Faure died while doing the deed in a whorehouse. Urban legend has it that his partner became hysterical, contracting her

BAWDY BALLADS "The Horizontal Bop," *Bob Seger*

continued on page 115

persona sabotages the mission at hand, which is to get to know each other well enough to see if you want to take things further. Besides, you run the risk of getting stuck with whatever pose you come up with. Telling her that you love Elton John may get you in good with her now, but you could end up having to smile through a lot of unbearably sappy songs for the next month.

Also see: attraction, blind date, dating, disability—hers, first time with a lover, infatuation, morning after, one-night stand

first lover

You may think of her as the first person you had sex with. Or the first you *tried* to have sex with. Or the first you had an ongoing sexual relationship with. Whoever qualifies as your first lover, she's more than a figure from your past. She's an archetype—for you and for your current mate.

Let your memories of her be fond. But beware the tendency to mythologize your first lover as some kind of lost ideal. Fact is, you were younger when you were with her. And it's tempting to look back on your younger days as nothing but happy and carefree, while conveniently overlooking the hassles, the insecurities, and the reasons why your first lover is not your current lover. Besides, if you're going to have such a rosy view of things, wouldn't it make more sense to aim it at your current life? Start by putting your past into perspective, realizing that what you remember today as pure excitement was mostly the excitement of discovery. Everything wasn't better then. It was simply newer.

We shouldn't have to tell you this, but when around your current lover, avoid the subject of your first lover. If it absolutely cannot be avoided, keep any reference lighthearted and brief. Never say anything that invites comparison between the two—even if it's favorable. Telling your current that she's a better lover than your first may seem harmless or even complimentary, but it suggests that the two are in competition. At the very least, it suggests that your first lover is still in the back of your mind somewhere. That's exactly the sort of notion you want to quash.

Also see: past partners—longing for, remarriage, virginity—hers

first time with a lover

It's not going to be the best sex you've ever had. It's definitely not going to be the best sex the two of you will ever have with each other. But if you go about it right, you're both still in for major thrills.

Danielle Steel fans may not like the idea (and what guy reads Danielle Steel anyway?), but it makes sense to lower your expectations about your first time with a lover. Think about what's really going on during the inaugural ball: Though the two of you are hot for each other, you're jumping in cold in regards to the complicated choreography of the sex act. You know little or nothing about each other's bodies, rhythms, signals, or preferences. At the same time, you both may be unsure of what's happening emotionally. Why are you doing this? Where is it leading?

Then there's the old bugaboo of performance anxiety. There's nothing inevitable about erection difficulties or instant ejaculation during an initial coupling, but it sure as hell can happen. The

F

situation is anxiety-provoking for her too. Odds are, she'll worry that she'll take too long to have an orgasm. Throw in the necessary details about contraception and safe sex, and you get something a lot different from the Hollywood ideal of the first time, with all that slow-motion schlock music, that perfect body harmony, and of course, that simultaneous orgasm.

Treat your first time with her as what it is: a time for talking—beforehand—about your expectations, about the meaning each of you attaches to your looming consummation, and about contraception and safe sex.

That gagging sound you hear is coming from a million guys demanding to know why, for chrissakes, we have to *talk* about everything. Can't we just get it on and not worry about anything?

Well, the very reason for having a pre-passion tête-à-tête is so you *can* get it on without worrying. You'll not only have a much better time during the action but also avoid that postcoital confusion where you both wonder what happens next. (Like, is somebody supposed to go home now?)

Besides, since when is it a chore to talk about sex with a woman you're attracted to? Get her on your lap, take turns putting lips to ears, and talk intimately and sincerely about what this upcoming sex means to each of you. How is that going to dampen the experience?

Is there a risk of blowing the sexual opportunity by understanding it better? Sure, but only because of what you discover via talk, not because you decided to talk. If there's a disconnect between you—say, you assume you're on the road to wedlock and she's only doing it to get even with her two-timing boyfriend, the current WWF champion—you're better off knowing that. Aren't you? You also may be better off getting the hell outta there.

Now, are you ready for a blasphemous piece of advice? Here goes: Your best approach to your first time with a lover is not to have intercourse with her. Simply agree to forget about the penis/vagina thing for now. This book is loaded with pleasurable and satisfying alternatives to intercourse. Explore some of them. Even without official intercourse, the excitement is still there. How could it not be when you're getting naked with a new lover?

This is action without the anxiety. Erection and lubrication don't matter all that much. Birth control and safe sex are easier to deal with in the absence of penetration. When you do other stuff, you get comfortable and familiar with each other's bodies even as you enjoy them for the first time. You learn each other's sexual language.

And by the time you do have intercourse, you'll be experts.

Also see: clumsiness, contraception, dating, first date, foreplay, morning after, one-night stand, safe sex, shyness, virginity—hers

flapper

A rebellious party girl with short hair and shorter skirts. Fanatic about the latest music. Couldn't care less about home, tradition, or accepted "feminine" behavior. A little cynical about the world. Daring in fashion. Into makeup. Most of all, she's firmly dedicated to sexual pleasure and freedom. Sounds like your ex-girlfriend, doesn't it? But as modern as she seems, the flapper was the young woman on the cutting edge of the Jazz Age sexual revolution back in the 1920s.

F

That revolution was as significant in its time as the one that started taking off in the 1960s. When it comes to sex, it's a pretty good bet that anything you think is new only updates something old.

Also see: sexual revolution

flirtation

You could move this term to the *H* section since it often follows the adjective *harmless*, as in "a harmless flirtation." Or put it under *J* since what we claim to be doing is never precisely "flirting" but rather "just flirting."

You may already know what a harmless flirtation with a new (or not-so-new) female friend is like. The eye contact is a little on the spicy side. Some suggestive smiles are passed. A few extra compliments get exchanged, with subtle but unmistakable sexual connotations. But that's as far as it goes. You both get a dash of excitement and a nice ego boost, with no cause for trouble on the home front if you're not single, and without unwanted expectations if you are. After all, you're just flirting.

Fair enough. But keep in mind that flirtation is not always frivolous. Sexually speaking, it's one of the initial stages of human courtship—the "Notice me!" and "I'm interested!" phases that any two humans must pass through on their way to sexual intimacy. The tools of flirtation tend to be nonverbal, such as eye contact to signal interest, or a smile to indicate a positive response. Even the ensuing small talk emphasizes tone over content—it's not what you say but how you say it.

And while the word *flirtation* may be English, the custom is followed all over the world, from the most advanced to the most primitive societies. Anthropologists suspect that some female flirtation gestures, such as the coy smile and the shampoo-commercial head toss, are universal. In fact, even some animals signal sexual interest with a toss of the head. See? Beasts flirt too.

When you flirt, you dabble in a powerful evolutionary strategy designed to grease the tracks for the express train to Sextown. If that's your destination, get on board and go for it. If it's not—if you're just playing around—remember that once flirting starts, applying the brakes isn't always comfortable or easy to do. Before you know it, the two of you are in a postflirtation phase of the courtship process—touching, synchronized body movements, caressing—and the whole thing is not as harmless as you intended it to be. That's why you should know your intentions and

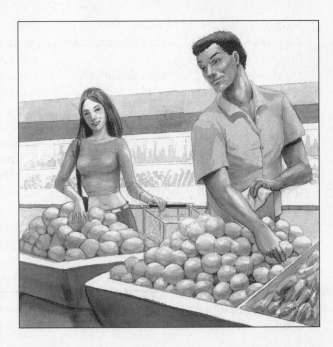

F

limits with a particular person before you start.

Also see: communication—nonverbal, courtship, eye contact, masher, meeting women, opening line, pickup lines, signals, slick

flogging

A whipping using a handheld instrument with several threads of leather dangling at the business end. The back or buttocks are usually the target. What does it have to do with sex? Plenty, for those who choose to explore the erotic possibilities of power exchange along with the increase in physical intensity that arousal's heightened pain threshold offers. As with any sado-masochistic sexual activity, flogging is always consensual, with agreed-upon limits and a safeword to stop the "punishment" when you've had enough.

Oh, yes. . . . The word is also a cheeky bit of slang for male self-pleasure, as in *flogging the frog*. So you can even flog and be flogged at the same time. Though it's probably not a good idea to literally flog your figurative frog.

Also see: bondage and discipline, dominance and submission, leather, paddle, safeword, spanking, whips

flowers

Give them. Give them often. Give them to a new lover after your first time. Give them to your wife of 30 years for no reason. Send them. Or deliver them yourself, by hand. Or have them waiting for her. Just make sure she gets them.

Flowers touch women deeply and never fail to accomplish great things. That's why any guy can score points with a simple bouquet. But you're going to do

better than that. You're going to learn to appreciate flowers yourself. Think about it. Flowers are essentially a plant's sexual parts—amazing and beautiful botanical sex organs with a thousand pleasing shapes and colors and fragrances. They're entry points into the world of the senses, of which women and sex are part. Truly know flowers, and your gift of these miracles turns into something much more powerful than a nice little gesture. You connect your humble little love affair to nature's great and beautiful sexual mysteries. So don't just give flowers. Make them part of your life. She will notice. And your life will be enriched.

Also see: birthdays, courtship, making up, romance, surprises

food

Don't dis the dinner date. It's a time-honored prelude to passion, and for good reason. Swapping food for sex has always been good survival business in the animal kingdom, where females seek males who can provide. We modern humans aren't so crude about it, of course, but it's still a fact that treating a woman to dinner gives the impression that you have means and that you're willing to share them with her.

Food is also a big player in the human courtship process because it's all about sensual cues. A meal for two triggers the senses—taste, smell, sight, even touch. In the right environment, eating is a ritual of allure and proximity, where the two of you face each other straight on and unwittingly synchronize your movements. That's sexy. Even the way your meal progresses—from appetite to anticipation to enjoyment to satisfaction—mimics the mounting excitement of you-know-what. So when it comes to seduction, food is your ally.

Hers too. It's an old saw, but women really do use food to seduce men. You can't assume anything, of course, but it's a pretty good bet that a new female acquaintance who invites you over for her beef bourguignonne has more than *her* beef on her mind.

There's no need to get postmodern about your dinner date when there's a hint of sex in the air. Forget the Nepalese folk food and seek out a white-tablecloth establishment where the whole idea is for the two of you to feel comfortable, waited upon, and good. Focus on the 10 senses (your 5 and hers), not the joint's reputation. And don't even think about splitting the tab this time. Right now, time-honored courtship ritual trumps more modern notions of equality.

Oh, yes. One more thing: Resist the urge to gorge yourselves. Overfilled stomachs have a way of snuffing out desire for sex. Moderately filled stomachs stoke it.

Also see: beer, courtship, dating, oysters, rituals, seduction, whipped cream

forbidden
See: taboos

foreplay
There's no such thing. The word suggests a pointless preliminary before the main event, like waiting in line to ride a roller coaster. But that makes sense only if you think of sex as no more than penetration and orgasm, with everything else as warmup. That ain't the way it is. Foreplay doesn't come before sex. Foreplay *is* sex.

You knew this in your early teens. With actual intercourse not in the cards, sex was a thrilling combination of kissing, touching, rubbing, squeezing, petting, and all those other interesting things humans do to pleasure each other and themselves. You didn't dismiss all this as just a prelude. It was *action*. It still is.

There are plenty of good reasons to make foreplay an extended action sequence. Yes, a big one is to help bring her along to full arousal. But this is no one-way street. The more turned on she gets, the more turned on you get. The result is an arousal feedback loop that the two of

115

F

Hot Dates 1933 A federal judge ruled that contraceptives served a medical need and that government had no place coming between a doctor and his patients.

continued from page 110

vaginal muscles to such an extent that **the prez's penis had to be surgically removed**.

Foreign Affairs
After a 7-year engagement, Kenya's Mohammed Aloo, 100, finally married his fiancée. Why the lengthy delay? It seems that **Aloo wanted**

his bride to finish grade school before the nuptials. She was 14 on their wedding day.

In Extremis
We should reconsider describing the well-endowed as "hung like a horse." Your typical stallion has an average erection of 2½ feet—a lot

True or Phallus?
There is an annual festival devoted solely to testicles.

BAWDY BALLADS "My Stove's in Good Condition," *Lil Johnson*

continued on page 124

F

you can exploit for extreme pleasure—regardless of whether you follow it up with coital union.

There's more. Foreplay fosters intimacy, which delivers big payoffs in an ongoing sexual relationship. It also creates that thrilling sense of cresting excitement that a lot of couples leave behind with their dating days. Then there's the obvious: Foreplay is your chance to enjoy, from top to bottom, that fetching female body to which you've earned access.

If you do proceed to the old in-and-out, generous amounts of foreplay will have made your erection and her orgasm more likely to happen. Concentrating on the pure pleasure of foreplay rather than the necessity of an erection or the desirability of an orgasm prompts the latter two to take care of themselves.

Nobody has come up with an all-purpose manual telling you what to touch, where to lick, and how hard to rub. That's a good thing, actually, because the key to foreplay is simpler than that. In fact, it comes down to two words: *Pay attention*. Let her pleasure be your guide. Experiment. If she doesn't let you know—via moans or words or arching her body toward you—whether something feels good, go ahead and ask if it does.

And pay attention to what feels good to you too. That arousal feedback loop is yours for the asking.

Also see: arousal, communication, stimulation, touch

foreskin

The fold of skin that covers the glans, or head, of the penis. Also called the prepuce (pronounced "PRE-pyoos"), the foreskin cooperatively retracts during intercourse, freeing the sensitive glans to head up the action. Some insist that the foreskin is a key instrument of sexual pleasure, but urologists are by no means unanimous in their assessments of its sensitivity. There's little doubt about the importance of foreskin hygiene, though. To discourage infections, it's important to pull back the prepuce and clean it regularly, especially after intercourse. Obviously exempt from this requirement are those men—including the majority of males in the United States—who have had their foreskins removed via circumcision.

Also see: circumcision, frenulum, hygiene, phimosis, piercing, prepuce, smegma

fragrances

Here's how to prepare your love nest for maximum olfactory impact before ushering in your new lady: Decide how much money and time you want to spend on fragrances. Then head to Kmart and spend that money on household cleansers, a broom, a mop, a bucket, and plenty of washcloths. Use the time not to introduce new odors into your bedroom but to clean out the entrenched ones—of dirty socks, forgotten underwear, stale beer, and long-lost pizza crumbs. Nothing else you could do would create a more enticing atmosphere for sex.

It's not that added fragrance doesn't help. On the contrary, it can boost the erotic environment. But it takes a subtle, knowing touch to make it work. And, frankly speaking, a lot of guys couldn't appreciate a fragrance if you squirted it up their noses. Women, however, know the difference between a sensual environment and a manipulative one. If you try to cover up peculiar odors, she'll be on to it. And if you overwhelm the air without putting much thought into it, she's likely to wrinkle her nose and ask, "What's that smell?" You'll have created distraction, not seduction.

So what's the right fragrance for sex? Ah, if only there were a one-scent-pleases-all answer, life and love would be a lot easier. Alas, smell is so subjective a sense that you can't predict her reaction to any one fragrance. Don't try. Do your homework instead. Get her talking about fragrances she likes. Ask her what she thinks as you pass by a particularly aromatic aisle in a department store. Poke around candle shops and perfume displays. She'll let you know the kind of scents she prefers. Once it's established that sandalwood incense turns her into a purring heat source, go ahead and light it up. Otherwise, less is more. You can't go wrong with a vase of sweet-smelling roses in a clean, well-ventilated bedroom.

The same subtle approach applies to your cologne or aftershave. A fragrance attracts women by insinuating, rather than announcing, itself. And whatever it is, it smells stronger and different to her than it does to you. Try this: Throw away whatever cologne you've been using. Buy another one that's twice as expensive. Then use half as much.

Also see: atmosphere, beds, body odor as an attractant, body odor—controlling, hygiene, perfume, pheromones, scents

free love

The term is 1960s retro; the idea behind it isn't. In a nutshell, those who advocated free love believed that any sexual connection should depend only on the (often spontaneous) decisions of the two (or more) people involved, and not on any social structure such as family, marriage, law, or religion. Practically speaking, today any sexual intercourse out of wedlock is an example of free love, though hardly anybody would call it that. So, even though the idea still has plenty of detractors, it's not all that radical.

Also see: flapper, promiscuity, safe sex, sexual revolution, STDs, wild women

French

No getting around it, our Gallic friends are the reigning champs in the world cup of sexual reputation. The very word *French* is synonymous with oral play, and the subtlest hint of a Parisian accent oozes seduction. What's with these guys? Are they really so much better lovers than we are?

Sexologists will tell you that certain Mediterranean cultures—France especially, but also Italy and Greece—are much more comfortable with eroticism than we Americans are. Unlike us, they're not the inheritors of a pleasure-denying puritan history. For centuries, France even boasted the freest flow of pornography, until the rest of the West caught up in the mid-1900s. And the French aren't as heavily bombarded with the media message that their sexuality is somehow subpar and will stay that way unless they buy lots more stuff. As a result, they have a more relaxed and open approach to things sexual. And it's precisely a relaxed and open approach that makes a good lover. So there you go.

You even see the difference in politics. A recent French president kept a mistress throughout his incumbency, and none of his countrymen (or -women) thought twice about it. A recent American president got a little on the side, and the late-night jokesters are still making a living off him.

This is not to suggest that you must enjoy pornography or condone adultery in order to catch up with the French. But it's worth knowing that you probably have more cultural sexual repression to overcome than they do. If they're winning, it's because the playing field isn't level.

Also see: bidet, femme, French tickler, ménage à trois, monogamy, politicians, Sade—Marquis de

French kiss

Any kind of mouth kiss that involves one or more tongues. So, contrary to a common assumption, French kissing refers not to a single act but to a glorious array of osculatory activities that range from the slightest touch of two tongue tips to passionate probing of seldom-explored regions of her mouth and beyond.

Frenching is a superb alternative to rushing into intercourse. Spend some time on it. Start slowly, with lips only. Wait for the kisses to deepen on their own before you introduce your tongue. Even then, do it as subtly as possible at first. To up the ante, let two criteria guide you: your sensations and her responses. Feel what's going on, and pay attention to the feelings. Improvise. Don't do things with your tongue simply because you'd planned to. Let the moment be your inspiration. Opportunities abound for two-way communication, a kind of lingual call and response. Go with it. Make it last. This is sex as intimate as intercourse.

Still, resist the temptation to just shove on in there. Many women love French kissing when they're ready for it, but everyone hates it when they're not. It's no fun when you're expecting a kiss and

get a simulated tonsillectomy instead. Follow the universal rule of lovemaking: Never insert anything into anything until both the inserter and insertee are clearly ready for it.

Also see: breath, foreplay, hickey, kiss, licking, lips, mouth

French tickler

If you ask for a French tickler at your friendly neighborhood sex shop, you'll probably get a condomlike slip-on with something rubbery or plastic protruding from the end to provide extra stimulation for your lover during intercourse. The problem is that what gets tickled is the inside of the vagina, which is far less sensitive to that kind of touch than the outer vulva and clitoris. So, a lot of sex toy aficionados prefer bumpy or fingery or shaggy attachments on a cock ring; its position closer to the base of the penis directs the ticklers to the outer vagina, where they do the most good. That's more in keeping with the original French tickler from days of yore, which used goat eyelids at the base of the penis to drive women wild.

Still, condom-style French ticklers can certainly lighten up the bedroom—especially the arty kinds with the ticklers shaped as demon tongues or gargoyles and the like. You can always don one and then use your penis to rub her clitoris before or instead of entering her. Just make sure you use a real condom underneath the toy version, if you need one.

Also see: cock ring, sexual aids, vibrator

frenulum

It's the small area of skin toward the front of the underside of your penis, where the head and shaft meet. In uncircumcised men, it serves as the attachment point for the foreskin. But we don't care about that; we care only about its extremely exquisite sensitivity. Your frenulum is a top-tier sexual pleasure zone. Consider it a primary target of the masturbating hand or the fellatio-performing tongue.

Also see: erogenous zones, fellatio, glans

frequency

Perhaps no sexual topic is more laden with myth and urban legend than the question of how often American men get laid. Consider that two of the myths—that we're constantly having sex and that we're a nation with undersexed wives—are largely incompatible (unless one argues that American men have constant sex with women who aren't their wives. But the surveys don't support that, either.)

One truism is that frequency declines with age—not with old age, mind you, but in a steady downward slope from about 30. Face it, you have a lot of other things to deal with. And your body tends to slow down as the mileage piles up. Bummer? Not if you look at it this way: While young men spend a lot of time seeking sex without getting enough, many middle-aged men spend less time searching and get all they want. Who's better off?

Another fact is that all the surveys in the world can't provide a number you can use as a frequency goal. Assuming you don't act compulsively, exploitatively, or recklessly, whatever amount of sex you truly want (rather than think you should have) is the amount that's best for you. But if you insist on some statistical guidance, an early sexual-frequency study by Alfred Kinsey came up with the following range for men: from one orgasm every 30

years to five a day. Your ideal frequency probably falls somewhere in between. Does that help?

Frequency becomes a real issue only when there's a desire discrepancy—that is, when you want it much more often than she does. Or vice versa, which is the case in roughly half of discrepancies. This is a problem that doesn't often resolve itself. You have to face up to it, and that means talking. One thing to consider before you start the conversation is that pronounced desire discrepancies are often not really about sex. Other power struggles, like money or division of labor, may be playing themselves out in the bedroom.

When you do talk about sexual frequency, make sure you put the whole range of sexual activity on the agenda. Don't define the problem as a question of having intercourse or not. With such a limited approach, you run the risk of one of you consenting to more sex as a chore or the other accepting deprivation. By including all the other stuff—from cuddling to massages to hand jobs to sex toys—you're much more likely to negotiate ways to make each other happy. And you may learn a thing or two about your partner's real desires.

Also see: aging, cystitis, marriage—lack of sex in, promiscuity, quality versus quantity, refractory period, withholding

Freud

The father of psychoanalysis and liberator of human sexuality (1856–1939). Sigmund Freud's world was one of unconscious motives, guilty secrets, and unspeakable passions and longings. He believed that your adult personality was shaped by how you progressed through five psychosexual stages of development: oral (the first year

F

of life), anal (from age 2 to 3), phallic (roughly from 3 to 6), latent (from the end of the phallic stage until puberty), and genital (from puberty on).

Before Freud, human sex was as taboo a topic in scientific circles as it was in polite society. With Freud, it became a legitimate subject of public inquiry. Because of him, we talk about it. And we talk about it with a vocabulary that he enriched, with such words and phrases as *libido*, *penis envy*, and *Oedipus complex*.

Like any pioneer, he sometimes screwed up. And like any century-old work, Freud's sex theories often don't hold up. Most famously, Freud's view of sex was so male-centered that some of it is now virtually useless in practice. Still, if it weren't for him, you wouldn't be reading this book.

Also see: dreams, Electra complex, hang-ups, libido, phallic, women

frigidity

Erase this one from your vocabulary. It's an outdated way of referring to what's really a range of conditions that have to do with female sexuality—mostly, difficulty in having orgasms or becoming sufficiently aroused. The conditions are still around, of course, but the word has fallen out of favor because it makes a statement about the woman as a human being instead of describing her treatable conditions. Your Kelvinator is frigid; your girlfriend isn't.

Finally—and we hate to bring this up—a woman's sexual-response problems may have something to do with her lover's skills. It's worth thinking about.

Also see: arousal, foreplay, clitoral orgasm, nymphomania, shyness, sex therapy

G

games

The kind with two winners, that is. Sex is supposed to be fun, remember? A good way to make sure it stays fun is to inject a dose of lighthearted play into the action. Adult sex games do a bang-up job of breaking down barriers to intimacy and expanding your sexual horizons.

The classic bit of fun is sexual role-playing. Choose personalities that have some erotic zing for you. Stay in character. And fill the final act with hot sex. Examples: You be the lecherous uncle and she the virgin. Or she the horny teacher and you the shy student. Add some costumes and take it up a notch on the fantasy scale—the pirate and the princess, the alien and the earthling. You may find yourselves enacting long-held erotic fantasies. And you may bring to the surface suppressed sexual potential. But forget all that stuff for now. Just play. Keep it light. Have fun. It's a *game*.

If you're like a lot of couples, you may need a little push before you're ready to let the games begin. That's where the booming business of adult board games comes in. They're short on rules and shorter on competition, so they're great for guiding the shy through sexual play they'd never think of themselves. Most board games just ask you to do little erotic things that seem silly but encourage communication, not to mention arousal. For example, a card may tell you, "Touch your partner somewhere you've never touched before." Or you may land on a square and find yourself instructed to spread some whipped cream where you'd like your partner to lick it off. See the potential?

Also see: body oils, bondage and discipline, boredom, costumes, dominance and submission, erotic literature, fantasies, fetish, laughter, phone sex, playacting, rough sex, sexual aids, striptease, teasing, variety, water sports, whipped cream, wrestling

G

gang bang

Two guys having sex with one woman is one kind of threesome or ménage à trois. Add at least one more man to the mix, and you got a gang bang. That slang term usually refers to several men having sex more or less simultaneously with one woman. When the sex is sequential—one guy after another—you're talking "train."

It's often assumed that a gang bang inherently exploits the woman involved. Also, the phrase *gang bang* has a harsh sound to it—after all, it's also used to refer to gang violence. But as an entirely consensual activity, this kind of group sex is a big turn-on for some folks, women included.

Notice we said "some," not all. The logistics of a threesome are complicated enough. Add other guys, and the whole thing is probably more trouble than it's worth. More important, the consent of all involved has to be achieved without a hint of pressure and must be rock solid. A gang bang should never even be considered if alcohol has been consumed. (Yet such an encounter rarely gets off the ground without alcohol in the picture.) Remember, from the point of view of a woman who feels coerced or taken advantage of, it's not very far from gang bang to gang rape.

Also see: alcohol, date rape, group sex, ménage à trois, pulling a train, rape, threesome

gang rape

Group sexual assault is such a despicable act that it may seem there's no further point to be made. There is, however, because guys can unwittingly do something that fits the legal definition of this odious crime.

Gang rapes often take place in a party atmosphere where the booze and testosterone are flowing freely. What's passed off as a frat ritual or a game is in reality a bunch of men taking sexual advantage of a woman, who's perhaps drunk or stoned and who's definitely in no position to consent or even communicate her nonconsent. Such a scenario has nothing to do with fully consensual three-or-more-somes that are mutually planned and enjoyed by all.

What it is, fellas, is rape. Now there's really no further point to be made.

Also see: fantasies, paraphilias, perversions, pulling a train, rape, sex offenders, violence

garter belts

They're simply old-fashioned belt-and-strap devices for holding up stockings. If you're anything like the rest of us red-blooded American males, you find them inexplicably exciting. Maybe that's because a garter belt so teasingly accents all of a woman's most feminine parts—her navel, her hips, her buttocks, and her thighs and the private spaces between them.

It also helps that modern women reserve garter belts for special occasions only. As practical pieces of underwear, they've never been very convenient. The clasps that attach to the stockings are ridiculously difficult to fasten, and they dig cruelly into the tender flesh at the back of a woman's thighs whenever she sits down. In fact, that's probably a main reason why practical-but-unalluring panty hose were invented.

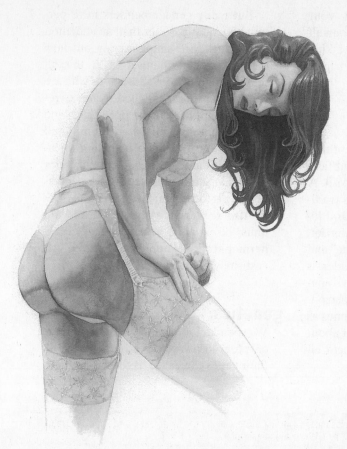

And even though most brides still wear garters, the old garter-and-bouquet-toss tradition is becoming less popular. Yes, some couples still trot it out. And some single women will still knock down the bridesmaids, the flower girl, and the groom's great-grandmother to snatch that wilted bunch of roses. But lots of other women are insulted by the implication that they want to catch the bouquet to catch a husband. They're also less than enthused about the other "prize" they win if that nosegay hits them—the chance to have a man they've probably never met stick his hands up their skirts in front of an audience of 100 and an obnoxious deejay making snide remarks.

We bachelors have never been all that into the ritual anyway. The main reason most of us participate is that it's held toward the end of the reception, after we've taken full advantage of the open bar. Plus, our athletic and survival instincts prompt us to stick our hands up in the air to catch any object that's hurtling toward our heads.

If you're the lucky guy who ends up with the garter in his fist, take it like a gentleman. Make eye contact with the flower-toting female as she perches on that banquet chair, and give her a congenial, conciliatory grin to let her know you're only going along with this public spectacle to humor the newlyweds. When it's time to do the deed, just get in and get out (you know what we mean). Slide the garter to just above her

So if your woman slips out of her party dress to reveal a garter belt, it's only because she knows it turns you on. It's her not-so-subtle way of letting you know that she wants your body and she thinks you're sexy. Dim the lights, put on a Rod Stewart album, and tell her she wears it well.

Also see: cross-dressing, lingerie

garters

These elastic bands bedecked with ribbons and lace were originally used to hold up hosiery. These days, the only time most women will ever wear one is on their wedding day.

knee—no farther—then extract your hands immediately. And remind yourself that at the next wedding, the bride hiking up her dress is your cue to take a trip to the men's room.

gender bender

People in this category don't accept that anatomy determines gender identification, and they don't care who knows it. A gender bender intentionally blurs traditional boundaries between male and female, in dress, demeanor, sexual behavior, art, even language (calling men "she" and women "he," for example). Gender is often bent for public consumption, sometimes entertainingly by female impersonators and drag queens and sometimes as an in-your-face political statement about the oppressive nature of society's rigid, either-or gender categories.

But many gender benders have personal liberation, rather than an audience, in mind; they're simply acting out how they feel about themselves. If this all seems a bit much for those of us who are happy with our assigned gender, remember that there have been times and places where women were considered guilty of blurring the sex boundary whenever they dared to have an opinion or enjoy sex. Sometimes, yesterday's gender-bending is today's mainstream thought.

Also see: androgyny, anima and animus, bisexuality, cross-dressing, drag, hermaphrodite, homosexuality, transvestism, yin and yang

genetics

We spend a lot of time blaming our parents for our own shortcomings. After all, their genes can cause us to lose our hair,

---

Hot Dates **1930s** In eight-page comic strips called Tijuana bibles, everyone from Dagwood and Blondie to Clark Gable and Joan Crawford had sex with reckless abandon.

continued from page 115

Answer:

True. Montana's Original Testicle Festival is dedicated to giving testicles their due. The event serves up the organs in many creative ways, including beer-battered and deep-fried. The "ball" gets rolling the third Thursday of each September.

bigger than the boys in the locker room, but much smaller than the elephant (5½ feet) and a mere fraction of the **10-foot average erection of the humpback whale**. So maybe the proper phrase is "He's got a wang like a whale"?

LEGAL BRIEFS

Baby, you can drive my car—but first you must have sex with me: A Wyoming man sued a woman for breach of contract, saying he agreed to give her a car worth $300 in return for a $100 payment and 50 sexual

favors. (For the math-impaired, **that's an average of $4 per sexual favor**.) The plaintiff said the woman defaulted after 33 installments. A judge tossed the lawsuit, deeming the contract illegal.

Seemed like a Good Idea at the Time. . .

In the 1940s, an American doctor named Walter J. Freeman **performed lobotomies on institutionalized homosexual men and women** to "cure" them of their sexual orientation. The draconian

---

BAWDY BALLADS **"Let's Do It,"** *Cole Porter*

continued on page 129

(except in the case of ear and nose hair—then they're responsible for our overabundance of it), drop dead of a premature heart attack, get fat, come down with diabetes, you name it.

Is there anything in our lives that is not directly related to our genetic makeup, or are we mere racehorses who fall or triumph according to our breeding? Turns out there is one very important aspect of you that has almost nothing to do with the blood in your veins: It's the way you love.

Researchers at the University of California, Davis, took a look at 445 pairs of twins. Seventy-five percent of the subjects were identical, or genetic, twins, who carry the exact same genes. The others were fraternal twins. The researchers rated all of them for six different styles of love and found that the genetic twins were no more likely than the fraternal twins to love in the same fashion.

What this means to you is that even if your parents were dysfunctional and wholly unable to love, that story does not necessarily need to be relived by you. There is nothing hardwired in you that prevents you from choosing another path. For many men, that's a large reason to rejoice. Carry on, wayward son.

Also see: chromosomes, love, PMS, sex offenders, sexual attraction, violence, zygote

genital warts

Meet the bug behind the most common sexually transmitted disease in the United States: the human papillomavirus (HPV), father to genital warts. And unlike bacterial infections (or that brother-in-law houseguest who finally gets the hint), this virus never goes away.

It's sneaky too. Many infected people never know they have it because HPV can stay hidden in their bodies without ever showing up as warts. And then they can unknowingly pass it on to someone else. In fact, here's a sobering thought: There's a one-in-five chance that the next woman you sleep with will have an HPV infection.

If it does show up as warts, they'll be little cauliflower-like bumps on your penis or elsewhere on your genital area. They can also show up around your anus and even in your mouth (you guessed it—they get there through oral sex). It's a good idea to have your doctor check you during regular exams, especially if you suspect that one of your partners may have had it. Periodic self-exams are wise too.

It was once thought that these warts were ugly but harmless. Not so anymore. Some strains of the virus have been linked to penile cancer in men and cervical cancer in women. And one recent small study found that genital warts increase men's risk of developing prostate cancer.

Currently, your only treatment option is to have the warts removed. A doctor can prescribe a medication that you dab on your warts a couple of times a day. If that doesn't work, he can fry or freeze them off in his office. The problem is, this solution works only for the visible warts—it won't eradicate warts hidden in the layers of your skin.

Researchers are still trying to find a vaccine for the virus. It's been a tough go since, as with the common cold, there are so many different strains.

If you want to avoid this lifelong hanger-on, your best bet is still a plain old condom. Even though condoms

G

won't entirely protect you—because warts can lie outside the boundaries of the rubber—they can reduce the risk substantially, especially for men. One study showed that failure to use condoms made men three times more likely to develop warts. In women, the odds were about half that.

Also see: papilloma, Pap test, penile cancer, STDs, warts

getaways

See: sex tours and resorts, travel as an aphrodisiac, travel—planning

get off

A common slang term meaning "reach orgasm" or "bring your partner to climax." For you history buffs, this definition dates back to 1867. Before that, *get off* meant "tell a joke or story." We're thinking that once the jokes turned dirty, one thing led to another—hence, today's definition.

By the way, getting off can refer to climaxing when either having sex or going it solo. This may be how the phrase evolved to also mean "perform a jazz solo."

Also see: clitoral orgasm, come, manual stimulation, masturbation, orgasm

gigolo

The character that Jon Voight played in the film *Midnight Cowboy* never had much success in his plans to become a highly paid gigolo in New York City. But that was in 1969—and a lot has changed with the new, service-based economy.

A gigolo, of course, is a male sex worker. It is not, as is sometimes thought, simply a guy who gets lucky often. And if you're pondering a sudden career change, it most certainly is a form of prostitution and thus is generally illegal in the United States.

Whom do these men serve? Their clientele consists mostly of upper-level businesswomen who are focused on their careers and don't have time for long-term relationships. They still want sex and intimacy, but they don't want some guy banging on their doors in the morning or calling them at work. (Is this starting to sound familiar? It should, since it's the very same thing we men have complained about throughout history.) A small percentage of clients are husbands who pay for their wives to get off. These husbands are usually either unwilling or unable to sexually perform themselves.

Speaking of performing, a lot is expected of gigolos. A woman wants a hard-on for her hard cash. It follows that most successful gigolos are sexually insatiable and able to get and keep erections with minimum stimulation—even if the woman they're with isn't somebody they'd normally pick.

Don't think for a minute that it's all fun and games. Husbands can, and do, walk in on unauthorized transactions. More than one gigolo has barely walked away from such a scenario. And, perhaps not surprisingly, a gigolo sometimes falls in love with one of his clients. Needless to say, it's often unrequited love, with heartache following shortly thereafter.

Also see: escort service, john, money, prostitution, satyriasis, trick

give head

This phrase started showing up in the early 1940s to describe oral sex. Even though it's widely used to signify fellatio, a man can also give head to a woman. That's because it refers to the head atop your shoulders, not the head of your penis.

Since the term encompasses your whole cranium, why not put your noggin to use? A lot of women find it erotic when you use your head with abandon during oral sex. Rest your well-shorn cheek against her when you need a break from tongue action. Rub your forehead over her. You can even run your hair across her. Yes, this will leave you with a sort of passion mousse, but it can be highly sexy: Rolling your dome around uninhibitedly shows you're really, really into giving her head.

Also see: cunnilingus, fellatio, glory hole, licking, oral sex, tongue

glans

The head of your penis. If you're circumcised, it's the ever-present helmet. If you're not, it's the part that turtles out to greet you when you're erect.

What's oddly cool is that your glans is made of the same tissue as a woman's clitoris. It's packed with nerve endings that account for most of the penile sensations you feel during sex.

Armed with this knowledge, ask your woman to dwell on your glans the next time she goes down on you. Request that she hold it in her mouth and toggle it with her tongue. Some guys even like to be chewed gently. Let's repeat that word: *gently.*

And if she gives you a hand job, request that each stroke pass over the glans. Many women grip too low on a man's shaft and don't stimulate the top part enough. Onward and upward!

Also see: circumcision, frenulum, lips, penis, premature ejaculation, reproductive system—yours

glory hole

If you're a miner, a glory hole is a large, open excavation in the ground. But to most men, the closest the term comes to mining is that it requires an operating shaft.

That's because it's a hole that's fashioned at waist level and just large enough to permit a penis to poke through. It allows someone on the other side to give you a hand or blow job while protecting both your anonymities. (It also gives you the option of "doing" a stranger.) You mostly see glory holes in adult video and toy stores, but sometimes they're a featured attraction at sex and fetish parties too.

Also see: fellatio, oral sex

gonad

The average guy thinks that this is simply his younger brother's first name. It's actually the scientific term for any gamete-producing gland. And a gamete is a reproductive cell. Which means either a sperm or an egg. Which means *gonads* refers to a woman's ovaries as well as a man's testicles.

So go ahead, call your little sister a gonad. Science is on your side.

Also see: ovaries, reproductive system—hers, reproductive system—yours, testicles

G

gonorrhea

Popularly known as the clap, gonorrhea warrants no applause. There are more than 350,000 new cases of the stuff in the United States every year.

You'll know that you're one of them if you experience the following symptoms: One to 7 days after intercourse with an infected partner, you notice a burning feeling when you take a leak. If you milk the shaft of your penis, you'll usually see yellow pus ooze out the end. Say hello to *Neisseria gonorrhoeae*, a sexually transmitted bacteria that's taken up residence in your system. You need to see a doctor pronto for some antibiotics.

Ignore gonorrhea, and you run the risk of becoming infertile. Even so, a lot of guys see the clap as no big deal—go on a round of pills, and it's gone. That may explain why the percentage of men with gonorrhea who get repeat infections within a year hovers between 17 and 22 percent.

The scary part of that attitude is this: Studies have shown over and over that being infected with gonorrhea makes it easier for you to catch the virus that causes AIDS. And the bacteria is growing increasingly resistant to antibiotics. Not such a harmless little bug anymore, huh?

The clap is almost entirely preventable with the use of condoms. Yet another very good reason to wrap your willy.

Also see: AIDS, ectopic pregnancy, epididymitis, IUD, NSU, STDs, urethritis, venereal disease

group sex

Synonymous with *orgy*, group sex has likely been around for as long as . . . well, as long as there have been groups. And sex. Ancient religions used group sex to worship fertility gods and to give widows and infertile couples a chance to carouse and conceive. The children born as a result of these gatherings were considered sacred in some cultures.

Even today, not all men and women view group sex as a mangling of morals. Millions of Americans take part in swinger activities that sometimes include orgies. And like the rituals of ancient days, these assemblies are grounded in rules and etiquette.

For example, if a couple opens their house to a group-sex evening, there are very explicit expectations upon the attendees. People cannot bang away willy-nilly at every opening that passes by. They must wait to be invited to join a grouping.

Drop by one of these events, and you might see a Mongolian cluster—a group with more men than women, where the women tackle several guys at once. Or you might spot a rainbow—a group with people of several ethnic backgrounds. Then there's the rowboat, where a woman climbs aboard a reclining man while giving head to two other men, one on either side of her.

If you're a bachelor, we hate to burst your rapidly inflating bubble, but single men are rarely welcome at group gatherings. Single women, on the other hand, are very welcome.

Also see: interracial sex, ménage à trois, swinging, threesome

grunting

We grunt at the gym to push through our last chinup. So it's only logical that we make similar guttural sounds during our bedroom workouts.

That said, there's a big difference between staged, exaggerated grunting and the sounds that are a natural part of lovemaking. We're not trying to give you stage fright; we're simply letting you know that the grunts that come out of every third-rate male porn star while he's hammering away are not what the typical woman wants to hear. His are faked and forced. Don't let yours be the same way. If you groan and grunt naturally, without thinking about it, fine; don't censor yourself. But if you consciously throw in a groan every now and then just because it's been a while since you've made a noise, save yourself the trouble. She'll see right through it. Besides, it means you're over-thinking things instead of just enjoying yourself.

Also see: communication—nonverbal, moaning, talking dirty, voice, whispering

G-spot

In the 1940s, German obstetrician Ernst Grafenberg began a controversy that continues to this day. He described an area in a woman's vagina that became known as the G-spot. Trouble is, nobody has ever really seen this purported center of sexual pleasure.

The reason the G-spot can be as elusive as the Loch Ness monster is that it's made of erectile tissue that can be felt only when a woman is aroused. So gynecologists are unlikely to come across it, because a pelvic exam is far from arousing, and medical ethics boards prefer to keep it that way. No autopsy has been able to confirm the existence of the G-spot, either.

So where is this legendary happy zone said to be situated? On the upper part of the vaginal wall, 1 to 2 inches behind the back of the pubic bone. It consists of nerve endings and blood vessels that, when stimulated, can grow to be as big as a half-dollar.

Not all women feel something when you stroke the spot; some feel that they need to urinate. But for those who respond well to G-spot wrangling, it can be a source of overwhelming orgasms—sometime even leading to the equally mythic female ejaculation.

You and your partner can figure out how responsive she is to G-spot simulation with a minimum amount of

Hot Dates **1930s** Thirty states passed mandatory sterilization laws for those likely to bear "socially defective" children.

continued from page 124

operation had the effect of turning them into asexual zombies.

Foreign Affairs
Hugh Hefner's got nothing on Hafiz Ghulam Qadir of Pakistan. In 1985, Qadir, who claimed to be 130, married for the third time. His bride was 37, while Qadir's oldest son was 90.

"I feel the vigor of a young man in my freckled body," Qadir told an interviewer for United Press International. We feel queasy.

In Extremis
As proof that today's seniors are more active than those of past generations, we have Flora: **At 83,**

True or Phallus
The average erect penis contains twice as much blood as a flaccid penis.

BAWDY BALLADS "Afternoon Delight," *Starland Vocal Band*

continued on page 136

G

spelunking: Next time you're deep into foreplay, lie face-to-face. Slide your index and middle fingers into the top third of her vagina. Feel for a rougher patch of skin in the above-mentioned location, and stroke it with your fingertips as if you were beckoning someone to come (which, in a sense, you are). If this doesn't produce any sensations of particular interest, wander around the area doing the same thing. She'll let you know if and when you strike gold.

The G-spot is slightly harder to hit during intercourse. The best positions for stimulating it are doggie style and woman on top.

Also see: clitoral orgasm, female ejaculation, necrophilia, Pap test

guilt

Most of us think we understand guilt: To wit, the anxiety we feel when we know we're doing something wrong. Simple, huh?

Not quite. The fact that you feel guilty does not, in and of itself, mean you shouldn't be doing whatever it is you're doing. There are women who feel guilty about having intercourse with their husbands, because they were raised to see sex as the dirty part of marriage. And there are recently divorced men who feel guilty about sleeping with women besides the ones who just dumped them. Indeed, some of us experience guilt anytime we do something enjoyable or anytime we chill out instead of being productive. (This, too, is often the legacy of overly austere religious educations or family traditions.)

The key to truly understanding these feelings is to separate raw guilt from le-

gitimate conscience. Does it make logical sense to feel guilty about the behavior that gave rise to the guilt? If so, it's your conscience talking, and you should consider listening. But if you constantly feel guilty about things that can't be logically explained—like the aforementioned guys who don't want to "cheat" on their ex-wives—you need to talk yourself through it. Or maybe talk things out with a trusted friend. As often as you need to. As often as he can stand it.

It sounds too easy, but it really does work. Unless the guilt is pathological, in which case—as we say many other places in this book—therapy may be the answer.

Also see: affairs, best friend's wife, compulsive behavior, emotions, extramarital sex, fantasies, fig leaf, hang-ups, hypnosis and performance enhancement, impotence, kinky, Madonna/whore complex, making up, paraphilias, perversions, phallic, religion, secrets, sex therapy, taboos

gusher

The late, great comedian Bill Hicks liked to joke that he'd wiped entire civilizations off his chest with a gray gym sock. Well, some days you can spread the polliwog empires across your torso, and some days you're lucky to fling a small village or two on your pubic hair. That's the difference between a gusher and a piddler.

It all depends on the amount of semen held under pressure in your testicles, prostate, and seminal vesicles. And that varies according to a host of physical and psychological factors. If you're too tired or too drunk, you're not going to set any new Olympic benchmarks for ejaculatory performance. And since semen is 95 percent fluid, even dehydration can make a difference. Your level of excitement also plays a huge role. If you're highly aroused by the sex kitten and her sister rolling around in your bed, the three of you may end up awash in the stuff.

For an objective reading of whether you've just scored a gusher, go dig around in the kitchen drawer for a measured teaspoon. If there's more spume than you can scrape into that, you've got a gusher on your hands, as it were.

A few final things to remember: Most women really don't care *how much* you come—they're more concerned with how long it takes you. And the amount of ejaculate you produce has nothing to do with how manly you are.

Now please, for the sake of muffins and cookies everywhere, go wash out that spoon.

Also see: cum, sloppy sex, wet spot

G

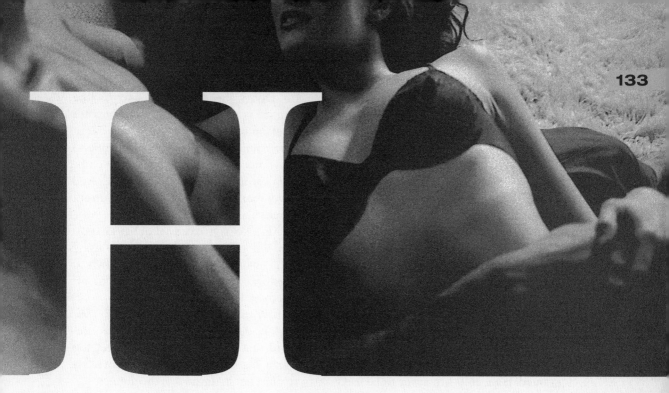

hair

Ever since evolution placed us at the top of the great global slag heap, we've been trying to figure out what to do with the stuff. Especially once we start to lose it.

So here's some refreshing news: Women don't care that much about the hair on the tops of our heads. Really, they don't. In a survey of 2,000-plus women, we found that only 1 percent named hair as the most attractive male feature. In fact, hair came in dead last among the 11 physical features we asked the women to rank. It turns out that women don't even care about a lack of hair. When asked, "If a man starts to lose his hair, what should he do?" a whopping 91 percent of women answered, "Don't worry about it."

It's a different story, though, when it comes to the various swatches, wisps, and tufts that sprout up across our bodies. Some women dig fur on your chest and back; others recoil. And you'd be hard-pressed to find a woman who's ambivalent about the burgeoning clumps of hair in your nose or ears.

Here are some handy-dandy tips on plucking, in the event you do decide to trim your bodily tresses.

• For eyebrows and ears, a technique called electrolysis permanently rids you of hair after a few sessions.

• For your nose, use scissors or a battery-powered nose-hair trimmer. Trim only those hairs visible at the openings of your nostrils. When using a battery-powered trimmer, turn it on before inserting it in your nose, and don't insert the blade more than ¼ inch. If you experience any soreness or scabbing, see your doctor.

• For your back and chest, you have a number of options. Shaving is the easiest but also needs the most maintenance. Waxing gives you a longer period of hairlessness, but it hurts like hell. Several rounds of laser treatments will thin your shaggy mane for good—at the cost of a cool grand or more.

Also see: beard burn, finasteride, hygiene, male body, pubic hair

handcuffs

How did something designed to subdue robbers, murderers, and maniacs ever find its way into the bedroom? It's quite interesting, really. Handcuffs give you unfettered access to the person before you. That's highly erotic to many men, and not a few women (especially if the guy is the one wearing the cuffs). This may sound like common sense, but we've learned not to take common sense for granted: Handcuffs are never to be used except with a willing partner. You may give handcuffs as a surprise gift to see how she reacts—though we'd caution you to lay some groundwork first in "casual conversation"—but the presentation of this gift should *never* take the form of slipping them on her in bed one night.

Lawyerly caveats dispensed with, let's get back to the merits of metal. Particularly for those deeply involved with the bondage scene, nothing compares to handcuffs. Unlike leather and ropes, nobody except David Copperfield is going to break free from a set of well-made manacles. That knowledge on the part of both parties only adds to the psychic kick.

Here's a quick user's guide: Go for high-quality cuffs from a police supply store. Cheap metal pairs like the ones you get at most porn shops can break or, worse yet, slip until they're so tight that they cause damage. That's also why you should double-lock cuffs—that's the setting where they won't tighten once they're in place.

Be gentle when you go to put them on. Don't sling them on her wrists like you see cops do on TV. These things are steel, and they can bruise the hell out of her. Your captive also should be able to move her wrists freely inside the cuffs. Don't worry; they'll still be secure. And never make her lie on the cuffs; it can cut off circulation.

Also, keep an extra set of keys handy. You'll doom your chances of ever using cuffs again if she has to truck down to the local garage to have them cut off after you lose the keys.

Last, make sure that you and your partner decide ahead of time on a safe-word that she can say if things get too rough. Just choose a word you're not likely to blurt out in the heat of the moment.

Also see: bondage and discipline, safeword

hang-ups

If you have sexual hang-ups, well then, lucky you. Seriously.

One of the remarkable aspects of sexuality and eroticism is that it serves as a window into your greater psyche. Look at hang-ups as a way to learn more about yourself.

Say, for example, you have a hang-up about going down on a woman, even if she's freshly showered. Regard this as an opportunity to delve into *why*. Do you think a woman's vulva is inherently dirty? When did you start believing that? What were the circumstances? Take a long, hard look at how you came to that conclusion.

You may discover that what you really have is a religious objection—which makes it a *value*, not a hang-up. If you've examined the issue and found out that it's a deeply held ethic, so be it. Explain that to your partner and let life go on.

Also see: Electra complex, fears/phobias, Freud, guilt, homophobia, Madonna/whore complex, religion, spectatoring

heartache

Love entails loss. It's the price of admission to what truly is the greatest show on Earth. Ultimately, through death or a parting of the ways, love carries with it heartache.

But maybe there's an even worse tragedy than loss—maybe it's when love is never found. You see, you cannot diminish your vulnerability to sorrow without diminishing your openness to the depth of the love that causes it.

Sadly, many people do make such a devil's bargain. To inure themselves against the consuming blaze of grief, they deliberately reduce their investment in love. And that is tragic beyond words. One of the noblest challenges of life is to choose, over and over, to accept the risk of heartache in order to love fully.

So, can we offer you ways to quickly fix the rupture in your chest? Sorry; only time will do that. Grieving likely will scour you clean again, but it will do so at its own pace. Give in to the sadness, understanding that this, too, shall pass.

You know that, intellectually. Think back to the heartache you've experienced in other areas of your life: the loss of a parent, a sibling, a friend, even a cherished pet. As wrenching as the feeling was at the moment, it eventually subsided. Sure, you still carry it with you at some level, and now and then that same ache—you know the one—flares up for a while, maybe when you visit a certain place or hear a certain song or channel-surf past a certain movie. But you survived that heartache, and you moved on.

During those times when you feel that you will go absolutely mad, we urge you to pick up a pen. Or a paintbrush, or a scroll saw, or a chisel. Work with your hands. Create something, anything. Pour your anguish into that. There's a reason so many songs and books and paintings are created from heartbreak: Great art comes from intensity, whether good or bad.

Also see: breaking up, death of a partner, depression, desertion, rejection—romantic, rejection—sexual, remarriage, secrets, single—suddenly, trust—rebuilding

heart conditions

If you're one of those guys who was hoping to go out with a bang, we're about to disappoint you. Fewer than 1 percent of the guys who drop dead of a heart attack do so during sex. And your overall risk of death while screwing is estimated to be one in a million.

Indeed, a British study of 918 men showed that sexual activity may even have a protective effect on men's health and hearts. The men in the study who had the most sex had half the risk of death from heart disease of their less-stimulated counterparts.

One reason why so few of us check out in the act is that most men with severe heart disease also have erection problems. But even if you've been diagnosed with heart disease and are still able to get hard, docs rarely ask you to abstain. At most, they tell you to take it easy and avoid anything involving trampolines.

One area that *is* a cause for concern: If you have been diagnosed with heart disease and are on nitrate-based medications such as Nitro-Dur (nitroglycerin), never take erection drugs such as Viagra (sildenafil). Combine the two, and you're headed for a potentially fatal drop in blood pressure. It'd be a damn shame to drop before the sex even gets under way.

Also see: DHEA, estrogen, impotence, poppers, progestin, smoking, steroids

hermaphrodite

About 1 out of every 2,000 children born in North America has ambiguous genitalia. That means that it's not clear at birth whether the child is male or female. Such a child—and the adult that the child becomes—is called a hermaphrodite, or intersexual.

Since the number of people born with this condition is surprisingly high, there's a chance you might become involved with an intersexual at some point in your sexual career. You may even have some interest in the subject already: There's a plethora of chicks-with-dicks porn movies on the market.

Those movies, though they may use the word *hermaphrodite* on their covers, do not feature true intersexuals. Usually, the men-women you see are pre-operative transsexuals—that is, men who are in the process of undergoing sex changes but still have their penises.

Hermaphrodites, on the other hand, often undergo surgery at an early age. Doctors make a guess at which gender seems most appropriate and then surgically remove what doesn't fit. Unfortunately, some intersexuals grow up feeling that the doctor chose wrong.

Also see: androgyny, anima and animus, cross-dressing, eunuch, gender bender, micropenis, transvestism, yin and yang

herpes

Think you know what someone with genital herpes looks like? Next time you're in a public place, count off four normal-looking people. One of them has it. That's right, almost 25 percent of Americans test positive for herpes simplex virus type 2. And that's not counting those with HSV-1, another type of herpes virus that generally just causes

---

Hot Dates 1938 A study of 1,300 college students found that one in four female undergraduates and one in two male undergrads were no longer virgins.

continued from page 129

Answer:
False. It holds a whopping eight times as much blood.

she arguably is the world's oldest porn star.

Asked by a writer for Salon.com whether she enjoyed her work, Flora unhesitatingly replied, "You'll have to speak up, dear. My hearing isn't what it used to be."

LEGAL BRIEFS
In Texas, a man was fined more than $400 for paddling the butt of his wife's lover but not meting out the same punishment to his wife. **The cuckold received a 30-day probated sentence** after being con-

---

BAWDY BALLADS "If It Don't Fit (Don't Force It)," *Barrel House Annie*

continued on page 143

cold sores around your lips but can also occur on your genitals. A type-1 infection can travel south via oral sex, and a type-2 infection can migrate north the same way.

Condoms offer limited protection against herpes because the virus can be shed from any part of the genitals, not just what's covered in latex. That said, as is stated on the package, condoms do *reduce* your overall risk of contracting sexually transmitted diseases, herpes included.

Obviously, your chances of being infected rise with the number of partners you've had. If you've slept with 2 to 4 people, your odds of carrying the virus are 20 percent. That jumps to 25 percent if you've had 5 to 9 partners, and 31 percent if you've had more than 10.

Here's the kicker: Most people who carry the virus don't know it. The symptoms can take years to show up—if they ever do. That's why some people who have been monogamous or celibate for a long period can suddenly find out that they have herpes.

When symptoms do occur, they include small sores and crusty, blisterlike lesions in the genital area; and itching or burning that can be mistaken for jock itch. The first episode is usually the worst and can be accompanied by flulike symptoms. Subsequent outbreaks are milder and generally clear up in about 10 days.

Given the statistics and the uncertainties, you might consider asking your doctor to do a diagnostic blood test at your next checkup. If you test positive, antiviral drugs can reduce or eliminate the painful outbreaks.

From there, it's a matter of responsibility: If you're positive for the bug, please, *please* warn potential partners. You're on the verge of giving them a life-long disease. Though you're most contagious when symptoms are actually present, you can pass on the virus even if you never have symptoms, or if you had just a single outbreak a decade ago. And even if you don't have serious symptoms, that doesn't mean that the person to whom you give it won't. For one thing, recurrent infections tend to be a lot worse for women than for men. At special risk are pregnant women and those with immune systems weakened by AIDS, chemotherapy, radiation therapy, or high doses of cortisone. For example, a pregnant woman can pass a herpes infection to her infant, causing critical illness or death. Infections have even been implicated in certain cancers, such as cervical cancer.

If your partner already knows that she's positive too, she'll probably be relieved to have found someone to whom she doesn't have to worry about giving herpes. In this situation, however, it's more important than ever to find out whether she's HIV-positive. Having sex with an HIV-infected person while either one of you is experiencing a herpes outbreak makes you up to 32 times more likely to contract the AIDS virus.

Also see: AIDS, condom, rashes, safe sex, scratching, STDs

heterosexuality

At a sex conference we once attended (yes, we actually get paid for such things), a woman stood up in the middle of a talk on sexual orientation. Here are her exact words: "Heterosexuality may be considered a simple lack of imagination."

H

Think of sexual orientation as a bell curve—you know, the thing you got graded on in college. At the far right end of the curve, you'll find hard-core heteros. At the far left end, you'll find firmly entrenched homosexuals, who are equally averse to the idea of having sex with women.

Most of us fall in the middle ranges. It's normal to have an occasional same-sex fantasy. It's normal to have an erotic dream where a guy suddenly shows up. It's normal even to have experimented with another man. This does not revoke your right to consider yourself heterosexual.

Also see: anima and animus, bisexuality, dreams, fantasies, homosexuality, kinky, prison, role reversal, threesome, transvestism

hickey

It's the reason turtleneck manufacturers will never go out of business—and it could be the reason you're not getting second dates, if you're still leaving them on women during first dates.

Also called a suction mark (by those of us past 10th grade), a hickey is, of course, that annoying red blotch that suddenly appears on you or your girlfriend after you've made out—which, if you're still leaving hickeys, you're probably still doing in the backseat of your car. The point of contact gets red because the suction breaks small blood vessels under the skin. Until it heals a couple of weeks later, a hickey becomes a virtual mood ring, changing from red to blue to brown to yellow.

To speed healing, use a topical cream containing phytonadione, a fancy name for vitamin K_1. The brand Dermal-K is available at health food stores.

Also see: biting, cars, erogenous zones, kiss, licking, mouth, tongue

Hite Report, The

A lot of dearly held—and plainly wrong—attitudes about sex got tossed out the window in the sexual revolution of the 1960s and 1970s. Part of the credit goes to Shere (pronounced as in Cher) Hite, author of *The Hite Report: A Nationwide Study of Female Sexuality.* Hite sent out questionnaires to 100,000 women and, in 1976, published the results of 3,000 of them in her book.

Some reviewers and fellow researchers took Hite to task for her lackadaisical statistical reporting, but that didn't stop the book from reaching the bestseller lists. For the first time, women had easy access to what other women thought about sex, and they found themselves reassured by the familiar complaints, opinions, and experiences they read there. Among other things, the report pointed out that women were largely dissatisfied with their sex lives—a revelation whose fallout we're still feeling today. Lucky us.

Hite also reported that as many as 70 percent of women do not reach orgasm during intercourse. Rather, for many women, it's direct clitoral stimulation that does the trick.

In 1981, Hite published a follow-up for men, *The Hite Report on Male Sexuality.* Not nearly as groundbreaking as her first book, it still shook a few trees by showing that we're not all that happy with our sex lives either. So there! The new report revealed that we brutes aren't quite as hung up on "getting in" as has historically been portrayed. In fact, Hite discovered that we enjoy a broad range of bedroom (and nonbedroom) activities. She also found that sex isn't just a youth sport—that even many older men have very satisfying sex lives.

Also see: menstruation, sex research

homophobia

It's been said that homophobia is the last acceptable prejudice. Indeed, in a 2000 Roper opinion poll, 42 percent of respondents felt that we, as a society, have gone too far in accepting homosexuals. And in a 1999 Gallup poll, 46 percent of people said that homosexuality is not an acceptable lifestyle.

Men are homophobic for three prime reasons: First, they're repressing their own interest in other men and lashing out at what they see as improper objects of their desire. Second, some homophobic men believe that that their religion condemns homosexuality. And third, other men are homophobic simply because they're ill-bred ignoramuses.

Those of us who don't fall into any of these categories (that's more than half of us, remember) have better things to worry about than what other guys are doing in the privacy of their own bedrooms.

Also see: Don't ask, don't tell; threesome

homosexuality

In the *Sex in America* survey, researchers found that 2.8 percent of men and 1.4 percent of women considered themselves homosexual or bisexual. But here's the interesting part: When the researchers asked how many respondents had ever

engaged in same-gender sex since puberty, the numbers shot up to 9 percent for men and 4 percent for women.

So there's a 1-in-10 chance that you've been sexual with another man at least once in your life. That warrants talking about. First of all, it doesn't mean that you're gay or even bisexual. It's quite normal for men who are as straight as a Kansas highway to engage in same-sex fantasies or behavior once in a while. On the flip side, it's not uncommon for gay men to acknowledge their homosexuality late in life—even after they've married and had kids.

You can see why the debate would rage on over whether people are born gay or whether it's a learned behavior. Our take on the subject? Who cares if it's one or the other? Even if it *is* a choice, who are we to tell you that it's not your choice to make?

Also see: anima and animus, bisexuality, drag, drag queen, dreams, gender bender, heterosexuality, lesbian, male body, outing, *Playgirl*, poppers, prison, role reversal, sodomy, switch-hitter, transvestism

hormone replacement therapy (HRT)

See: estrogen, testosterone replacement therapy

hormones

When you call somebody hormonal, generally—and stereotypically—you're referring to a woman. But you, sir, are a brimming stew of hormones yourself.

Though for men, testosterone is the lead dog in the pack, it's far from the only one. Others include cortisol, epinephrine, and norepinephrine. These babies are responsible for the old fight-or-flight response. They also rise in response to caffeine or nicotine.

Here's an interesting fact: Adrenal hormones such as those listed above play a big part in enhancing memory. Because they get released in response to emotions and stress, you stand a better chance of learning and remembering something new if you're in a moderate state of emotional arousal, not relaxation. So those arguments you used to have with your high school girlfriend right before math class actually did you some good.

Believe it or not, men's hormone levels are also more unstable than women's. Theirs fluctuate more on a monthly basis; ours are all over the map *daily*. That's why we can be royally pissed off one moment and, 5 minutes later, it's water under the bridge. Women get the oft-used term *bitchy* to describe their mood swings. We get the more forgiving *mercurial*.

Also see: DHEA, estrogen, hysterectomy, infertility, menopause—yours, micropenis, pituitary gland, postpartum depression, PMS, progesterone, progestin, prostate cancer, smoking, testosterone, witch's milk

horny

If we have to tell you what this word means, we'd like to welcome you back from your coma. So let's move on to the effects of horniness, which are many.

The most obvious thing you already know about horniness is that, for many men, it's difficult to control. Case in point: When men in a study group were told to consciously suppress sexual arousal while watching skin flicks, they couldn't do it.

This lack of control over horniness is pretty universal. An unfortunate 54-year-old farmer by the name of William McCavanagh found this out the hard way. Police discovered his beaten, dead body after he wandered into the woods one fine day. The assailant? A horny buck who didn't appreciate having his rutting season interrupted.

It follows that horniness makes us do stupid things. Like walking alone at night to visit the red-light district in crime-ridden Mexico City. Like groping a co-worker in the conference room. Like hitting on your wife's best friend.

When such urges strike, it's time to take matters in hand—literally. The quickest way to relieve yourself of the cloudy judgment that comes with horniness is to masturbate. Do it before your wife's best friend comes over. Do it before you go out with a hot business acquaintance on company time. Do it before you leave for Mexico City.

Also see: arousal, randy, road erection, wet dreams, wife's best friend

human papillomavirus (HPV)

See: genital warts

hump

Back in the early part of the 20th century, *hump* entered the lexicon as a synonym for "have intercourse." It can also refer, derogatorily, to a female sexual partner. Use at your own peril.

Also see: dry hump, X-rated

hung

It sounds as if it were a fairly recent addition to the English language, but this adjective describing someone with a large penis has been used since the 17th century. It's commonly used in phrases such as *hung like a horse*. And in gay parlance, a woman is *hung like a doughnut*.

You may wonder if your wand qualifies. Try this: Immediately after you pop an erection, hold a tape measure along the topside of your mast, from base to tip. If it reads 6½ inches or longer, it's official: You're hung. The farther above that number you get, the deeper into the category—so to speak—you get.

Okay, Mr. Ed, now what? As you may have experienced already, the larger you are, the fewer women you can fully penetrate, given that there's a finite amount of space in a vagina. When your large member slams against a woman's cervix, the sensation she feels is akin to what you endure when you have a nut bumped. So with length comes responsibility.

Particularly if you're with a small-framed woman, don't immediately start pile driving her. Ease your way in slowly until you find out how shallow the waters lie. If you find yourself striking bottom more often than is comfortable, roll over onto your back and suggest that she straddle you. That position makes it easier for her to control how far you slide in. Ditto when she gives you oral sex.

And if you're not certifiably hung? Good news: The most pleasure-sensitive part of the vagina is its outer third—the area you're best-suited to please. Another interesting, uh, tidbit for average guys: When a woman is first aroused, her vagina expands to accommodate an object of undetermined size. After a few minutes of thrusting, it contracts to fit more snugly around the penis. Works for us.

Also see: cervix, micropenis, packing, penile enlargement, size—penis, vaginal injuries

hygiene

Women hate dirt. It stands to reason that the one thing women hate even more than dirt itself—with a consuming passion—is dirty men. If you want your sunny personality to shine through enough to win you some major sack time, you first need to ensure that she doesn't have to rummage through a layer of topsoil to get to you.

Here's a cleanliness to-do list for the man who has sex on his mind.

• Take a shower. Women delight in the scent of a freshly washed man—butt and balls included. If you're uncircumcised, draw back your foreskin and soap yourself off. Sound obvious? Then why do women complain about male hygiene as much as they do? More to the point, why do they react with near ecstasy when they find a guy who actually smells decent?

• Brush those teeth. Early A.M. sex ain't gonna happen if you blow a mouthful of morning breath in her face, so get up a few minutes early, empty your bladder, and hit the Colgate. Incidentally, nighttime sex, too, becomes iffy when your mouth smells like a bad tooth.

• Groom those fingernails. Make sure they're clean and trimmed. A grubby paw doesn't inspire passion in anyone except a female mechanic.

• Remember your other appendages. Smelly feet, socks, or shoes are going to send her running for the air freshener. You shouldn't have to worry about this (and neither should she), given the vast array of foot powders and absorbent insoles out there nowadays.

• Ditto on earwax. The women we talked to all agreed: It's the *anti*aphrodisiac. (Ear hair isn't far behind.)

• Watch what you wear. It doesn't matter how clean your skin is if the stuff you cover it with is filthy. Sure, clothes are meant to come off, but you'll never get that far if she's been staring all evening long at that brownish, unidentifiable stain on your sweater.

• Finally—and we agree that it's not fair—to her, *wrinkled* equals *dirty*. Learn to iron, stud.

Also see: beard burn, bidet, body odor—controlling, breath, douche, dressing you to look sexy, fragrances, hair, pubic hair, scratching, sexual etiquette, short-arm inspection, smegma, sweating, underwear

hypnosis and breast enlargement

Sounds strange, doesn't it, that hypnosis could have an effect on the size of a woman's breasts? Well, there's actually some science behind it, albeit a little out-of-date.

Two small studies during the 1970s found that some women could indeed pump up their busts via hypnosis. In one, the 22 volunteers saw an average 1.4-inch increase in size. In another, the 13 participants averaged more than 2 extra inches of breast size—that's about two cup sizes. Of course, it didn't work for everyone, and at the time, breast augmentation surgery was rapidly taking hold, so hypnosis paled by comparison. These days, with the news reports of implants that leak or become encased in scar tissue, some women have been looking for more natural ways of busting up.

It's doubtful that your missus will find a qualified hypnotherapist who does breast enlargement sessions in-office, but there are a number of guided-imagery and hypnosis tapes for sale on the Web. A few things to consider: Hypnosis is a largely unregulated field. Look for a tape put together by a psychologist or certified clinical hypnotherapist. It's not an ironclad guarantee, but it'll boost your odds of getting a quality product.

Oh, for those of you who fancy yourselves armchair hypnotists, merely standing over your drowsy partner and chanting "Your eyes are getting heavy—and so are your breasts" likely won't cut it.

Also see: breast enlargement, dressing her to look sexy, hang-ups, implants, penile enlargement, sexy, size—breasts, third-degree cleavage

hypnosis and penis enlargement

It's wishful thinking if you believe that you can enlarge your penis through hypnosis. Funny thing is, that's kind of what hypnosis is: concentrated, wishful thinking.

Alas, there are no studies that we know of that have examined whether hypnosis can make your dick suddenly morph into King Richard.

So if you opt to purchase one of the few hypnosis cassettes geared toward penis enlargement, make sure it has a money-back guarantee. To find out what's on the market, just type *hypnosis and penis enlargement* into an Internet search engine.

Also see: hung, micropenis, penile enlargement, penis pump, priapism

hypnosis and performance enhancement

We tend to forget that there are aspects of personality beneath everyday awareness. That's what hypnosis is for—to connect with parts of you that reside in corners you're unaware of.

Often, you suffer with the results of ignoring your internal workings: in erection problems that have no medical cause, in phobias that seem to come from nowhere, in hang-ups that hinder your love life. For many men, hypnosis can help.

If you leave a splinter in your foot, the area around it won't heal. Hypnotherapists tackle that idea with a technique called regression to cause. After putting you in a light trance, they help you backtrack to the psychic splinter, if you will. Then they try to help you remove it.

Many times, especially when dealing with sex, they find a lot of built-up guilt around issues that you may not even remember. And guilt has a remarkably dampening effect on sex lives. Release that guilt, and you find your performance once again unimpeded.

Remember, though, that about 20 percent of people won't go into a trance. Generally, those are the highly rational, logical folks who feel a need to be in control at all times. The other 80 percent should look for a psychologist or psychi-

atrist who does hypnotherapy, or a certified clinical hypnotherapist.

Also see: dreams, emotions, fears/phobias, guilt, hang-ups, impotence, performance anxiety, sex therapy, wild

hypnosis and seduction

Though women have been known to become mesmerized at the sight of a dangling Rolex, if you're hoping to merely cast an entrancing eye upon a woman and have her rip open her bodice . . . well, we regret to inform you that hypnosis doesn't work that way.

That myth came from the days when hypnosis was considered a form of mind control akin to brainwashing (like the classic Reggie Jackson "I must kill . . . the queen" scene in the movie *The Naked Gun*). It's better, and more accurate, to think of it as a form of mind *persuasion*.

If you want to use a hypnosis-like technique to seduce a woman, try this: Take advantage of her aural inroads. Many women, you see, are far more influenced by sound than by sight when it comes to sex. So tell her a story.

H

Hot Dates | **1940s** This was a great decade to be a man: DuPont introduced nylon stockings, and the French named a skimpy bathing suit after the atomic-bomb test site Bikini Atoll.

continued from page 136

victed of trespassing and assault for the attack on the phone-company employee who'd enjoyed his wife.

The judge in the case said he consulted with 200 to 300 people in the community and found that most thought the husband should also have paddled the wife. By not doing so, the husband failed to apply equal

justice under the law, the judge concluded.

Seemed like a Good Idea at the Time. . .

In the Middle Ages, a husband leaving home for an extended period might lock the little woman into a partial or full pudenda. And no,

True or Phallus?
The slang term *nookie* comes from the Latin word *nokeria*, meaning "valley."

BAWDY BALLADS | "My Ding-A-Ling," *Chuck Berry*

continued on page 148

Tell her in picturesque detail about the trip you took to a tropical isle. Or, if your parole conditions have kept you closer to home, talk about an incredible meal you had at a dimly lit French restaurant. Use sensuous language; describe the softly caressing breeze, the musky flavor of the wine, the way you were absorbed by the incredible presentation of the food. Keep your voice low, as if you were having a hushed conversation in bed. Keep it up for 5 minutes or so.

If you do it well, her eyes will seem far away as she lets herself be "spellbound" by your storytelling. When you're done, she'll smile lazily and find herself in a strangely erotic frame of mind.

Then it's your turn to be mesmerized.

Also see: phone sex, politicians, power, seduction, sweet talk, travel as an aphrodisiac, voice

hysterectomy

The surgical removal of the uterus (sometimes including the cervix, ovaries, and fallopian tubes) via an abdominal or vaginal incision. The word is based on the Greek root for "uterus" or "womb," which is also where the word *hysterical* comes from. This is no coincidence. In fact, throughout the 19th century, hysterectomies were a popular "cure" for women deemed hysterical or neurotic.

There are, of course, legitimate reasons for hysterectomy, including fibroid tumors, advanced pelvic infection, and an assortment of other uterine problems. But as many as one-third of the hundreds of thousands of hysterectomies performed every year, usually on women in their early 40s, may be unnecessary. For that reason, your partner should always get a second opinion before going under the knife.

Sex after recovery from a hysterectomy should be as good as ever for both of you. Better, in fact, because whatever made the operation necessary should no longer be bothering her. And unwanted pregnancy is no longer a concern.

Among the few negative side effects are hormone problems that can result from a hysterectomy in which the ovaries also are removed. The two of you need solid, specific information from her doctor so you can handle the changes and keep your sex life steady. Also, such a gynecologically drastic operation may make her feel that she's less of a woman. Disabuse her of this real but unfounded fear. Tell her in no uncertain terms that her femininity has nothing to do with her plumbing. Then take her into the bedroom and prove it to her.

Also see: estrogen, mastectomy, menopause—hers

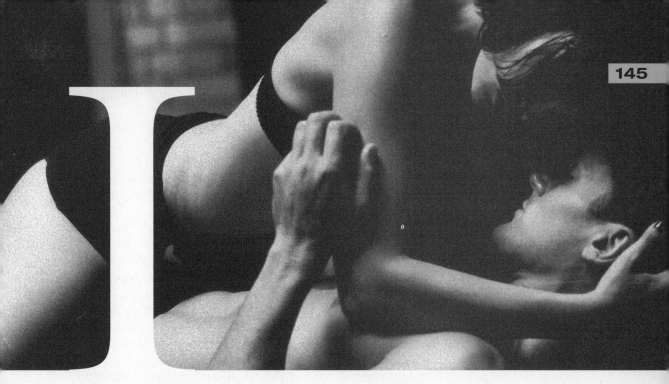

implants

Sacs filled with one of two substances—silicone gel or saline solution. By far the most common of the two, saline implants make up 97 percent of all faux breasts inserted these days. Silicone suffered from a tarnished image a few years back when researchers thought this type of implant could lead to breast disease. Though a number of studies have since shown there is no clear connection, saline remains the stuffing of choice.

Do implants feel like real breasts? Well, the newer-generation models aren't as rigid as lore would suggest. And yet. . . . An Australian woman reportedly survived a bar shooting when an errant bullet ricocheted off her implants. Does that tell you something?

Also see: breast enlargement, breast fondling, media, size—breasts, third-degree cleavage

impotence

This word meaning "lack of power" is the one that most men use to describe an inability to have erections. While such a problem is indeed serious, it hardly makes one powerless. So instead let's just use the term preferred by the guys in white coats (and some former presidential candidates looking for second careers as TV pharmaceutical pitchmen): *erectile dysfunction*.

Erectile dysfunction, or ED, has a less permanent ring to it—as well it should. Just about every man who once had erections and who's still taking breath can regain his former capacity. He just has to be willing to work for it.

That said, the 20 million to 30 million men in the United States who experience ED will not all take the same route back to firmness. That's because the underlying reasons for the condition vary from person to person.

Once upon a time, it was believed that long-term erectile dysfunction was "all in your head," albeit the wrong head. For some of us, this is still true. Performance anxiety, stress, and guilt are leading psychological causes of ED. Even sleeping with a woman you find intimidatingly attractive can leave you with a soft-on.

Today, however, docs know that ED often stems from a physical problem, especially if your dysfunction has grown steadily worse over the years. The culprit can be anything from diminishing testosterone levels to undiagnosed heart disease. In the latter case, your ability to get stiff is among the first things to go when your arteries clog up. Consider your flagging member an early warning system—one that your life may depend on. Erectile problems can also indicate adult-onset diabetes, so a full checkup is in order.

Whatever the case, the boys with the Bunsen burners have developed some bang-up drugs to help. Most famous is Viagra (sildenafil). The drug works in 70 to 75 percent of men, even if their ED is psychological in nature.

Urologists do say that too many men use Viagra incorrectly. First and foremost, you won't get top results from it if you take it with a fatty meal. That means no burgers, steaks, or corn dogs for a couple of hours before and after you pop one. Have a salad with fat-free dressing or a light pasta dish as your precoital repast.

And remember that Viagra doesn't "give you" an erection, it creates the ideal physiological conditions for one. You still need to be in an arousing environment. That means that you can't just toss down the little blue pill and go watch the Cowboys play—unless you spend most of your time ogling the cheerleaders.

Also see: anticipatory anxiety, arousal, body fitness, erection, erection difficulties, fertility, papaverine, penis pump, performance anxiety, prostate cancer, refractory period, sex—lack of, smoking, weight loss, yohimbine

incest

Every society on this planet regards incest as taboo. We all know the technical definition: sexual relations between persons who are so closely related by blood that their marriage is illegal or forbidden by custom.

Though all cultures have issues with such behavior, no one is quite able to explain why. Some think it's because inbreeding leads to genetic defects. Others say the sexual jealousy it creates would cause catastrophe within a family. Yet others believe that it's shunned because it would keep groups from intermarrying and forming important alliances.

None of this quite explains the predominant emotion provoked by the word *incest*: horror.

And the results of incest can indeed be horrifying, especially if the transgression occurs between an adult and a child. One study found that most women who had experienced incest during childhood were extremely fearful of their ability to protect their own children. Many of them were handicapped by their anxiety, sometimes withdrawing entirely from the world in order to keep their kids safe.

It's estimated that 20 percent of all women have had at least one incestuous experience before the age of 18. Some are the victims of sexual predators—male or female—who can't be trusted around any defenseless kid.

In other cases, incest begins as a father's misunderstanding of his daughter's actions or requests. Take the example of a 9- or 10-year-old girl who's still young enough to have few inhibitions about nudity. She may innocently flit around your house in her underwear. To your adult mind and to the hardwired beast within you, her behavior may come across as sexual, maybe even flirtatious. But—and we say this as clearly as we can—it is not.

You're her father, and she trusts you. If you violate this trust, you will never get it back. And she will live with the results of your actions, often permanently. You, in turn, will discover how truly deep the pit of guilt can be.

We're not condemning the fleeting sexual thoughts that you may have. They're more common than you may realize. You just can't act on them.

Also see: compulsive behavior, fantasies, innocence, *Lolita*, paraphilias, pedophilia, perversions, sex offenders, sex therapy, taboos, underage

infatuation

A stool requires three legs for stability. Remove one and you fall on your ass. So it is with love. The three supports are thus: passion, intimacy, and commitment. Subtract any of them and what gets crushed may be your heart.

Infatuation is one of these shakey constructions. It's what you get when you're awash in passion but bereft of intimacy and commitment.

A relationship based solely on passion is hell-bent for destruction. With the elation comes incredible jealousy. Simple quarrels can threaten the solidity of your relationship. And when the physical attraction fades somewhat—as it always does—the two of you start looking elsewhere.

That's all fine and dandy if you're just in for the short haul, but if you aspire to more—and find yourself continually falling into relationships that sound like our one-legged stool—you need to work on your commitment and intimacy skills.

Also see: commitment, companionship, intimacy, jealousy, love, morning after, passion, sex symbols, sexual attraction

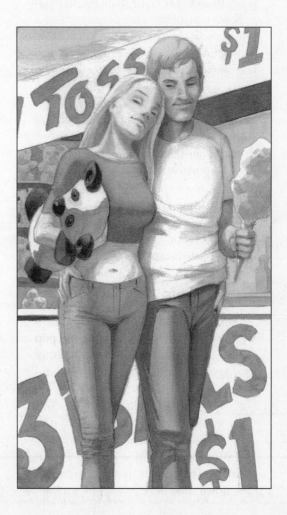

infertility

With all the things that can (and do) go wrong with the human reproductive system, it's amazing that any of us was ever born. Once upon a time, it was automatically assumed that problems with fertility were the woman's fault. Science has shattered that misconception. About a third of the time, it *is* the woman who's having trouble. Another third falls squarely upon the shoulders of the man. And the final third of infertile couples owe their woes to mixed causes.

Because we're all guys here, we're going to concentrate on male infertility. It happens when some disorder or combination thereof prevents your sperm from getting the job done. Usually, the problem is treatable. A big exception is testicular damage that shuts down sperm production. This can be caused by chronic infections, trauma, undescended testicles, or some other condition. Once that factory is closed, it can't reopen. You're the equivalent of a postmenopausal woman.

But usually, the problem is low sperm quantity, poor sperm quality, or both. A low sperm count is defined as fewer than 20 million healthy tadpoles per ejaculation. Smoking, prolonged illegal drug use, chronic alcohol abuse, poor diet, unrelieved stress—all the usual sins—sabotage sperm production.

But you're probably not going to go from infertility to fatherhood just by getting sober and eating more vegetables. Lots of physical disorders in the genital area contribute to male infertility. One is varicocele, a condition in which varicose veins allow blood to pool in your testicles, raising the temperature of your scrotum and thereby killing sperm. It's commonly described as a "bag of worms" that feels like it's attached to one of your balls.

Another problem you may encounter downtown is damaged sperm ducts, which could be a genetic mistake or the result of scarring from a sexually transmitted disease such as gonorrhea. Less commonly, hormonal irregularities—

Hot Dates **1939 to 1945** During World War II, 50 million condoms a month were handed out to servicemen overseas. That amounted to 8 per soldier per month.

continued from page 143

Answer:
False. It's derived from the Scottish word *noke*, meaning "recess" or "crack." So stop a Scot and thank him for his invention.

those aren't wrestling holds, but rather what we've come to know as chastity belts.

The metal plate of a partial pudenda (from the Latin *pudere*, "to be ashamed") covered only the vulva area and contained a vertical slit through which the wife could urinate. To further discourage paramours, **the device had metal teeth, which were often spring-loaded**.

The full pudenda prevented both vaginal and anal entry. In addition to the tiny urination slit, it had a rear opening that was larger, but not so large that one could have intercourse—or defecate without causing an ungodly mess.

Foreign Affairs
On the grounds of the swanky Hilton Hotel in Bangkok, Thailand, sits a shrine containing **dozens of colorful**

BAWDY BALLADS *"My Pencil Won't Write No More," Bo Carter*

continued on page 163

such as high levels of prolactin or low levels of the thyroid hormone—cause sperm problems.

Fertility disorders are usually a combination of several of these factors, and the diagnosis is rarely simple. If you and your missus have been unsuccessfully trying to conceive for at least 6 months, find a fertility specialist. It takes only one of your millions of sperm to fertilize an egg, and advances in the treatment of fertility problems mean docs can offer all sorts of ways to make sure a strong, lone soldier completes the humanitarian mission.

Also see: boxers or briefs, eunuch, fertility, sperm count, testicles—undescended, testicular trauma

injuries

Football, hockey, and sex are all full-contact sports. And in the rough and tumble, people get hurt. Fortunately, you can gird yourself for the gridiron of love with a little knowledge.

Most sexual injuries are self-inflicted, as in the case of the genius who tore off his left testicle masturbating against the drive belt of running machinery. To make matters worse, he attempted to close his torn scrotum with a staple gun. (You'd think the desire to keep things like staple guns away from your scrotum is instinctive, but apparently not.)

We know you'd never do anything that dumb, but lots of your brothers have fallen victim to unorthodox masturbatory practices. So, say, if you're stuck in a hotel room with a blue movie and a free hour, don't use hair gel, shampoo, or any other stand-in lubricant to grease your pole. Many household products are caustic: You could end up with severe burns.

And, like your sleeping wife, your penis does not respond well to hurried attempts at penetration. If you try to thrust before you're fully erect, you can bend or buckle it, causing a penile fracture—and trust us, you don't want to experience the pain that comes with that. Such damage can also happen when a woman is on top, you slip out, and she slams back down again. (Mention this danger in passing when she's bucking wildly away.) If it happens, get immediate treatment or you might end up with Peyronie's disease, a permanent bend of the penis.

Finally, show a little patience when you wake up with a piss boner. It's tempting to force it down toward the toilet and have at it, but you run the risk of straining the suspensory ligaments that provide leverage for your erections. Keep doing this and you can end up with a pecker that points downward even when fully erect.

Also see: athletic sex, back, boxers or briefs, cars, chains, cock ring, danger, disability—overcoming, flogging, hickey, hung, klismaphilia, K-Y jelly, lubricants, ointments, outdoors, Peyronie's disease, phalloplasty, road head, rough sex, rug burn, safeword, suppositories, testicular trauma, vacuum devices, vaginal injuries, whips, wrestling, zippers

innocence

A word much intertwined with the idea of youthfulness and wholesomeness, innocence speaks directly to many men's deepest sexual urges. We are greatly stirred by the sight of a fresh-faced, chaste young woman who has yet to be burned and hardened by an endless parade of rogues.

What is it that attracts us so much? Theories abound, but it may be that we're just biologically programmed to respond to youth and health. Innocence captures the essence of those. Young women are historically and physically less likely to carry disease and more likely to have healthy babies. And that's all our genes and loins care about.

Our heads are a different matter. Adult men—yes, that's you—need stimulating conversation, shared history, and common ground to forge a successful relationship. It's hard to get that solely from the face of innocence. And the drive that seeks out innocence often fails to recognize things like legal age of consent, student/teacher protocol, and such. Just ask Roman Polanski.

So enjoy innocence. But don't become so wrapped up in its pursuit that you fail to check in with the streetwise part of yourself that knows when you're crossing the line.

Also see: incest, *Lolita*, pedophilia, underage, virginity—hers, young women/ older men

Internet dating

If you're online, you know how easy it is to come across sex-related material. You also know how easy it is to have cybersex while plugged in. Whether it's actually a woman on the other end of the modem is another discussion entirely.

What we're interested in here is slightly different: What are the ramifications of meeting sex partners over the Internet? Glad you asked. As it turns out, getting your rocks off with someone you met online can be even riskier than picking someone up from the population at large.

When researchers looked at a group of people who visited a Denver public-health clinic, they found that 16 percent of them had used the Internet to hunt up sex partners. Of those, 65 percent got lucky. Or unlucky, depending on how you look at it: Finding a partner on the Web (just like finding a partner in a bar or club) made it more likely that those people came down with a sexually transmitted disease.

Why? Because the anonymity of the Web makes it a likely haven for casual-sex seekers. You can meet up with a person, have sex, and never know anything more about each other than your handles, so to speak.

Here's a big shock: People who have lots of casual sex tend to have more STDs than those who don't.

Already, online chat rooms have become the singles bars of the present day. Now they also have the potential of becoming the STD bathhouses of yesteryear. That doesn't mean that you should regard all the people you meet online as lepers, just that you should approach cyber-initiated physical encounters with your eyes at least as open as your fly—and take appropriate precautions.

Also see: communication, compulsive behavior, cybersex, matchmaking services, meeting women, personal ads, safe sex, singles scene, STDs

interracial sex

First off, we take issue with this phrase. In the words of some forgotten wise man, there's only one race: the human race. We put the entry under this heading simply because the term is in common usage, rightly or not.

So what should you expect if you date a woman of a different ethnic background than yours? It's a valid question because of all the myths and stereotypes out there. However, there's little merit to any legends you may have heard about the strange and exotic sexuality of women from other cultures. Women all across the globe are built fundamentally the same.

Unfortunately, one thing about inter-racial relationships *is* different from same-race pairings: the way many ob-servers perceive them. Even in this day and age, you'll get quizzical looks, at the least, and threats, at the most—particu-larly if you're a black man dating a white woman. You might also have to contend with being ostracized by members of your own family.

The quizzical-looks scenario is easier to deal with: Let people look, as long as they remain respectful. If they get rude, your best bet is to just walk away and comfort your partner. Never debate the point with an aggressive, hostile stranger.

If family members turn away from you, it's a tougher haul. There really isn't anything you can do except hope that they'll eventually outgrow their bigotry. They might not, at which point you have a choice to make.

Also see: mail-order brides, preference, sex tours and resorts, taboos

intimacy

You hear a lot about women wanting more intimacy from their men, but what the hell does that mean? Well, according to the triangle theory of love, intimacy joins passion and commitment as one of three key ingredients in a complete, abiding love. It means that you feel free to talk about

anything. You're patient and under-standing with each other.

As long ago as prehistoric times, women satisfied the need for intimacy by congregating with other women and chatting happily while their men went out to hunt, gather, and visit Paleolithic strip joints.

Nowadays, thanks to the liberation movement, your woman's support system is all off at work. Inevitably, she turns to you to sate her intimacy needs. And you're just not that well-equipped to deal with it.

The best thing you can do is spend a half-hour or so every day just talking with her. About anything. Ask her how her day was, tell her how yours was, talk about what she'd like to do this weekend. It doesn't matter. To her, talking freely is a sign that everything is okay. So put your newspaper aside for that 30 minutes and play the part of a whiskered old woman. Maybe it's not as much fun as the strip

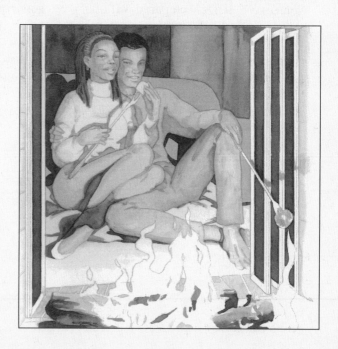

joint, but it has its own quieter rewards, and we can almost guarantee that she'll show you greater interest and appreciation in return.

Also see: afterglow, commitment, communication, companionship, desertion, discretion, drugs, empty-nest syndrome, estrogen, fantasies, foreplay, games, love, lovemaking, partner, passion, pregnancy, rear entry, rituals, secrets, sixty-nine (69), surrogate, trust—rebuilding

IUD

Back in the 1970s, the use of intrauterine devices for birth control plummeted amid reports of widespread pelvic inflammatory disease as well as grim tales of the grisly miscarriages of unplanned pregnancies. All of the problems were traced back to one kind of IUD—the Dalkon Shield—but the contraceptive method never recovered from the bad press. Today, only half of 1 percent of women use IUDs, compared with 17 percent who take the Pill.

That's unfortunate, because 5 percent of women on the Pill will get pregnant in any 1 year. Fourteen percent of couples using latex condoms will have a baby on the way in that same year. The two types of IUDs still on the market are much more effective, largely because there's not as much chance for human error as with the other methods.

An IUD is a small, T-shaped device inserted in a woman's uterus. The more effective type—just 0.8 percent of women using it get pregnant each year—is sheathed in copper. The other one, which has a 2 percent annual failure rate, contains progesterone, a female hormone. Though the exact mechanism is unknown, both seem to work by preventing sperm from joining with an egg or by preventing a fertilized egg from adhering to the uterine wall.

The copper one can stay in for up to 10 years. The progesterone one needs to be changed annually. IUDs are best for people who are in long-term, monogamous relationships. That's because some sexually transmitted diseases, such as gonorrhea and chlamydia, can lead to pelvic inflammatory disease in IUD users.

Also see: pelvic inflammatory disease, progesterone, STDs

Janus Report

In the early 1990s, sex researchers Samuel and Cynthia Janus published *The Janus Report on Sexual Behavior*, a far-ranging look at modern-day sexual beliefs and practices. It was the first sex study done since the pioneering clinical research of William H. Masters, M.D., and Virginia E. Johnson, Ph.D.

Among the highlights of the Janus' findings: Almost 90 percent of surveyed married men said their favorite way to achieve orgasm was through intercourse. Only 75 percent of married women felt the same way. Sixteen percent of married women said oral sex was their favorite way to get off. And 7 percent of wives preferred to masturbate.

Here's a heartening fact from the report: 56 percent of married men and 49 percent of married women felt that it was important that their partners be open to sexual experimentation. Among divorced women, that number jumped to 58 percent. So you've been officially notified that women are as sexually experimental as men. Put that knowledge to use.

Then there are data on the number of people who have had sex for money. Take note that people who identified themselves as ultraconservative were more likely to have reported making such a transaction than were ultra-liberals.

The Janus Report is of particular interest to statisticians, but it's not too eggheaded for the average guy to enjoy. If you want to take a look at what your fellow countrymen are up to, the book is still widely available. Read it with a nice divorcée. . . .

Also see: sex research, talking dirty

jealousy

There she is, across the room. Talking to another guy. Worse yet, another handsome guy. (We're assuming that you're handsome too; if we're wrong, you're even worse off than we thought.) And damned if she isn't laughing, touching him on the forearm the way she used to touch you.

On the other side of the world, in the Polynesian Islands, the Kiribati people know what you're feeling. They call the worst form of jealousy *koko*, "a murdering thing."

While jealousy is a normal emotion, no one disputes that it can have a destructive effect. In one survey of 651 university students, more than one-third said that jealousy was a significant issue in their present relationships, causing problems ranging from loss of self-esteem to bitter arguing to stalking. It can also cause the very thing a jealous man fears the most: the departure of his woman for another man. That's the irony.

Intense jealousy can strangle a relationship to the point where it can no longer survive. If you pound on her emotionally every time she wears a sexy dress, is a little late getting home, or goes out drinking with friends, you're setting yourself up for a fall. That doesn't mean you can't *feel* jealousy. You just have to keep it in check. Even little passive-aggressive remarks—"Wow, that must have been some line in the supermarket"—can take their toll, depending on the situation and the woman.

What do we mean by "depending"? Simply that jealousy is a paradox. Much like alcohol, it's poisonous when taken to an extreme (or, for some people, to any degree), but in moderation, some people think it can act as a love balm. One study of married couples showed that 40 percent of the women had used jealousy to test their husbands' commitment. For example, your wife may have smiled at another man in full view of you. Or she may have deliberately not answered your phone call when you were expecting her to be at home.

Maybe she was trying to get a rise out of you. In her mind, a jealous reaction is proof positive that you still want her. To her, indifference is deadly—a sign that you want out of the relationship. So, if you should pick up on these little cues, go ahead and address the issue head-on: Ask her if she's feeling neglected. Does she need something you're not giving her? Just be cool about it. No physical aggression, ever.

Also see: best friend's wife, bimbo, dressing her to look sexy, commitment, emotions, marriage—open, past partners—dealing with, past partners—talking about, polygamy, secrets, swinging, threesome, topless bar, travel ruins relationships, trust—rebuilding, wandering eye, wild women

job loss

Work defines men. What we do, and how we provide for our families, is tied closely to how we feel about ourselves. And when we lose our jobs, we suffer from far more than the lack of our paychecks. It's as if we've been held up for scrutiny and judged as substandard.

If this happens to you, how can it not have an effect on sex? It affects *everything*. Depression sets in. Feelings of worthlessness plague you. You're angry and uncommunicative. You may even experience temporary erection problems. Hardly an ideal situation for sex.

How can you ride out any shortcomings in the sack until you find another job? Shake things up a little bit by getting away somewhere. If your checkbook doesn't quite say "Europe," hike up into the nearest hills for a couple of days. Use this time to renew, not stew. Figure out your action plan in the clearness of a new place. As an added bonus, this simple change of scenery may provide enough head-clearing distractions to make you forget your woes and rediscover your sexual energy. Remember that this is a temporary situation—at work and in the bedroom. Don't give it any more weight than that. Above all, remember that your wife is your ally, not your enemy. Don't take out your frustrations on her, and she'll help see you through it.

Also see: boss's wife, emotions, financial difficulties, performance anxiety, size—wallet, stress

john

We're going to tell you how to be a good one—that is, a good customer of a prostitute. Let us preface this discussion by reminding you that in this country, prostitution is legal only in a select few counties of Nevada. Every day in the United States, men get busted for approaching prostitutes or decoys. So we're going to assume that you're just about to head into one of Nevada's 30 or so legal brothels and you want some advice on how a decent john acts.

In large part, the way you treat a pro determines the quality of service she provides. Yes, we know, she's just acting anyway. But you want her to turn in an Oscar-winning performance, and nobody wins an Oscar when they have no motivation to play the part. By being a decent guy and following a few etiquette tips, you make the whole experience that much more worthwhile.

Two things are important above all else: Be sober and be clean. That means take a shower and brush your teeth just as if you were going on a date. Remember, too, that flattery is a time-honored ritual, even in situations like this. Don't go overboard with it, but mention how nice she looks or that she has great hair or eyes.

Just before it's time for the main event, offer to give her a brief shoulder or back massage. Not all prostitutes go for this, because it puts them in a position of vulnerability. Those who do will appreciate it. She's probably stiff and sore: They aren't called working girls for nothing.

When you're in the middle of the act, don't insist that she tell you over and over again how much she likes it. Yes, as we said, she's playing a role—which, after a few times, gets really tiresome for her. She'll end up rolling her eyes—in impatience, not ecstacy—and freezing up on you.

Finally, if you plan on frequenting this particular lady or establishment, tip her when it's over, even if it's only 20 bucks. It's a virtual guarantee that she'll remember you next time and go out of her way to please you.

Also see: playacting, pulling a train, sex tours and resorts, trick

J

SPECIAL REPORT
Jobs and Sex

We sex-book publishers can talk about cum etiquette and kinky positions all day long. It's what we do. The rest of you are better off keeping sex talk (and even this book) out of the office.

Much as we hate to put a damper on anything sex-related, the simple fact is this: Sex and work are like plutonium and neutrons—mix the two, and you'd better be ready for the cataclysm that follows. A single wrong move on the job can leave you screwed, sued, unemployed, and a whole lot poorer, as a certain drug company CEO learned when he had to pay $3.6 million out of his very deep pockets to a secretary who alleged that he groped her and demanded sex.

We're guessing you probably don't have $3.6 million laying around for just such an occasion, so do yourself and your career a favor. Keep reading.

sexual harassment

You think this charge is leveled only against presidents and Supreme Court nominees? Think again. About 15,000 such complaints are filed with the federal government's Equal Employment Opportunity Commission annually. In one survey of 2,757 adults, 45 percent of female respondents said they'd been harassed on the job. Not surprisingly, in nearly every case the harasser was a man.

Now, most of us are decent-enough guys. We don't go around fondling our female co-workers or purposely trying to make our colleagues feel uneasy. But sexual harassment is sometimes referred to as an eye-of-the-beholder offense, meaning that even if *you* don't think you're doing something improper, *she* might cry foul. And she might be on solid legal ground, at that.

The fact that sexual harassment is also one of those unfortunate transgressions that carries a stigma makes it doubly important for you to know the laws. That way, if you're ever wrongly accused, you'll have some idea about how to erase the huge blot the charge can put on your career.

To get the lowdown, we sought legal counsel. No, we're not fond of lawyers, either, but they sure come in handy when translating legalese into plain English. Here's the advice we got from several leading attorneys, among them Gloria Allred, who's filed high-profile harassment suits on behalf of numerous women. Hey, if you want to know what the other side is thinking, you go to the source, right?

Simply defined, sexual harassment is any kind of workplace communication that's sexual in nature *and* inappropriate. More specifically, sexual harassment is anything communicated at work that meets the following criteria. (For the record, *communication* refers to anything you say, e-mail, leave on voice mail, or even tack to your bulletin board.)

• The comment, joke, or advance must be unwelcome. So if *she* asks *you* to meet her in the storage room in an hour, you're generally off the hook. We say "generally" because you'd have to prove that she did the propositioning, if she ever brought suit. And that still may not save your job. She may claim later—especially if you're her boss—that she felt pressured to go out with you or to con-

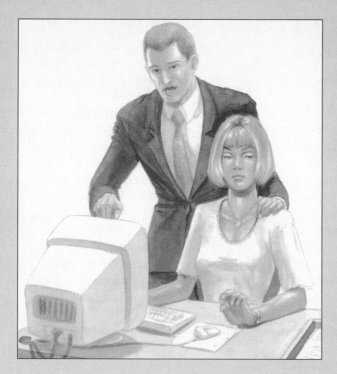

gory may be repeated requests for a date or frequent comments about copy-room-Carrie's legs. Also bear in mind that you don't have to make the comments about Carrie's legs in front of Carrie herself to be deemed guilty. Anybody who overhears you—even a male co-worker—could take umbrage and lodge a complaint.

As for severe (and we really hope we don't need to tell you this), a one-time grope of your intern's buttocks would be enough to get you fired on the spot.

• The content has to be either sexual in nature or hostile and directed at someone specifically because of her sex. Discussing your morning roll in the hay over a business deal falls into the sexual-in-nature category. So does telling a co-worker she looks delicious. Even, be warned, if you say it only with your eyes. As for treating colleagues differently based on gender: You're looking for a lawsuit if you habitually berate your female subordinates while showing leniency to your male office cronies.

As if these criteria weren't enough, there's also another category of infraction all its own: third-party harassment. This involves indirect communication that creates what is called a hostile environment. Think of it as polluting the office air with sexual innuendo. A *Playboy*-centerfold screen saver, raunchy jokes told in an open cafeteria, phone sex within earshot of others—all these things can make colleagues feel uncomfortable in their own work spaces.

tinue dating you after she lost interest. Further, though most employers allow interoffice dating, your company may have a stern policy prohibiting you from dating people who report to you or even people who don't report to you but who are lower in the pecking order. It's a good idea to check with human resources before you make dinner plans.

• Many courts take the complainant's gender into consideration, so if the target of the alleged harassment is female, the suspect behavior need be offensive only to a "reasonable woman." That means you can't use your own sensitivity meter here. (There's that eye-of-the-beholder thing again.) One good tip: Ask yourself whether your words or actions would offend your mother or sister. We're assuming your mother and sister aren't named Hefner or Guccione.

• The behavior has to be either "pervasive" or "severe." In the former cate-

(continued)

SPECIAL REPORT
Jobs and Sex (cont.)

J

To review, then, and to help you avoid getting a reprimand instead of a raise, we've boiled down the legal gobbledygook to six rules of thumb. (We know, you only have two thumbs. But we thought "rules of finger" sounded silly.)

1. Never make lewd comments or jokes with punch lines about a pubic hair in somebody's Coke.

2. Stash your nudie magazines at home; and drink from your Three Stooges cup rather than from the boob mug that pours fluids from its nipple.

3. Refrain from complimenting a co-worker on her looks or wardrobe. Focus your praise on workplace issues: "Brilliant idea!" "Stellar presentation!" Leave "Astonishing ass!" for the women you meet in bars. And even then, we're not sure it's such an inspired thing to say.

4. Never tell her (or even imply) that dating you would be a smart career move. That's classic quid pro quo harassment— "Do this, get that"—which is every corporate defense attorney's worst nightmare.

5. Don't stare at her breasts or crotch when talking to her. Avoid up-and-downing her body with your eyes. While you're at it, watch your own body language; for instance, if you're not wearing underwear, keep your legs closed during one-on-one meetings with female staffers.

6. Finally, keep your hands to yourself. Yes, we know you're not going to insert your thumb in her vagina as a way of showing her what a nice job she did on that presentation. But realize also that even those "harmless" pats on the shoulder could make her uncomfortable enough to schedule a consultation with attorney Sue Yerassoff.

dating a co-worker

Given what we just got through telling you, we're going to assume that the co-worker in question isn't your boss or your employee. That said, it makes sense that you would, at some point, want to mix business with pleasure. You spend most of your waking hours at work. Besides, you have a lot in common with your colleagues: similar career interests, the same lunch hangouts, the same dragon-lady boss. It's not surprising, then, that 70 percent of all workers have either dated or married someone they met at their jobs. In fact, there are 10 million new office romances every year, making the workplace the top spot where couples meet today (aside from college).

Still, the office romance has its own set of challenges. You have to stop flirting with the other girls at work. Guys who used to be cronies forget to mention they're grabbing brewskies later on. Your colleagues may resent the "unfair advantage" your new alliance has created. They may also hate being a party to your flirtations or love spats. (Hey, if they wanted to see that crap, they'd watch *Ally McBeal*.) Not to mention that if things end in a breakup, you have to see your ex every damn day.

If even these petty particulars don't discourage you from dating the gal down the hall, you still need to protect yourself from a harassment charge and from certain other pitfalls of the office romance. Here's how.

• Stay on the level. Date only your peers. Dating up or down—even, again, if it's entirely consensual—puts you especially at risk. As her supervisor, you can't possibly be objective when evaluating her work performance. (And if things go sour, she'll resent being evaluated by you and hunt for signs of unfairness in your ratings.) If you're the one who's lower on the totem pole, work mates will think you're sleeping with the boss to get ahead. Or some head.

• Know your company's climate. While fewer than 1 percent of companies have formal anti-dating policies, a handful go so far as to require top execs and their office love interests to sign contracts stating the relationships are "welcome and nonharassing." Even beyond such issues, many employers despise the way office romances affect esprit de corps and overall workplace chemistry.

• Be direct. Don't ask her to dinner on the pretense of discussing the Ungerman account and then slip in a kiss. Tell her up front that you're interested in her for nonbusiness reasons.

• Ask just once. If she says no, don't assume she means "Ask me again another time." A lame excuse—"I have to bathe my cat"—should be taken as a no. Aside from making you look desperate, asking repeatedly opens you up to a possible harassment suit.

• Don't keep the romance a secret. First of all, you're probably not fooling anyone; you're just making the relationship seem clandestine and suspicious. People will think that the two of you volunteered to work together on that Ungerman account to fan your love flames, not to further corporate goals. No need to take out an ad in the company newsletter. Simply drop a subtle hint to a few colleagues, and trust us, the news will spread faster than you can say "water cooler." If, despite all our warnings, the two of you have a boss-subordinate relationship, tell your human resources department as well.

• Be discreet. Treat each other like professionals at the office, saving the hot-and-heavy stuff for after hours. Don't grab and gloat (not even just to the guys at lunch). No touching, flirting, or closed-door meetings. Watch the body language and bedroom eyes. Also, be very careful about the messages you send to each other through e-mail and voice mail. In case you were wondering, your company has unfettered legal access to all such messages sent and received on company time and property. Thirty-nine Dow Chemical Company factory workers found that out the hard way when they were fired for sending obscene jokes and pictures through the company's e-mail.

doing it on the job

One reason that so many of us were utterly fascinated with Bill Clinton's Oval Office antics is that, truth be told, we too have fantasized about scoring more than an attaboy in the boardroom. Surveys show that about 10 percent of office couples have copulated in their place of business. One poll found that the most popular spot for at-work sex was on the boss's desk.

As enticing as that may sound, we suggest keeping your fantasy in your pants. Obviously, if you were to actually get caught, you'd be in trouble. But realize, too, that even if you're just overheard or suspected of eating something besides lunch on your lunch break, thin-skinned (or jealous) co-workers may accuse you of creating a hostile environment. None of this will look good on your résumé.

So we end by repeating the advice with which we started: Concentrate on work at work.

Joy of Sex, The

When British gerontologist Alex Comfort died in early 2000 at the age of 80, he left a joyful legacy—specifically, *The Joy of Sex* and its racy siblings *More Joy of Sex* and *The New Joy of Sex*.

Upon its 1972 release, the original *Joy of Sex*, known for its erotic sketch work, made Comfort a household name rivaled only, perhaps, by Hugh Hefner. If there was an overriding message to Comfort's work, it was this: Remove the grim, pinched mask from sex and delight in it. "The day may come," Comfort once said, "when we regard chastity as no more a virtue than malnutrition."

Sales of the landmark book suggest that the world had been starved for such an affirming view of sexuality: More than 12 million copies are in circulation.

Also see: erotic literature, *Kama Sutra*, sex education, sexual aids, sexual revolution

J

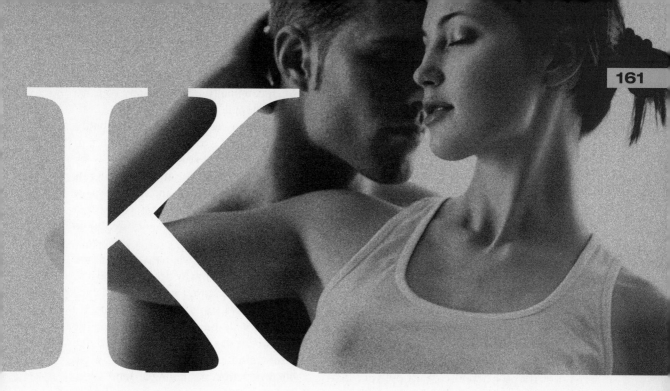

K

Kama Sutra

Probably the world's oldest and most widely read sex book, the *Kama Sutra* was written sometime around the 5th century by the Indian sage Vatsyayana.

Kama refers to one of the ancient responsibilities of men in their roles as heads of households: pleasure and love. In other words, a properly educated man of society should know how to take the skin boat to tuna town. Or something like that. *Sutra*, in case you're wondering, loosely translated means "teachings."

Old though it may be, the *Kama Sutra* is far from dated in much of its material—with a few notable exceptions. One is the advice on how to keep your woman from going astray: Sprinkle a monkey-dung potion on her head.

Likely the most famous part of the book is its extensive collection of sexual positions. One of our favorites: A woman lifts her legs up and crosses them while her lover is inside her. It's known, surprisingly enough, as the tight position.

If you and your partner are in a bit of a rut, or if you're feeling sexually playful, pick up a copy of the book and give things a shot. But hold the monkey dung.

Also see: erotic literature; *Joy of Sex, The*; piercing; tantra; variety; yin and yang; yogi

Kegel exercises

You know to do chinups if you want stronger biceps. You know to do leg presses if you want to increase your vertical leap on the ball court. But did you know that certain exercises can improve the quality of your erection and your ejaculatory control?

They're called Kegels, named after Los Angeles doctor Arnold Kegel, and they target your pubococcygeus, or PC,

K

muscle. That's the muscle directly behind your testicles that you used to use when you wrote your name in the snow and didn't want the letters connected to one another.

Chances are, you never really thought about this before. So do it now. Use two fingers to press on the flesh behind your testicles. (Helpful hint: Don't do this if you're at work and the boss is watching.) Next, do what you do to stop the flow of urine when the cops cruise by. Feel that jump? That's your PC muscle.

An ideal workout is to tense like that for 1 to 2 seconds, 20 times in a row. Do this 3 times a day for 3 weeks. Boring meeting? Do your workout. Stuck in traffic? Pump your PC.

After the 3 weeks are up, put your PC to the test. You can try this with either a woman or those fingers again. Either way, bring yourself to the point of orgasm, then clamp down with your PC for 10 seconds or so. If the muscle has become strong enough, you'll cut yourself off from ejaculating. It's tough to do at first, but with practice and finesse, you'll eventually be able to go as long as you want.

Also see: multiple orgasms, orgasm—delayed, PC muscle, premature ejaculation, size—vagina

kids

You may have heard that Norplant, IUDs, and the Pill are among the most effective forms of birth control out there. Hogwash. As any father will tell you, having a couple of kids is the most successful way to prevent future pregnancies.

We talk about the lack of sex in marriage elsewhere in this book, so let us turn your attention to another important aspect of parents and sex: what to do when you finally get some—and your kid walks in on it.

Too many couples handle this badly. Dad gets angry over the interruption of his blue-moon event; mom covers up quickly and loses the mood. What gets forgotten here is the implicit message that's passed on to the hapless child: that sex is bad, a guilty secret nobody should know about.

Since you know what an ounce of prevention is worth, why not head down to the hardware store for a hook and eye? You deserve some privacy. If your kid makes a walk-on appearance anyway, be cool about it. Calmly say that you'd like a few minutes alone with Mommy. No big production, no flailing around.

Later that evening, when you're tucking your kid in, explain that you and Mommy were simply loving each other. Talk about how adults sometimes like privacy, and take the opportunity to answer any questions.

Also see: afternoon delight, appointments, breastfeeding, contraception, empty-nest syndrome, fertility, incest, marriage—lack of sex in, past partners—dealing with, pedophilia, pregnancy, quickies, sex education, time-saving tips, underage

kinky

The two most common questions sex therapists hear are "Am I kinky?" and its polar opposite, "Am I normal?" In fact, if there's anything weird about Americans' sex lives, it's their obsession with sexual normalcy.

A big chunk of this obsession comes from our society's puritanical attitudes toward sex. Think back to childhood and puberty for a second. You learned to hide your 7-year-old boners. You got a guilt trip thrown your way if you went out on a hot date. And God forbid your mother walked in on you jerking off.

Add the fact that school sex education is largely a lesson in biological plumbing—that is, if you get such education at all. Some school districts either ignore sex or tout the unlikely goal of abstinence. So it's not surprising that—denied access to role models, sex information, and realistic guidance—so many of us wonder whether we're normal.

So let us shed some light on whether or not you're kinky. Some wise and thoughtful person once said: If you use a feather, that's erotic. If you use the whole chicken, that's kinky. Not a bad guideline to go by.

Beyond that, "normal" is largely irrelevant. You will *always* find someone who shares your sexual interests. Yes, there will be fewer available partners the farther out the bell curve you get, but the advent of the Internet has made it easier than ever to find those people.

And, yes, you will always find some people who think you are kinky. Hell,

some people will tell you that anything other than missionary-style intercourse is kinky. If you're going to feel anything about that, feel sorry for them . . . and then ignore 'em.

Also see: abnormal, fantasies, paraphilias, perversions, taboos, variety

Kinsey

He was a biologist who changed the way we think about sex, simply by researching it. Alfred Kinsey was zealous enough to interview tens of thousands of people about their sexual practices, an unheard of undertaking in mid-20th-century America. He was dedicated enough to stick close to the scientific method (though not sufficiently close for his detractors). And he was brave enough to publish the stunning results in 1948 as *Sexual Behavior in the Human Male*, a work so influential and controversial that it's simply referred to as the Kinsey Report. That book (along with his subsequent *Sexual Behavior in the Human Female*) intrigued and inspired the nation and rode America's interest to best-sellerdom.

Hot Dates 1939 to 1945 During World War II, 650,000 illegitimate children were born in the United States and another 333,000 were born in Britain.

continued from page 148

phalluses made of everything from **Styrofoam to concrete** and ranging in length from a few inches to 10 feet. The Thai people leave the shafts as offerings to a female spirit in an effort to ensure future prosperity. Be sure to have your travel agent request a dick-view room.

In Extremis
Though, admittedly, she had some help from silicone injections, San Francisco topless dancer Carol Doda stunned her fans in the weeks following her 1964 debut as **her bust swelled from 34 to 44 inches**. "I expand with the heat," she explained to

True or Phallus
Snakes do not have penises.

BAWDY BALLADS "Torn between Two Lovers," *Mary Mcgregor*

continued on page 170

Kinsey's work showed what seems obvious today—that there's a whole lot of sex going on out there that doesn't conform to "acceptable" standards. For example, he confirmed for the first time that lots of people have sex before marriage, that women like oral sex, and that every part of the body is an erogenous zone for at least some people. Obvious stuff? Maybe today. But it was only hearsay before Kinsey made it official.

As it turns out, Kinsey would have made a heck of an interview subject himself. Despite his image as a conservative, bow-tied professor, he reportedly paraded around nude on scientific expeditions and engaged in an ongoing ménage à trois with his wife and male research aide, among sundry other randy pursuits. But this side of him merely validates his life's work. Modern sex research started with this courageous pioneer's discoveries.

Though the good doctor died in 1956, the Kinsey Institute for Research in Sex, Gender, and Reproduction, which he founded in 1947, grinds on at the campus of Indiana University in Bloomington.

Also see: bestiality; frequency; Freud; *Hite Report, The*; Janus Report; Masters and Johnson; ménage à trois; nymphomania; sex research; zoophilia

kiss

Want to know how important a kiss is? Forget to give your wife or girlfriend one the next time you head off to work. You'll find out soon enough.

You might be surprised to learn that kisses also have a role in sex. Forgive us our sarcasm. A common complaint among women is that guys are only interested in kissing for the 5 minutes immediately preceding the unclasping of the bra.

The unfortunate thing here is that some women see kissing as a barometer of a man's ability to make love. If a woman tells her gal pals that her ex was a lousy kisser, all her friends immediately fill in the blanks and figure that's why she dumped him.

Good news, though: Perking up your pucker is among the easiest things to do. Mostly, it requires the simple knowledge that your woman wants you to do more of it. She wants a kiss in the middle of the day, for no reason. She longs for a passionate lip lock that takes

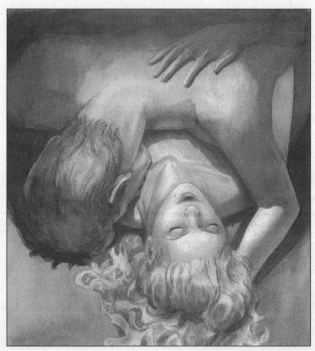

her back to your courting days. She expects a quick smooch as you walk out the door, every time you walk out the door.

Once you've got that down, the technique is pretty easy. Develop a sense of playfulness with your lips. During sex, vary the speed of your kisses—some short, some long and lingering. Toss in a few tender ones, and then brush them out of the way with brazen, forceful ones, paying attention to her reaction. Once you're done with her mouth, never forget that the rest of her body likes to be kissed too.

Kiss her fingers, her throat, her shoulders and back. Explore with your kisses, loitering at the places that elicit happy noises. Don't ask her for a performance evaluation. Just relax and enjoy it. She'll comment on your abilities soon enough.

Interesting, gratuitous fact: A kiss burns between 6 and 12 calories. If you average 9 calories per peck and pucker up thrice daily, you'll kiss 9,855 calories goodbye every year.

Also see: afterplay, beard burn, biting, breath, foreplay, French kiss, hickey, licking, lips, mouth, thrush

klismaphilia

Don't clench up now: Klismaphilia is the sexual enjoyment of enemas. An enema, of course, is a procedure whereby various types of fluid are squirted up your butt. The fluid's subsequent expulsion cleanses the colon of feces. A cool enema can lower a fever, and a warm one can treat hypothermia.

There is, however, an entire subculture that has taken enemas from the prep room to the rec room. An aficionado seeks out an "enemate," someone with whom to give and receive these flushings. Sometimes, there are overtones of dominance and submission: The person receiving the enema is tied up and forced to hold it (a particularly difficult thing to do) until the administrator gives permission to let go.

What motivates those who partake of this particular fetish? The anus is rich in nerves, as evidenced by the fondness among many for anal intercourse. In men, the prostate receives some stimulation from an enema, which in itself can be a pleasurable thing.

While it would be easy to take a whatever-floats-your-boat attitude here, you should know that the practice is not without risk. If you use a sharp enema pipe, you run the risk of puncturing your bowel wall. When one of your enema solutions is wine or some other kind of booze, be especially wary. If the dose is off, you could end up dead from alcohol toxicity. And just think of how your obituary might read. . . .

Also see: anal sex, bidet, bondage and discipline, dominance and submission, douche, fetish, prostate, rectum, sodomy, sphincter, suppositories, water sports

K-Y jelly

The grandpappy of sexual lubricants, K-Y jelly was originally designed to ease the entry of your doctor's fat finger during prostate exams, and for related gynecological uses. It wasn't long before it found its way into bedrooms.

The good thing about K-Y is that it's widely available in drugstores, in supermarkets, online, and even at some convenience stores. Since it's water soluble, it doesn't break down a condom like petroleum-based lubes do.

The bad things: The original formulation is not spermicidal (though you can buy K-Y Plus Nonoxynol-9), and no type of K-Y prevents the spread of sexually transmitted diseases. It's also heavy and greasy, and it dries out quickly after you put it on. You have to keep adding more if the use to which you're putting it lasts more than a few minutes—as we all hope *you* do, of course.

Also see: anal sex, lubricants, vaginal moisture, whipped cream

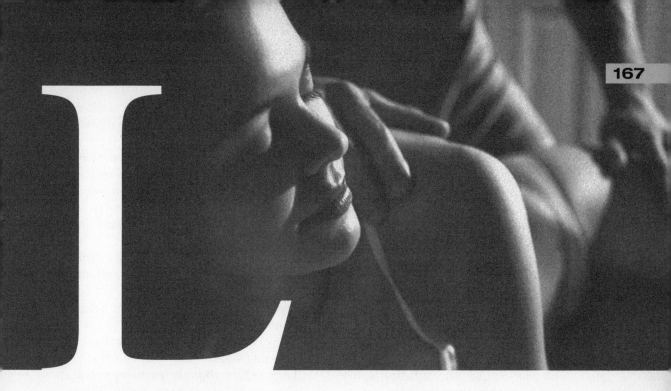

L

labia majora and minora

Time to brush up on your Latin. *Labia* translates to lips. *Majora* and *minora* mean big and little, respectively. Thus, when you peer at a woman's genitals, you see one set each of big and little lips.

The labia majora are the ones that form the outer part of her oyster shell. Unless she's shorn clean, their outer surfaces are covered with pubic hair. When she's aroused, they swell noticeably and get a puffy sort of feel.

The labia minora are the ones you spy when she parts her legs widely. In crude colloquial terms, they're sometimes called piss flaps because they enclose her urethra, the hole from which she urinates. They also form a cover for her vaginal opening.

Her little lips are too often overlooked in the mad stampede for the clitoris. Too bad, because they're packed with nerve endings and highly sensitive to a knowing touch. They also contain an opening called the vestibule, through which a lubricant is secreted to ease your passage into paradise valley.

You can put this insider knowledge to use next time you're headlong into foreplay or even giving her a massage. Gently use your fingertips to knead her lips. Squeeze and tug her labia minora softly, pulling them outward and rolling each one delicately between your fingers.

Also see: afterplay, arousal, clitoris, cunnilingus, erogenous zones, foreplay, lubrication, massage, piercing, prepuce, pubic hair, pudenda, shaving, urethra, vagina, variety, vulva

lace

What's so nice about lace? A better question would be: What isn't nice about lace? This fetching, flimsy fabric

L

is perfect for bras and panties and garter belts and just about anything else that could adorn her flesh. Perhaps the most alluring aspect of lace is that it's full of holes. It covers her modestly . . . except where it allows her skin to peek through.

Lace dates back to at least the 16th century, when Holy Roman emperor Charles V brought lace-making courses to the schools and convents of the Belgian provinces. Now you can see why it often signifies innocence, purity, and femininity. And why it's so erotic when a woman uses the material of chastity in a decidedly non-chaste manner.

If the two of you want to venture a bit closer to the edge of kink, strips of lace happen to make nice, soft restraints to gently bind her wrists or ankles.

Also see: aphrodisiac, bondage and discipline, cross-dressing, dressing her to look sexy, fetish, innocence, leather, lingerie, silk, transvestism, underwear

latex

You may think of latex only as a wonderful alternative to smelly oil-based paint. And the handyman in us salutes you. But if you'd get out of the workshop more often, you'd find out that latex has also made its mark on the fetish scene.

Popular in Europe, latex has been making a transition to the United States because of its remarkable abilities to enhance the human body. If you've ever squeezed into a wetsuit, you know how nicely synthetic rubber sucks your gut and butt into place. Latex-wear is kind of the same, minus the dorky flippers. (The fact that you need to slather your body with baby powder or a water-based lu-

bricant before donning latex attests to just how tight a fit it is.)

It also gives you a sense of sexual empowerment. Unlike leather, another popular fetish-wear material, latex is nonporous and traps body heat and perspiration. When that layer of sweat develops underneath it, latex becomes even more sensual as it slips against your body—a turn-on in and of itself for many latex fetishists.

Latex-wear is among the few truly unisex items in the erotic wardrobe, lending it a feeling of futuristic androgyny. More fetish stores are beginning to carry latex, and there are also many Web sites that sell the gear. Just be sure that your partner is not allergic to latex before you ask her to wear that shiny, black cat suit. Latex sensitivity is a nasty allergy—potentially fatal—and it's more common than you may think.

Also see: androgyny, bisexuality, body oils, bondage and discipline, condom, costumes, dry hump, fetish, kinky, leather, male body, scents, silk, sweating

laughter

Next time you have a stack of old *Playboy*s, a box of tissues, and a day with nothing to do, go back through the last decade of centerfolds. Specifically, check out the turn-ons and turn-offs listed on the Playmate data sheet.

Over and over, you'll see a sense of humor or the ability to make her laugh listed as a Bunny turn-on. The lack thereof often makes it onto the turn-off section. This holds true, too, for the few women left in America who haven't been in *Playboy*.

Perhaps more than anything else, women love funny men. If you can make a woman laugh, your chances of getting her into bed increase dramatically. So let this be a wake-up call to your sense of delight and playfulness. Don't be afraid to crack wise or poke fun at yourself.

Note that we said poke fun at *yourself*, not at her. Guys like to good-naturedly mock each other. It's a way of keeping our egos in check and our priorities straight. Women do not share our enthusiasm for this. If you tease her about her butt, her job, her cat, or anything or anyone else she cares about, be prepared for an unfriendly response. Yes, it's a double standard. Accept it and live with it.

As long as you obey the above rule, you should never hesitate to laugh in bed. If you're in the midst of sex and you and your partner can laugh because of something you said or did together, it's an excellent indication of your comfort level. Taking things too seriously can turn sex from a joy into a task. Laughter takes the pressure off.

Also see: afterplay, boredom, clumsiness, communication, desperate, farting, moaning, performance anxiety, sexual etiquette, smiling, stress, teasing, turn-ons

leather

Men are a reflective sort. We lie awake at night pondering the true nature of the universe and why virtually any woman looks good in leather. Here's some help with the second question.

Leather's appeal begins with its smell. To many sniffers, it conjures up images of animalistic sex and forbidden desires. It's the quintessential symbol of wild behavior. And that's why every badass from James Dean to the Fonz has draped himself in rawhide.

Leather also symbolizes power and domination, especially in the fetish community. As with any fetish-wear, it means different things in different contexts. If you're in an all-leather outfit wielding a whip, you're in charge; subtract the whip and add a collar and chain to that same outfit, and she's probably going to be in charge (and likely holding the whip).

Even if you're not into leather as a fetish accessory, it can still have a place in your sex life. If you'd like to put more skin into your bedroom but you don't want to freak out your partner, start out slowly. Many couples begin with the purchase of a pair of leather pants or a skirt. Underwear is optional. Once she gets into the groove with those, go for the full monty: leather bra, panties, and garter belt.

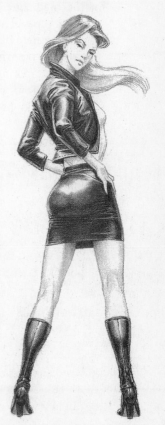

Also see: animals, bondage and discipline, athletic sex, cock ring, dominance and submission, dressing her to look sexy, dressing you to look sexy, fetish, lace, latex, paddle, playacting, randy, rough sex, scents, sex symbols, silk, tattoos, underwear, whips, wild

legs

Is it the way that they move, the way they feel, or where they lead? Whatever the reason, men have long been fascinated with women's legs and the panty hose commercials that glorify them (except that one with Joe Namath—that just creeped us out).

Throughout history, legs have symbolized power and strength in both men and women. Fortunately, women have been more expressive in displaying that power through fancy shoes and revealing dresses.

Contrary to most of those hosiery ads, the type of leg that men find most attractive is not stick-shaped. According to a 2000 survey of readers of the magazine *Leg Show*, the most popular type of woman's leg is a curvaceous one. Curvaceous legs have full thighs tapering to the knees and full calves tapering to the ankles. Think Marilyn Monroe. In second place came a thick, heavy leg; think Betty Grable or Marlene Dietrich. Coming in third was the long-and-thin supermodel leg.

You know, of course, that some guys identify themselves as breast men, ass men, or leg men. Some experts believe that these preferences are rooted in our early childhood experiences. We attach significance to a body part that stimulated us sexually before we knew we were being sexually stimulated. So a guy may become a leg man if as a child he was, say, pleasantly bounced upon his mother's knee. Other experts believe that it's a biological reaction, a matter of hormones.

Regardless of the reason for your fascination, there is a plus to loving legs. You might more easily get away with ogling: It's harder to get caught when you're staring down.

Also see: beauty, body shapes, fetish, garter belts, garters, muscles, ogling, preference, sexual attraction, sexy, turn-ons, wandering eye

---

Hot Dates **1944** The rate of venereal disease skyrocketed after news reached U.S. troops that the drug penicillin could cure syphilis and gonorrhea.

---

continued from page 163

Answer:
False. Actually, each snake has two. But, in a remarkable show of self-restraint, he uses only one at a time.

reporters, whose interest had been piqued by the hordes swarming the Condor Club to catch a glimpse of Doda's burgeoning boobs. Doda, who later insured her breasts for $1.5 million, received a Business Person of the Year Award from Harvard University for her "asset management."

LEGAL BRIEFS
A 45-year-old Tennessee woman and her 26-year-old son pleaded no contest to incest after admitting they were married to each other. **The woman also pleaded guilty to bigamy,** as she'd married her son while still wedded to her fourth husband.

Seemed like a Good Idea at the Time. . .
Never lecture a Nicaraguan prostitute about safe sex. When researchers made condoms available

---

BAWDY BALLADS **"Why Don't We Do It in the Road?"** *the Beatles*

continued on page 175

lesbian

Slip any porn film that caters to straight guys into your VCR, and you're guaranteed three things: cheesy guitar riffs, bad lighting, and lesbian sex scenes. But wait a second: Isn't this supposed to be *straight* porn?

Since well before the days of celluloid sex, men have found girl-meets-girl get-togethers highly stimulating. There are a bunch of possible reasons. Number one is that women's bodies are beautiful and exciting to us. Pile on a few extra, and that's a bonus. Number two is that witnessing "forbidden" love is a major turn-on. Number three is that each of us fantasizes about finding himself in the middle of said lovely ladies. And, finally, some guys may like watching sex but don't really want to see another guy's butt in the action.

As for whether women enjoy watching two of their own kind, well, that's a completely individual matter. Some gals like watching other gals gettin' it on: They may appreciate the beauty of the female form as much as you do, or they may be turned on by the raw sexuality of the acts on screen, regardless of the genders involved. Others can't relate and are just bored; they'd rather fast-forward to the scene where the brawny plumber shows up to lay some pipe for the lonely housewife. And of course, there are ladies who think it's gross, at best, or unnatural and sinful, at worst. You should be able to figure out how your own woman feels shortly after the action starts, assuming you're not too preoccupied by the breathtaking cinematography itself.

Getting back to masculine interests, here's the bad news about lesbians: Odds are against your getting to join in if you meet a real-life couple. Lesbians in their 20s might be experimental, especially if they're determining whether they're bisexual or not. But once they hit their 30s and pair up, you'll be about as welcome in their bedroom as Jesse Helms.

Also see: AC/DC, bisexuality, dildo, femme, gender bender, hermaphrodite, homosexuality, switch-hitter, threesome, voyeurism

libido

A Freudian term for our sex drives and instincts.

Famed psychiatrist Sigmund Freud believed that the libido is the most basic and powerful human drive and that it develops in several stages: oral, anal, and phallic. The oral stage occurs in infancy, when children are interested in sucking and other mouth-related activities, such as spitting up on you. Freud labeled the period when children are toilet training, between the ages of 2 and 3, the anal stage. And finally, as youngsters enter pubescence and discover their genitalia, they go through what Freud called the phallic stage.

Contemporary psychology has jiggled Freud's beliefs, as his theories are focused primarily on biology and downplay other factors like cultural and social influences. Modern shrinks agree that the biological side is important: Hormones influence the basic human drive to reproduce and affect how we feel pleasure. But the way in which you act on those drives and emotions is determined in large part by your childhood experiences, family beliefs, and surrounding societal values. In other words, as with most things sexual, libido is determined by both the physical and the mental.

Also see: anima and animus, compulsive behavior, dreams, Electra complex, Freud, hormones, religion, sex drive

L

licking

Good lovemaking is like indulging in a gourmet meal: You don't dive right into the main course. To take a tortured metaphor a tad further, think of your penis as the filet mignon and your tongue as the oysters Rockefeller. The meat is probably the most satisfying, but the oysters make the whole experience that much more memorable.

Now that your mouth is watering . . . good spots to lick on a woman? Well, all of them really, but look for the less obvious to add a little variety and make your woman moan with surprise. Nipples and clitoris are the old standbys, with her neck coming in a close third. But what about a gentle swoop around her inner thigh? You can even slide up the length of her arm, slowly and carefully, and see how she responds.

Use just the tip of your tongue when you're venturing into new territory. It's much more subtle and erotic. A full-tongue slobber will make her think she's in bed with a Saint Bernard.

Some other places to try: Licking a woman's underarms can be incredibly arousing for her. Or, you may want to try the soft spot behind her knee. If she's not ticklish, and if she hasn't been wearing hiking boots all day, a well-placed tongue along the sole of her foot can also be cool—or hot.

And keep in mind, she's not the only one who reaps the benefits—arousing your lover is also arousing for you.

Also see: biting, breasts, cunnilingus, French kiss, hickey, kiss, mouth, oculophilia, oral sex, rimming, sexual etiquette, tickling, tongue, whipped cream

lingerie

Pavlov's dog had its bell. Men have lingerie. Both result in the same behavior: drooling and a wild thrashing at the leash.

Without question, many men's favorite erotic aid is lingerie. It turns your good girl bad quicker than you can say crotchless cat suit. Because men tend to be visually oriented, the ocular delight that is lingerie plays right up our sexual alley. But don't think for a minute that it always has to be in plain sight. Our imaginations rev into overdrive when we know that a woman in a conservative business suit has a wicked-looking garter belt on underneath.

Note, though, that she wears lingerie largely as a gift to you. That's not to say she doesn't enjoy looking sexy for you—she does, and knowing that you find her sexy can get her hot. But her erotic fires are stoked more by aural and sensual experiences. That's why so many women go nuts when you talk to them during sex or give them precoital massages.

So the task of buying lingerie, especially the first few times, will probably fall to you. Here are some pointers.

• Make sure first that the timing is right; lingerie is definitely not a third-date gift.

• Find out her proper size. We can't stress enough how important this is. If she tries on something that pulls where it's supposed to push—or if she fails to fill the cup size of the garment you picked—you'll be sitting alone with your purchase while she weeps her way through weight-loss or breast-augmentation ads.

• With that in mind, you may want to get her a camisole or silk robe on your initial attempt. These are more forgiving of errors in sizing. And don't be shy about asking for help at the lingerie store. Most of the women who work there are expert in figuring out sizes from the pictures you draw in the air.

- If you're too shy to even enter the store, try a mail-order catalog or a Web site. (Believe it or not, these are not just for your personal viewing pleasure—they actually sell stuff.)

- Finally, go for quality. Yes, it'll probably get torn after you have at it a few times, but nothing makes a woman feel cheaper than lingerie in a plastic Wal-Mart bag. Choose silk or satin garments. Avoid bright colors like pink or red or, worst of all, baby blue. Start off with black or a subtle gray.

One final suggestion: Avoid buying her lingerie every birthday, anniversary, and National Prune Week. Lingerie is best given for no special occasion because, really, it's a gift for you. You wouldn't want her to give you a nose-hair trimmer for your birthday, would you?

Also see: birthdays, boxers or briefs, bras, costumes, dressing her to look sexy, garter belts, lace, latex, leather, makeup, romance, sexual aids, silk, striptease, thongs, undressing

lips

There's a sexual triumvirate of highly sensitive spots on your body: your glans, your fingertips, and your lips. A lot of guys forget about that last one, but lips are blessed with thin skin and a high concentration of nerve endings.

That's a good reason why you should spend some time dwelling on hers. Trace them with your fingers. When you French kiss, let the tip of your tongue wander gently along them. Maybe try tickling them with a feather.

Use your own lips to explore her body. Don't feel obliged to dart your tongue out all the time. Let her pubic hair tanta-

lize you as you brush your lips over it. Meander along the different textures of her body: the smoothness of her stomach, the rougher skin on her knees, the sharp prickles of her eyelashes. Pay attention to the different sensations.

For best results, be sure to groom around your lips. If you have a mustache, trim it well back so you don't scour her. And do something about your chapped lips. A dab of the lubricant you have by the bedside will take care of them in a hurry. If perchance you don't have any, rub your finger against the side of your nose or forehead to borrow some of the skin oil there. Transplant it to your lips. Just make sure she doesn't see you doing this.

Also see: beard burn, cunnilingus, erogenous zones, foreplay, French kiss, glans, kiss, licking, mouth, ointments, oral sex, tickling, tongue, whispering

Lolita

A classic novel by Vladimir Nabokov. The title character, the stepdaughter of narrator Humbert Humbert, is a girl on the verge of womanhood. The story centers around the stepfather's unsuccessful struggles to control his desire for the blossoming young beauty. Humbert says, in one spot, "Every movement she made, every shuffle and ripple, helped me to conceal and to improve the secret system of tactile correspondence between beast and beauty—between my gagged, bursting beast and the beauty of her dimpled body in its innocent cotton frock." These are the over-the-top words of a man destined to make a very bad judgment call.

The name *Lolita* has become synonymous with any charming young woman

L

L

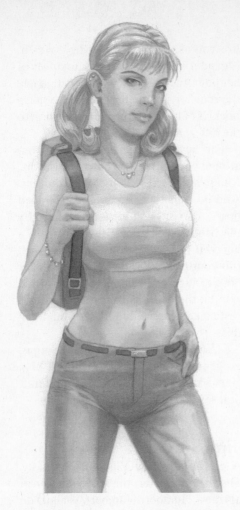

who inspires lust in an older man. Fantasies about Lolitas are widespread. Acting on those fantasies is generally illegal. Instead, why not go out and buy a cheerleader outfit for your wife or girlfriend?

Also see: costumes, Electra complex, erotic literature, fantasies, pedophilia, innocence, playacting, pornography, puberty, sex offenders, taboos, underage, young women/older men

love

Shakespeare wrote 154 sonnets on the subject; Woody Allen made 34 films about it in 35 years; Barry White explored the feeling on 30 albums and counting. There's been a lot of talk about love, and no one has ever gotten it completely right. Of course, that won't keep us from taking a stab at it, however inept that stab may be.

Love is a deep and abiding attraction based on trust, desire, admiration, and respect, all of which are mutual. So much for the clinical definition. Part of the problem with love is that it is many things all wrapped up in one thin word.

We expect love to be unchanging; it's not. We demand love to be impervious to all affronts; it isn't. We insist that love be the balm for all wounds; it can't be.

That's not to take away from the powerful force that actually is love. We just need to let it be what it is, rather than what we misconceive it to be. So, then, expect love to change. You'll want to roar from the rooftops when you first fall in love. Over time, that passion will mellow; and love will become a quieter, more thoughtful thing—not necessarily better or worse, just different. It's the difference between a summer storm and a breeze that carries the smell of autumn.

Know, too, that love is not invincible. If you do enough crappy things to each other over time, love will die—or be overwhelmed by so much hurt that what you feel mostly about each other, despite the love, is sadness. Common decency is the water that nourishes love's roots. Neither will love make all the wrongs in the world right. Anyone who has a difficult, challenging child knows this. You can love the little beast all you want—he'll still be a beast. But you'll love him anyway if you don't expect love to turn him into something he's not.

We can tell you how we feel on the subject, but don't let your inquiry stop there. In fact, let this be your foremost accomplishment in life: to know that every year brings you a greater understanding of that crazy thing called love.

Also see: attraction, emotions, free love, heartache, hormones, infatuation, marriage

lovemaking

Many guys know all about casual sex and are pretty good at it. But knowing *only* about casual sex is like spending your vacation in Athens without ever seeing the Parthenon.

Sex without love is screwing. Sex with love is lovemaking. There's a big, big difference. There's a feeling of godliness in good lovemaking that can't be achieved with a stranger or a casual acquaintance. There's trust and communication and a strange feeling that you're building on something, *toward* something beyond an orgasm. Indeed, in real lovemaking, the orgasm isn't even the point—it's the

closeness, the idea of sharing a knowledge of each other, a sublime intimacy that is reserved for just the two of you alone.

Here's something to try next time you're in bed with the woman you love: Spend more time than ever making eye contact. Don't just look at each other, look *into* each other. And when you reach orgasm, keep your eyes open and locked on one another. You may each catch a glimpse of the other's soul.

Also see: emotions, eye contact, intimacy, *Kama Sutra*, one-night stand, passion, soul mates, spiritual sex, zipless sex

lover

There's something most men would dance for joy to hear from their partners—and it's not their correct name. It's "You're the best lover I've ever had."

The problem is, though one woman may find you to be a gentle, considerate lover, another may write you off as an underwhelming Milquetoast. While one may think you're a champion bull, yet another may consider you a brute. There isn't one single formula you can follow to

Hot Dates 1940s FBI director J. Edgar Hoover and his 60,000 recruits kept sex files on everyone from senators and foreign diplomats to First Lady Eleanor Roosevelt.

continued from page 170

to 6,463 couples checking into 19 different motels in Managua, the capital of Nicaragua, about 61 percent of hooker/john couples used the prophylactics, compared to 20 percent of couples who exchanged body fluids but no money. When health brochures were also left in the motel rooms, however, **the rate of condom use among working girls actually dropped**.

Foreign Affairs

Here's an annual ritual for which we hope we are never chosen: **The Ethiopian Konso circumcise three**

True or Phallus ?
The nipples of a human male can produce milk.

BAWDY BALLADS   "Lay, Lady, Lay," *Bob Dylan*

continued on page 182

guarantee that you'll hear those magic words drip from every partner's mouth.

The trick is to find out exactly what your current partner thinks are the essential ingredients of a good lover. This, of course, means talking to her about it and paying careful attention to the way she responds to your natural impulses. Great lovers are flexible (philosophically as well as physically). They willingly adapt to each partner's preferences, finding a happy medium that pleases both parties. Lousy lovers are guys who say, "This is my style; take it or leave it"—and then are surprised when ladies leave it.

Also see: dreams, fantasies, past partners—talking about, preference, techniques

LSD

There's always someone who thinks you can enhance sex with drugs. In some cases, that belief may be true. But not with LSD. Sorry, Mr. Leary.

Sometimes called acid, LSD can produce both emotional and visual hallucinations and wide-ranging feelings, from confusion to despair to thinking you're an orange that everyone wants to peel. Moods can shift quickly, unpredictably, and violently. Needless to say, there's not much snuggling going on when you're tripping.

Some people think that a good trip can lead to highly spiritual experiences. That's a theory you might be willing to test when you're 20 and single and you have brain cells to spare, but older guys probably don't want to be hopped up in some farmer's field hoping for a sighting of the Buddha.

Also see: aphrodisiac, drugs, spiritual sex

lubricants

When it comes to both cars and sex, lubricants are your best friends. Sometimes, women just aren't wet enough on their own. Other times, you might be engaging in anal sex, an avenue that produces no slipperiness of its own. Another night, you just might be too much of a stallion for her and need a little grease to ease your way in.

Sex lubricants can be water-, silicone-, or petroleum-based. If you use condoms, go with one of the first two types; those that are petroleum-based—like baby oil, mineral oil, or petroleum jelly—will break down the latex in most prophylactics. Water-based varieties wash off easily; while silicone-based products are waterproof, so you can use them in the shower or for other splashy fun. Silicones also absorb more slowly into the skin, which means you don't have to replenish as often.

In our own test runs, we found ourselves partial to Astroglide for all-around use. It's a water-based lubricant, but it doesn't dry out as quickly as others of its ilk. Plus, it was discovered by a scientist who was working on creating slippery compounds for the space shuttle, and we're all for supporting NASA. You can find it at most pharmacies.

Also see: anal sex, body oils, condom, massage, ointments, vaginal moisture, whipped cream

lubrication

There are several ways to know when you've turned a woman on. Some are subtle: Her breathing gets heavier; she may emit a sultry noise or two; her nipples harden. Some are less subtle: She calls your mother to tell her you won't make your curfew. But perhaps the most obvious—and certainly the sexiest—is that warm, wet feeling she gets between her legs. For once, you know what she's feeling without her saying a word.

Lubrication is a woman's arousal response, just as an erection is a man's. Some women respond more quickly than others, and the amount of lubrication varies greatly among women. That said, the first thing to suspect if she's drier than a good martini is that you've short-changed yourselves in the foreplay department. Go back at least one base.

Of course, there are other factors that are beyond your control. Dehydration—such as that caused by a long, late night of drinking—can affect a woman's ability to generate juice. And if you're in the middle of a sexual marathon, she may simply dry up after a while. That's not because she's losing interest; her body just can't keep up.

Also not a reflection of your abilities is the simple fact that vaginal wetness is linked to the female sex hormone estrogen. When estrogen levels fluctuate—for instance, after child-birth and during breastfeeding or menopause—it's more difficult for a woman to get wet on her own, even when she's turned on. For all these situations, a good store-bought lubricant will work wonders.

Also see: arousal, breast-feeding, estrogen, female ejaculation, foreplay, marathon, medications, menopause—hers, sloppy sex, vaginal moisture, wet spot

lust

Haul out your holy books for a second. For our purposes here, we're going to define lust in the biblical sense. Don't confuse it with passion. Think about it in terms of virtue and vice—virtue being self-control and self-preservation, vice being the uncontrolled, self-destructive drive for sex. Hence, lust.

Part chemical and part mental, lust can lead you to some of the worst decisions of your life. It's an emotion that creates new rules for you—or, more accurately, that prompts you to ignore all the old ones. It scoffs at common sense, morality, and commitment. Many acts of infidelity are attributable to lust.

Unless you're of uncommon moral fiber, it's often too late to try to deal with lust once you're in its grasp. You need to create an avoidance strategy. Why? Because infidelity is one of the most common reasons that people get di-

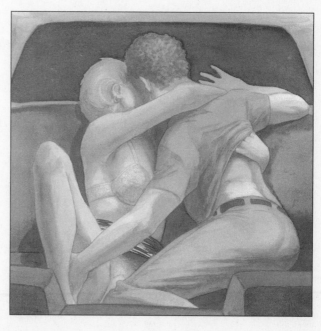

vorced. Even if you're single, a drunken one-night stand with someone in your department is a surefire way to create hassles at work.

Rule number one? Don't put yourself in situations where you may do something you'll regret. If you're on a business trip, for instance, don't get drunk in the hotel bar and talk to the attractive young woman on the stool next to you. Don't party with female co-workers after the convention ends. Okay, maybe you can't or don't want to get out of all social obligations, but you can at least limit the amount you drink. Better yet, masturbate in your hotel room just before you head out. It'll relieve a lot of the libidinous pressure. Just wash your hands before you go to dinner with your client.

If you do find yourself in a dangerous situation, the only way out is sheer strength of will. There will *always* be a Jiminy Cricket moment early in the lustful event, when your conscience pokes its nose in. Listen, listen, listen. Consider all that you have to lose for a few minutes of pleasure. Think about your wife and kids. Envision what life would be like at work on Monday—or in the unemployment line on Tuesday.

Also see: alcohol, affairs, best friend's wife, boss's wife, commitment, date rape, first time with a lover, horny, monogamy, one-night stand, passion, randy, travel— loneliness during, wife's best friend

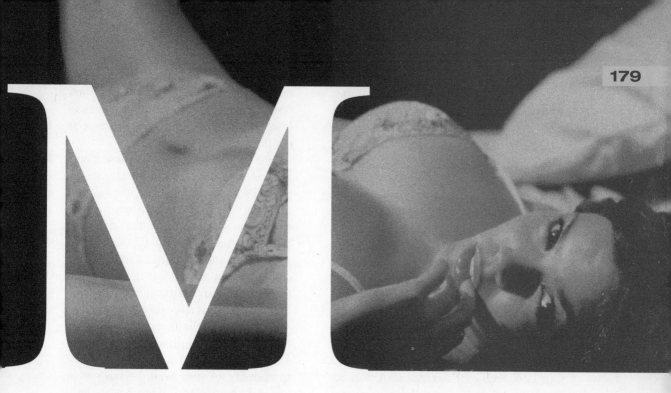

Madonna/whore complex

There are two types of women: Ones that you marry and ones that you screw. Right?

If you're nodding, watch out. You just tested positive for the Madonna/whore complex. It's basically when men want virginal saints as mothers to their children but uninhibited sluts as their bed partners.

According to sex therapists, this isn't all that unusual. Here's how it often plays out. A husband and wife have a wildly enjoyable sex life. Then she gets pregnant. Once the baby arrives, the husband no longer feels comfortable with their unconstrained sexuality. So he restricts their sexual interaction in order to keep her firmly planted in the Madonna category, taking the symbolism of her motherhood to an extreme. So, say they both enjoyed oral or anal sex before the kid entered the scene. Now, he considers those activities "too dirty" for her. As a result, their sex life becomes less satisfying for both of them.

It goes without saying that emotional tensions run high when one partner wants to box in the other partner's desires and personality. And it's this combination of emotional and sexual disquiet that often makes couples seek counseling.

It's not an easy problem to treat since it involves a lifetime of deep-seated religious or cultural values and beliefs. But neither is it impossible to change. You'll need a good marriage counselor or sex therapist who counts this among his or her specialties.

Also see: breastfeeding, divorce—issues that lead to, empty-nest syndrome, hangups, marriage, missionary position, prostitution, sex therapy, sexual revolution, sloppy sex, wild women

mail-order brides

The practice of ordering wives through the mail began in colonial days, when

M

lonely male settlers sent love letters to their women back in the Old Country, convincing many a female to follow them overseas.

These days, many American men still look abroad for a broad, though not due to a lack of local women. Tired of what they consider this society's overly opinionated, independent women, they see foreign brides as more submissive and loyal. Often, they're right. On the flip side, women from other cultures often see American men as less dominant and more financially secure than their own countrymen. These women are also right, in many cases.

How prevalent is marriage by mail? Exact numbers by nationality aren't kept, but in the 5-year period from 1992 to 1997, tens of thousands of American men found mates through international matrimonial agencies.

A word to those to whom all this is starting to sound pretty good: Some so-called marriage services are shams. Typically found on the Internet (what a shock—a scam on the Internet?), they deliver nothing but empty promises, though your money order—for what could be thousands of dollars—is safely cashed in a foreign land. Make sure you check the reputation of any company you deal with. See if you can talk with some, ahem, satisfied customers.

Also see: courtship, escort service, Internet dating, interracial sex, matchmaking services, meeting women, sex tours and resorts

mail-order medications

Flip through virtually any major newspaper, magazine, or tabloid, and you'll find a slew of advertisements for medications available by mail or via the Internet. Viagra (sildenafil), of course, is our main concern. With a quick and simple credit card charge today, you can have a bottle of Pfizer's finest in your mailbox tomorrow.

The companies that make these transactions are supposed to screen for people who shouldn't take Viagra. You fill out a questionnaire, a doctor ostensibly reviews it, and he either approves or denies the application. Uh-huh. When we ordered some, we found at least one company that mailed out the pills even though we indicated health problems that might kill us if we took Viagra.

Excuse our bluntness: It's dumb to order prescription drugs without a prescription. Sure, we want you to take responsibility for your health—your sexual health, in particular. But much as we hate to admit it, the system currently in place to supply consumers with these powerful meds is there, generally, for good reason. With the number of drugs now on the market, the number of people taking multiple drugs, and the risk of potentially fatal interactions between antagonistic drugs, it seems just plain foolhardy to play doctor. At least this version of the game.

Oh, and if you're under the impression that drug interactions come into play only when you're 75 or older, think again. There are plenty of drug combinations that can put a 20-year-old out of commission faster than you can say, "Viagra and nitroglycerin." Nor do both drugs have to be prescription medications. Take Tagamet HB 200, for example. Mixing this over-the-counter antacid with Viagra can cause unpleasant side effects such as headache, nasal congestion, upset stomach, and leg cramps.

Your family physician knows your medical history; these salesmen don't.

Plus, if you have difficulty getting erections, it could indicate underlying heart disease. You need to see a real, live med school graduate for treatment. So go ahead and order books, CDs, and power tools through the mail. Just leave the prescriptions to the docs and pharmacists.

Also see: heart conditions, impotence, medications, urologist

mail-order sex products

We'll be the first to admit it: We hate going into adult shops. And we do that kind of thing for a living. Considering that you don't even get paid to do it, you probably hate it even more than we do. It's no wonder. Most sex shops are dank, ill-smelling pits manned by questionable fellows in ratty T-shirts and suspiciously stained pants.

Fortunately, there's an alternative: the postal system. In fact, you can do more through the mail than Ted Kaczynski ever dreamed. Here's a short list of sex-related products you can have delivered directly to your door: condoms, videos, fetish-wear, toys, lingerie, lubes, the smaller species of livestock. Okay, we're not sure about that last one, but we've made our point.

There are drawbacks to ordering through a catalogue or Web site. For one, you can't judge quality or sturdiness very well. To offset that, make sure there's a generous return policy—you may pay a little more for the products, but it'll be worth it when you don't get stuck with something sitting unused under the mattress.

Also, know the reputation of the firm you're dealing with. Scam artists love both the mail and sex products. They

bank on the fact that you'll be too embarrassed to complain to the authorities about getting ripped off when you pay for a $200 anal intruder that's never delivered.

Here are a few companies that we know to be good: Xandria Collection, Good Vibrations, Adam & Eve, Blowfish, and Eve's Garden. They all have extensive collections of high-quality sexual products, and they offer decent-to-excellent return policies. Each has a Web site or catalogue.

Also see: erotic films, pornography, sexual aids

makeup

You've seen them. You've been smeared by them. Heck, you've probably even dated them. They, of course, are the Tammy Faye Bakkers and Mimi Bobecks of the world—the women who do not wear makeup so much as bathe in it.

The way a woman wears makeup is as personal and particular a decision as the style of clothes she wears, the breed of cat she prefers, the sort of men she chooses. Put it this way: It's as important to her as the kind of car you drive is to you. That car is your own form of makeup, albeit a bit looser fitting.

So what happens when you find yourself romantically engaged with a woman who uses a trowel rather than a powder puff? Or one who believes that frosted, blue eye shadow is to be applied from the hairline down? How about one who makes you check street corners to see if she's loitering longer than propriety dictates?

Here's exactly what you can do about it—and what you should *not* do. Mention how you feel, preferably without refer-

M

ring to circus clowns or the red-light district. Keep in mind that she may cake it on because she lacks confidence in her own natural beauty. Say something like, "You know, you look even more beautiful without all that stuff covering up your pretty features." Or, "I think you look best after a shower, before you put your makeup on." Compliment her on her beautiful eyes. Her full lips. Her sparkling, seductive smile. Do this not just once but over and over again. She may need repeat flattery to shed the cosmetic industry's powerful influence and to gain confidence in her unadorned looks.

If she blames her heavy-duty look on her stuck-up older sister who never taught her to properly apply eyeliner, treat her to a professional makeover at a day spa, where she can learn some tricks of the cosmetics trade.

What you can't do, of course, is demand that she wear less makeup. Ultimately, it's her face and her decision.

Hopefully, a nudge in a more natural direction is all she needs.

Also see: body image, cross-dressing, dressing her to look sexy, media

making up

Well, you could simply tape a peace treaty to her windshield. But if you want a more personal, tried-and-true method of making up, you need to learn the fine art of apology.

If you've screwed up, express your sincere remorse. Don't make excuses for your behavior; just take your lumps and eat your crow. And ask her to kindly accept your apology. She may not oblige—at least not at first. If she does, though, a lot of the steam will go out of her anger.

Even if you don't think that you were at fault, consider that an apology needn't be an admission of guilt. Sometimes it can just be a way of saying you're sorry that things are difficult or

Hot Dates 1952 A former GI underwent the first publicly acknowledged sex-change operation. He went to Denmark as George Jorgensen and returned as Christine Jorgensen.

continued from page 175

Answer:
True. Baby boys sometimes leak milk from their nipples. It's a reaction to maternal hormones still in their blood.

grandfathers from priestly families. Only the tips of the foreskins are cut off, but the men—who wear skirts during the ceremony—are banned from further sexual intercourse and thought of as women. Some become transvestites. The custom may have originated as a way of preventing older men from siring children who would have too high a social status—in the Konso culture, a family's status increases as its patriarch ages.

There's a loophole, however, that would make us get serious about saving money. If the chosen men don't want to participate in the ritual, they can hire stand-ins. You don't know what true poverty is until you live in a place where guys are willing to take that job.

In Extremis
One of the biggest—in every sense of the word—male porn stars was John

BAWDY BALLADS "Banana in Your Fruit Basket," *Bo Carter*

continued on page 187

that you're having a misunderstanding or that she's so hurt by whatever happened.

This distinction is important to bear in mind when you're wrapping your lips around an apology. If you don't think you've done anything wrong, don't feign regret just to put an end to the arguing. Your hollowness will shine through. All you need to do is show concern over the rough patch the two of you have hit.

In any case, give the relationship some time to return to normal. You're dealing with another human being, after all, and it takes a while for our emotions to swing back to level. The last thing you want to do is berate her for continuing to act "weird" just 5 minutes after you've apologized. Unless you want an entirely new argument on your hands.

Also see: arguing, communication, sweet talk, trust—rebuilding

male body

What do you consider an example of a great male body? A *Men's Health* magazine cover model? That statue of David? Well, the truth may be closer to Mick Jagger than to Michelangelo. At least to women.

While it's safe to say that many women *are* attracted to the finely chiseled look of a gym rat, not all have such lofty expectations. In fact, there is a surprising array of body flaws that certain women find downright charming.

Take the humble honker. Or maybe not so humble, because some women think a large nose on a man is sexy. They may conclude that you're more masculine if you sport a good-sized beak—a delicate button nose simply looks more feminine.

Then there's the Budweiser belly. Not all women are searching for rock-hard abs. Some prefer the softer look of a man who enjoys life and the good food it has to offer. Plus, it makes them feel that they don't have to starve themselves to stay skinny for you. It goes both ways, right? Right?

Short stature is another thing that's attractive to some women—especially to petite women. Imagine having a guy's sternum pressed into your face every time you had sex. That's what small women contend with when they date tall guys. They may prefer being able to look into your eyes without developing cricks in their necks.

And don't forget the scar, the lifelong reminder of battles fought, swords crossed, and seesaws tumbled from. A scar makes you appear mysterious, adventurous, rugged, unafraid to look after your woman when the going gets tough. Make up bawdy tall tales about how you got it, and consider incorporating them into your lovemaking fantasy play.

Finally, and perhaps most important, here are two words on baldness: Sean Connery. Many women find status attractive, and nothing signifies wisdom, maturity, and life experience like a smooth, shiny pate. You sabotage that when you futilely try to disguise it with a comb-over or ponytail. Cut your remaining hair short, and enjoy having women seek you out.

Also see: abs, body fitness, body shapes, Electra complex, erogenous zones, hair, power, preference, muscles, reproductive system—yours, sexy, size—nose

male pill

Since the 1970s, headlines have been blaring claims such as RESEARCH ON

MALE PILL INTENSIFIES and THE MALE PILL IS ON THE WAY. Yet here we sit, decades later, with only condoms and vasectomies as efficient forms of male birth control.

Why is that? Ask a hard-core feminist, and she may say it's because there aren't enough women scientists, men don't want to be responsible for contraception, and on and on. The truth, though, is rooted more in biology.

A woman releases one egg a month. A man can produce a million sperm per hour. Which do you think is easier to stop?

So it doesn't appear that anything new will be—ahem—coming down the pipeline anytime soon. British researchers are among those still working feverishly on a male pill; they've managed to reduce fertility rates in male mice by 90 percent by deactivating certain proteins on the vas deferens (the tube that carries sperm). But for those of us who aren't rodents, that option is, at best, years away.

Also see: condom, contraception, oral contraceptive, Pill—the, sperm count, vasectomy

manual stimulation

Today, many male gynecologists will examine a patient only if another staffer is in the room. It's a common practice intended to protect both parties. It guards the doctors against frivolous lawsuits, and it defends the patient by making sure that a guy doc doesn't simply reach down and massage her naked genitals till she reaches orgasm.

Up until the 1920s, such manual stimulation was an accepted therapy also called medical massage. It was used to treat the female "disease" known as hysteria, whose symptoms included anxiety, insomnia, irritability, heaviness in the abdomen, water retention, and a loss of appetite for food or sex.

At this point, we figure, you're asking yourself two questions: One, aren't those complaints an awful lot like your girlfriend's PMS? And two, why couldn't you have been a doctor back in the Roaring Twenties? Seriously, though, in the Western world, physicians through the ages believed that a lack of sexual gratification caused such discomforts. And since female masturbation was considered indecent and itself detrimental to health, doctors were forced to "treat" single, presumably celibate women themselves—that is, until the electro-mechanical vibrator was invented in the 1880s for the very purpose of giving docs a break. (Yes, really.)

Married women diagnosed with hysteria were instructed to go home and have sex with their husbands, a prescription that no doubt had helpful hubbies encouraging their wives to ask the doctor for advice at every opportunity.

Also see: clitoral orgasm, get off, hysterectomy, masturbation, PMS, sex therapy, surrogate, vibrator

marathon

A sexual session that lasts all night long. In our dreams, anyway: Actually, anything over 2 hours will get you up on the medal podium.

Considering that the average man lasts 14 minutes during sex, you have some training to do for this Olympic event. For a few days in advance, prepare for the meet with a workout called the Semans Stop-Start Method. Begin by manipulating yourself up to a "light-duty" erection. Then consciously let it fade. Next, massage yourself into a second, fuller erection, and forfeit that one too. Finally, get yourself completely erect and let your member stretch out to its full length (after first clearing away adjacent furniture, of course). Stroke to the moment of inevitability, taking careful notice of how it feels, then let it fly. Why all the trouble? Because we've heard that this routine teaches you where your point of no return is so you know when to back off during the actual marathon. That, friend, is the key to stamina.

Let's move on to the heat itself. The first thing you can do to run out the clock is loiter during foreplay. Try using your head—literally. A lot of guys tire out quickly while performing oral sex. For endurance, stick your tongue straight out and close your mouth around it. Then swivel your entire head while keeping your tongue still. It'll save your tongue by putting the brunt of the work on your neck muscles.

There are a couple of additional tricks for lasting longer during intercourse too. Change positions several times, for starters. Each time you do, you delay ejaculation a little bit more. You may also want to turn to the scissors—a position where your partner lies on her back while you lie on your side, facing her. One of her legs goes between yours and the other goes up in the air, supported by your arm. You enter her from the side. It's the least stimulating position known to man. That doesn't mean it feels bad, it just means you're likely to hold on longer before crossing the finish line.

Finally, remember that it ain't over until the fat lady sings—or at least falls asleep. (Note: This applies to slim women as well.) Keep kissing, nuzzling, caressing, and even softly licking her until she drifts off. You win.

Also see: afterplay, foreplay, masturbation, orgasm—delayed

marijuana

True, the relaxed, feel-good effects of piping some reefer may help put you in the mood for sex, not to mention heighten the whole sexual experience. The high may even prolong your erections. But the negative effects far outweigh the positives. Studies show that smoking pot on a regular basis can quickly make your sex life go to pot, even if you're a 20-something stud. One New York City pharmacist found that 10 percent of young men who had smoked marijuana at least 4 days a week for 6 months were completely impotent.

Weed can not only wilt your willy but also make making a baby really tough. While we're all for try, try again, at some point we'd like to actually succeed at planting our seed. Pot attacks fertility in a couple of ways. First, it can decrease testosterone levels, which in turn lowers sperm count and sex drive. Research has shown that weed may also damage sperm, making them unable to fertilize an egg. (Sharing doobies with your woman, by the way, can do double damage: Pot reduces her fertility as well, perhaps by inhibiting ovulation.)

Also see: drugs, infertility

marriage

Don't believe the doom and gloom coming from some misguided quarters of the population. Guys in barrooms and

M

holier-than-thou preachers love to disparage the state of American wedlock. But two Harris polls beg to differ: Of the 1,000 polled each time, more than 95 percent of those who were married said they felt good about their marriages. Less than 5 percent said otherwise.

And some researchers believe that men, particularly, are better off married than single. Wedded guys have longer lives, better health, and higher earnings than single men. More to the point of this book, they also have more gratifying sex lives. For one thing, they have sex more often than bachelors, simply because there's always a woman right there next to them in bed. And all that boot knocking may actually be behind some of marriage's other benefits, since having sex on a regular basis contributes to a healthier prostate, better-quality sperm, less stress, less chance of becoming impotent, and an expanded sense of well-being.

This is not to say that the marital bed is a bed of roses. If you honor your marriage vows, it's always the same woman right there next to you, and familiarity and routine can be the death of sex. This is due in part to a psychological phenomenon called sensory adaptation. You know what it is, even if you haven't heard the term before. It's when a stimulus that is constant and unchanging simply begins to disappear over time. Like when you jump into a cold lake: Eventually, it doesn't feel so chilly. Or when you live next to a pulp mill: After a while, you don't notice that your neighborhood smells like a dog fart. The entire human nervous system evolved to notice change and contrast in the world and to ignore nonessential background noise.

Since the average couple beds each other some 2,640 times over the course of a 25-year marriage, it's a challenge of the highest order to keep things full of change and contrast for that many rounds of nuptial nookie. Your wife becomes white noise, bursting back into your sensory awareness only when she takes off her ratty old nightshirt and puts on that skimpy, hot-pink number.

So go buy her an electric-blue number and a majestic-purple number—and pick up a pair of silky black skivvies for yourself. Set up a pseudocampsite in the middle of the living room once in a while. Encourage her to style her hair differently now and then (instead of griping when she comes home with a new hairdo). Go down on her while she's talking on the phone to a telemarketer. (Did a woman ever have a better reason for brushing off a nuisance call?) Do all these things and more to keep your conjugal union intense, to keep it varied, and to make sure your senses don't have a chance to fatigue.

Throughout this book, there are lots of other tips and suggestions to help you. Keep reading and put our advice to good use. Otherwise, you may find yourself in one of the 40 to 50 percent of marriages that end in divorce.

Also see: affairs, appointments, boredom, commitment, courtship, divorce—issues that lead to, extramarital sex, frequency, guilt, kids, mail-order brides, ménage à trois, monogamy, monotony, piercing, polygamy, remarriage, romance, routines, trust—rebuilding, wife's best friend

marriage—lack of sex in

First the days trickle by. Before you know it, they've become weeks. Surely they can't become months? Sadly, they can and sometimes do. And the thought occurs to you: Nothing is permanent but woe.

Such is the life of a man in a near-sexless marriage. How you got there is anyone's guess. Maybe she has some deep-seated aversions to sex that she was able to hide in the courting stage. Maybe she's just tired—worn out from work, housekeeping, and childrearing. At this point, you don't care what the reason is. All you know is that you're not getting any.

Your desire remains mountainous. It smacks you when you catch a glimpse of her exiting the shower, when you kiss her goodbye a touch longer than usual, when you briefly snuggle up together in those moments before sleep. And, man, it stings when she shoots down your advances.

Your first challenge is to avoid getting surly. We know how difficult that can be when you feel cheated, trapped in a marriage with someone who makes you feel ugly every time she shrugs you off. But here's the problem: If you get angry and bitter, you reinforce her negative feelings about sex. And you create even worse odds of her accepting your advances next time.

You need to strike a bargain with her. Tell her without rancor that you dearly need to feel that you're still a functioning man. Ask her if she'd mind setting aside 5 to 10 minutes to lend a hand. Or a mouth. What you're after here is anything but intercourse.

This will accomplish two things: By nixing intercourse, it relieves her of the need to feel sexually aroused and participate more actively. Also, it goes a long way toward satisfying your need to have sexual contact with your wife. Plus, every once in a while, seeing you get excited will make her hot, and she might join in. (That's gravy; don't assume it's a given.)

Our advice here is by no means comprehensive, nor is it the answer that will solve your problem long-term. It's merely a stop-gap measure until you both discover and deal with the underlying cause, which will require some work and understanding on both of your parts. The fact is, there are many reasons why a marriage may suffer from sexual drought—

M

Hot Dates **1957** The U.S. Supreme Court ruled that for a work to be obscene, it had to be "utterly without redeeming social importance." Prior to this ruling, any work depicting sex could be considered obscene.

continued from page 182

Holmes, who rose to fame in the 1970s. When erect, his penis was estimated at anywhere from 12½ to 15 inches in length. Holmes himself said it was "**bigger than a pay phone, smaller than a Cadillac.**" (We wonder if that would include the mid-sized Catera.) Holmes was said to have had sex with 14,000 women in a career that spanned some 2,000 porn shorts and features, including gay films. He died of AIDS in 1988.

LEGAL BRIEFS
A man in West Virginia was sentenced to 90 days in jail after pleading guilty to a misdemeanor battery charge for sneaking into a

True or Phallus?
The Barbie doll was modeled after a German sex doll.

BAWDY BALLADS "Nobody Does It Better," *Carly Simon*

continued on page 194

and some of those reasons may even lie with you. If your sex life doesn't improve and you're still going crazy, ask your wife to go with you to therapy. If she won't go with you, go alone.

Also see: abstinence, boredom, frequency, monotony, rejection—sexual, romance, sex drive, travel—returning from, withholding

marriage—open

In the 1970s, this term captured the Me Generation's emphasis on pleasure. It refers to a situation wherein spouses allow themselves the option of having sex with people to whom they don't happen to be married.

How does this differ from adultery? Both spouses have full knowledge of their partner's escapades—no secret midnight phone calls or immediate showers upon returning from "working late." You may think that jealousy would tear such marriages apart, but statistics seem to tell a different story. One small study published in 1986 concluded that couples in open marriages were no more likely to divorce than were couples in traditional, sexually exclusive unions. Open marriages that did break up were those that became open only in an effort to "save" already-troubled relationships (an interesting take on the old "I think we should see other people" line). People with defunct open marriages almost always blamed their divorces on issues other than extramarital sex.

For a couple who are able to buck the usual expectations of sexual exclusivity in wedlock and who have a solid emotional bond, an open marriage seems to be a way to satisfy their desire for occasional other partners without having to lie and skulk around in secret. They value honesty, openness, and sexual diversity more than monogamy.

Also see: affairs, divorce—issues that lead to, extramarital sex, jealousy, ménage à trois, monogamy

marriage proposal

Back in 1952—in other words, before the sexual revolution and the women's liberation movement—a Gallup poll asked married couples whether the husband or the wife had popped the question. The job had fallen to men 82 percent of the time. Only 9 percent of women had asked to be betrothed. (In case you were wondering, the remaining 9 percent arrived at the decision together.)

Fast-forward past the above-mentioned societal events to 1997, when Gallup asked the same question again. And the result was . . . drumroll, please! . . . identical. Despite all the lip service given to equality in relationships, proposing marriage is still very much a man's job.

So you may as well be good at it. And, really, a well-considered proposal can be a lot of fun for you too. It's the first step in the grand adventure of your life together. If you treat it as such, you'll have a timeless story to share with your friends, your families, and someday, your own kids.

Since it's the most important question you'll ever ask (except for "You *are* on the Pill, right?"), put some real thought and effort into planning it. There's nothing wrong with the old-fashioned, get-down-on-your-knee "Will you marry me?" But if you're looking for a real tell-it-to-the-grandkids sort of experience,

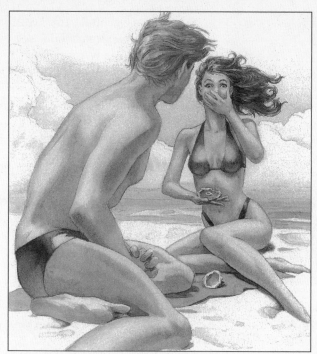

sexual advances. To the police, a masher is a guy who masturbates in public or otherwise sexually harasses women.

How will you know if you're coming off as a masher? Well, in the latter case, you'll have your penis in your hand and there'll be a busload of shocked theater-going blue hairs in front of you. The other case is more complicated. Here are some signs that she's not buying what you're trying too hard to sell.

• She stops smiling or looking you in the eye.

• She crosses her arms or legs.

• She orients her body away from you, or even starts moving away from you.

• She pulls a .357 Magnum out of her purse and fires a warning shot between your knees.

If you see more than one of these behaviors, back off and go read our entry on *flirtation.*

Also see: begging, clumsiness, communication—nonverbal, desperate, exhibitionism, onanism, opening line, paraphilias, pickup lines, rejection—romantic, rejection—sexual, sex offenders, shyness, unwanted advances

consider individualizing the proposal. If she's a scuba diver, propose underwater with your waterproof pen and pad. If she's a knitter, knit a scarf with your proposal on it—even if it looks like hell.

To really impress her, do something that she knows makes you uncomfortable. If you hate the limelight, make your proposal very public. Note, though, that the reverse doesn't hold true: If *she's* shy, *don't* flash her picture on the JumboTron while you get down on one knee. This is not the time to push her limits. You'll have a whole lifetime to do that.

Also see: romance, surprises

masher

There are two meanings of this word, neither of them flattering. In a social context, a masher is a guy who makes painfully awkward or aggressive romantic and

massage

There are tons of books out there on how to give a massage. It's a field of study all on its own. Our advice for you is not so much how to do it but that you *should* do it. One survey of more than 2,000 women asked what was guaranteed to turn them on. Massages came in a very close second, losing out

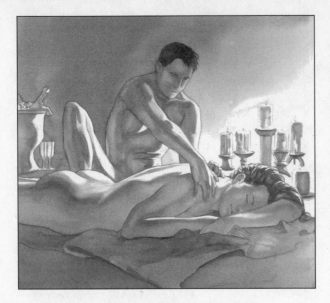

M

Leave her genitals for last. Let the momentum build so she's already ready to explode by the time your fingers hit her trigger.

If she's fast asleep by the time you get to her nether lands, let her simply bask in the afterglow. We promise that she'll thank you later.

Also see: back, body oils, brothels/bordellos, cramps—leg, feel up, G-spot, john, labia majora and minora, manual stimulation, mons pubis, performance anxiety, scents, skin, sweating, touch, tickling

only to the potent trifecta of candlelight, music, and a roaring fire. Imagine your chances if you combine all of the above. . . .

You don't have to be named Sven to give a passably good massage. The mere act of touching her all over goes a mighty long way. Bear in mind, too, that many men go at a massage as if they were tenderizing beef. Women don't want a physical-therapy session, so tone it down to a gentle stroke. As with intercourse, she'll let you know if she wants it harder.

Feel free to stroke her entire body, not just her back. Massage her face, hands, feet, even her scalp. Use wavy strokes rather than straight up-and-down ones. This keeps her nerve endings guessing at what's coming next, making them much more excited. And don't forget the parts of her body that rarely get touched, such as the backs of her knees and the undersides of her arms. Since they're normally ignored, a little attention will be highly stimulating.

mastectomy

Will you ever have to deal with your partner losing a breast? The sad fact is that one in eight women will have breast cancer during her lifetime. While not all of those women will undergo mastectomies, they'll still have to live with the possibility that the disease will return.

Putting aside our usual glibness, ponder for a moment the role of breasts in a woman's life. They've been objects of male attention ever since she hit puberty. They've nurtured her children, excited her partners, led her entry into every room. She's fretted over their size and whether they've aged well. They're the very essence of her womanhood. To bring it home: Can you imagine how horrifying it would be to not only learn that you have a life-threatening illness but also lose something so closely aligned with your sense of genderhood?

Whether or not she chooses breast reconstruction surgery, you're going to have to deal with the emotional fall-out. We ask you to employ your finest sense of compassion and decency. Many women worry more about how their partners will view them without breasts than about dying from an awful disease.

Do everything you possibly can, say anything you can possibly think of to re-assure her that you will always find her beautiful and sexy. Tell her that it would be impossible for *any* kind of surgery to diminish her in your eyes.

Yes, you will be caught up in grief too. Your woman's breasts have been a big part of your life. Let yourself mourn them, but remember that you come second in this situation. She needs you now like never, ever before. Be there for her.

Also see: breast cancer, breasts, hys-terectomy

Masters and Johnson

Two of the most important researchers in the field of sexuality are William H. Mas-ters, M.D., and Virginia E. Johnson, Ph.D. Say their names with due rever-ence.

The two hooked up back in the late 1950s and spent the next 10 years wiring up copulating couples in the lab and recording every shake, rattle, and roll. The result was the book *Human Sexual Response*, a classic in the field. Over the ensuing 25 years, other important books followed: *Human Sexual Inadequacy* and *Human Sexuality.*

Masters and Johnson also pioneered therapeutic remedies for premature ejac-ulation and erection problems—tech-niques that sex therapists still use. They also came up with something called co-marital therapy, in which a struggling couple is treated by two therapists—one man and one woman. This approach, which offers two professional perspec-tives and a real-life human relationship that patients can observe, is often quite effective.

The two researchers were married in 1971. Turns out that comarital therapy didn't work for them. They split in 1993 but continued to collaborate profession-ally up until Masters' death in 2001.

Also see: erection difficulties, impo-tence, premature ejaculation, sensate focus, sex research, sex therapy, sexual revolution, spectatoring

masturbation

As young men, we learned to toggle our switches in secret. We hid behind locked bathroom doors or waited impatiently until we had the house to ourselves. Then there was that one time when Mom walked in on us, scarring us for life. . . .

Despite our guilty furtiveness, we still manage to free willy on a regular basis: About half of all men, married or not, admit to masturbating once a week or more. Women aren't far behind: 45 per-cent say that they take a trip down south at least once a month.

We wouldn't presume to tell you how to masturbate; surely you've mastered the art by now. What we *would* like you to consider is coming out of the closet. Or garden shed, or whatever other locale you've chosen for your surreptitious pleasure.

Imagine how liberating and sexy it would be to masturbate openly in front of your partner: You'd take what had been a guilty secret these many years, bring it out into the open, and embrace it, together. Many women find it highly arousing when a man is that comfortable with his sexuality. It also cracks the door open for her to be more revealing of herself with you.

Apropos of which, encourage her to allow you access as she masturbates. You'll get a front-row seat for the best possible lesson on how to manually stimulate her. Watch what she does, and copy it next time it's your turn to play with her.

Note, though, that autostimulation is not something you do with someone you've just met: That's not erotic. It's just downright creepy.

Also see: begging, compulsive behavior, manual stimulation, masher, marathon, onanism, phallic, premature ejaculation, puberty, religion, road erection, travel—loneliness during, vibrating sleeve, vibrator

matchmaking services

Back when divorce was still a source of shame and dishonor, Jewish families usually turned to a *shadkhan* to find spouses for their children (hence, that annoyingly catchy "Matchmaker" song from *Fiddler on the Roof*). The *shadkhan* ferreted out the personal strengths and weaknesses of each potential mate so that all couples were as compatible as possible. For their services, *shadkhanim* were paid a percentage of the brides' dowries.

Sadly, wherever there's good money to be made, a shady underbelly appears. The ranks of matchmakers who were interested mostly in turning a profit began to swell. And so the profession was sullied.

That stigma endures. Many of us see matchmaking services as solely for the desperate, the gruesome-looking, the chronically unemployed, the losers of the world. That perception is overly pessimistic. What such services do is simple: They weed out potential dates that pose a high probability of driving you to drink—or to drink more than you would normally drink, anyway.

You want kids? They won't match you with anyone who doesn't. You dream of taking a year off to sail around the world? They won't set you up with someone who can't leave dry land without barfing. You think the best things in life are free? They'll exclude women who spend every spare moment at the mall. Do you have any idea how many random, pointless dates it would take to rule out these incompatible females by yourself? Well, okay, you probably do.

The service you choose can cost anywhere from a few hundred bucks to several grand. (We're not talking about personal ads here, which are often a matter of only a few dollars.) The most comprehensive type is known as an introduction service. It's for people looking for long-haul partners. Others, including video- and computer-dating services, are geared more toward casual daters.

Alas, like the *shadkhanim* of ill repute, there are those who want to fleece you by preying on your loneliness or boredom. Here's what to ask.

• How long have you been in business?

• How many of your clients are in my age range—and how many are women?

• What is your rate of success?

• How do you define success?

• What are the fees, and what do they include?

• How many matches do you promise and over what period of time?

- Who owns the service, and what is his or her background?

If you find yourself on the receiving end of a hard sell and end up getting pressured into signing up, check with your state's consumer-protection agency. Some states allow you to cancel a contract like this within 3 days of initiating it.

Also see: blind date, dating, first time with a lover, Internet dating, meeting women, personal ads, singles scene

mating

The next time a woman blows you off at a club, don't take it personally—unless you haven't brushed your teeth since the Carter administration. The dating rules, rituals, procedures, and frustrations that we regard as unique to humans are, in fact, hassles that our brothers in the animal kingdom have been dealing with since, well, forever.

All the pageantry surrounding mating has a purpose beyond just confusing us to the point of crushing beer cans against our foreheads. Due to their smaller size and more limited strength, females of most species are more vulnerable than males, especially during copulation. Toss in the fact that most males are especially aggressive when they're hunting for mates, and you can understand why females may be a little wary of males in general. Mating rituals serve to reduce that mistrust and hostility. They slow things down long enough for a female to decide whether she really wants to mate with you and, more important, whether it's safe to do so. Sobering, huh?

So study the human mating game. Learn the social skills you need to charm women and put them at ease

around you. We've peppered head-start lessons throughout this book. But keep a supply of empty beer cans handy, just in case.

Also see: animals, courtship, dating, desperate, no, rejection—sexual, rituals, signals, unwanted advances

media

There's a phenomenon in psychology known as the validity effect. It's been around a while. The Nazis called it the Big Lie.

Basically, the validity effect says that if you repeat even the basest untruths on a grand scale and with great frequency, eventually people will believe you. Advertisers know this. That's why everywhere you look, you see ads for products promising eternal youth, and happiness in a soda can.

So what does that have to do with sex? A great deal. Have you watched a movie lately, seen a prime time TV show, skimmed a magazine, flipped through a newspaper? Of course you have. And in the process, you've been bombarded with our culture's manufactured ideals of women and sex, among other things.

Women take these messages to heart. Again and again, they see scrawny models juxtaposed with weight-loss ads. They see hair dyes, body creams, cellulite-removal goo, vaginal deodorant spray, and endless racks of clothes in a size four.

Understand why she might be reluctant to show you her body? Everywhere she looks, she's being told she doesn't measure up. She has flabby thighs, a too-small bust, the wrong color hair. She's ashamed of the way she carries herself, the way her teeth look when she smiles, the way she smells, for God's sake. That's a hell of a burden to bear over the course of a lifetime.

Sadly, there's not much you can do to stop these media messages, unless you're Ted Turner. And if you are Ted, we have one message for you: Stop messing with women's heads. We're all paying for it in the bedroom.

If you're just a work-a-day Joe, there *is* something you can do for your woman on a personal level. Understand that she's being conditioned to feel crappy about her body and sexuality. Tell her again and again that she's gorgeous. Tell her you love her womanly curves, the way her hair looks when it's mussed, her intimate smells and tastes. Maybe one day she'll believe you and accept what you say as the Big Truth. Whether or not she ever thinks that the rest of the world

finds her beautiful, at least she'll know that the one special man in her life does.

Also see: beauty, beefcake, body image, French, relaxation, sex symbols

medications

Something is wreaking havoc in the sex lives of men everywhere—and it's not the National Organization for Women. It's medications.

There are well over 100 different types of medications that can foul up your frolicking. Some wilt erections. Others zap desire. Still others delay or inhibit ejaculation. And some freaky ones cause retrograde ejaculation—a condition where your semen ends up in your bladder.

Among the culprits: antidepressants such as Prozac (fluoxetine) and Paxil (paroxetine), ulcer pills such as Tagamet

Hot Dates 1960 The FDA approved the first oral contraceptive and, in doing so, set off a 20-year sexual revolution. By 1966, six million women were taking the Pill.

continued from page 187

Answer:
True. She was a likeness of Lilli, a German doll made in the 1950s. The doll, in turn, had evolved from a 1952 German cartoon character also named Lilli, who was a gold-digging trollop. Hmmm. Like mother, like daughter?

house and licking a woman's leg while she and her hubby slept. **The woman said when she awoke she felt "something wet"** on her leg. Her husband then awoke and chased the man out a bedroom window.

Seemed like a Good Idea at the Time. . .
Never let it be said that Madison Avenue spares any effort in its pursuit of bad taste. In the 1950s, a print ad showed **a short-skirted Native American woman rising from a makeshift**

hammock fashioned from a bedsheet. In the hammock lay a fatigued Native American man. The caption: A BUCK WELL SPENT ON A SPRINGMAID SHEET.

Foreign Affairs
This practice has long been out of fashion, but at one time in Thailand and Myanmar (formerly Burma), men walked around with as many as **a dozen metal bells—some as big as chicken eggs—placed under the skin of their penises**. Better than a gold watch was to receive from the

BAWDY BALLADS "I'd Love to Lay You Down," *Conway Twitty*

continued on page 203

(cimetidine), cholesterol drugs such as Lipitor (atorvastatin), drugs for lowering blood pressure or preventing seizures, even anti-inflammatory drugs such as Motrin (ibuprofen). And that's just a sampling.

Here's the double whammy: After a drug has done a number on them in bed once, a lot of guys worry that it'll happen again: They end up with performance anxiety and drooping danglers.

Fight back! Start by asking your doc for a different prescription. If our medical system is nothing else, it's flexible. Chances are excellent that there's another drug that won't get you down. In the unlikely event that there's no alternate drug, ask about trimming the dosage. Sometimes this does the trick. In other cases, your body gradually adapts to the medication and erection problems fade away. You can also fight fire with fire by turning to erection-enhancing pills such as Viagra (sildenafil).

But you know one of the best courses of action? Modify your lifestyle. Specifically, exercise, eat right, and relax. Dropping pounds through proper nutrition and moderate exercise lowers cholesterol, shaves off blood pressure points, and even lifts depression. And reducing the stress in your life goes a long way toward fixing what ails you. Result? Check with your doctor; you may not need a lot of those medications anymore. The only one who loses out is your pharmacist . . . and he's got a store full of medications to lift his own sagging spirits.

Also see: contraception, depression, drugs, erection difficulties, erection—firmer, finasteride, injuries, mail-order medications, papaverine, Prozac, retrograde ejaculation, sex drive, sickness, sperm count, STDs, stress, supplements, testosterone replacement therapy, urologist, vaginal moisture

meeting women

When looking for a woman, you do all the (supposedly) right things. You frequent the nightclubs, chat up the tight-bodies at the gym, and even let your mom set you up on blind dates. Yet the best opportunity for hooking up with a compatible mate may come along in a chance encounter: You spy an amazing woman in a public place and can't keep your eyes off her. A quick finger check reveals no glittering rings. So, naturally, you do nothing. You let the moment slip by. You just stand there and, in an instant, your potential soul mate walks out the sliding door . . . crosses the parking lot . . . puts her groceries in the trunk . . . starts her car . . . and drives away, never to be seen again.

We know; we've done it ourselves, many times. By the time you scan your brain for something to say and pluck up the courage to act, the moment has passed. An old adage tells us that luck favors those who are prepared. So be a Boy Scout.

That means that the most important thing to do when running into the supermarket is simply appear presentable. You don't have to put on a top hat and tails; just look clean. Otherwise, though you're a wonderful guy, she may not be able to get past the fact that your hairy nipple is poking through the tear in your oil-caked sweatshirt. Also make it a habit to run a comb through your hair before leaving the house.

When you do approach her, give up on trying to sound witty, clever, and erudite. You'll freeze up or sound rehearsed. Say something open-ended and matter-of-fact.

M

If you're in the cereal aisle: "It's hard to find cereal that's good for you yet doesn't taste like sawdust." If she responds with a smile and a comment, extend your hand and say, "Hi, my name is Bruno." (Do this only if your name is Bruno.)

Still too complicated? Try, "I was trying to think of a great way to start a conversation with you, but I couldn't. So I thought I'd just say hello." She'll most likely appreciate the no-bull approach.

If the two of you hit it off and she seems interested, offer her your business card or e-mail address. Don't ask for her number; she's not likely to feel comfortable giving it out to a guy she just met. Count it as a plus if she offers up her e-mail address. From there on out, it's up to her.

Also see: bars, clumsiness, desperate, matchmaking services, ogling, opening line, pickup lines, singles scene

ménage à trois

A French phrase that literally translates into "household of three." In the strictest sense, it describes a living arrangement between a married couple and an extra man or woman who has a sexual relationship with one of the spouses. More commonly, it refers to a threesome.

While a ménage à trois is a favorite fantasy of many men (and women), in practice it's a different story. The Kinsey Institute for Research in Sex, Gender, and Reproduction, in Bloomington, Indiana, says that only about 3 percent of married men and 1 percent of married women have had sex with one other partner while the spouse was present. And the majority of those folks said that they've done it only once.

If you are thinking of having a ménage à trois, remember that it is never something you want to spring on your partner or decide to do when both of you are drunk or stoned. It requires serious discussion to avoid any morning-after regrets.

Also see: extramarital sex, French, group sex, Kinsey, marriage—open, polygamy, sloppy seconds, threesome

menopause—hers

Part of our mission in this book is to dispel myths, fables, and misconceptions. And if there's one thing that needs correction above all others, it's likely the swirling misinformation surrounding female menopause.

Perhaps you view your partner's approaching menopause with dread. You expect her to transform from a vibrant, erotic woman into an irritable, asexual shrew. She's probably fearing the same thing, especially if she's between the ages of 45 and 55, the years of typical menopause onset.

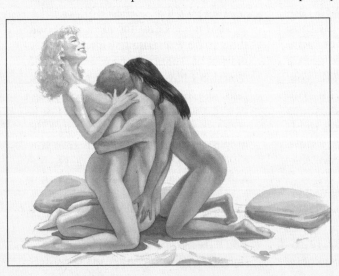

Menopause is exactly what the word suggests: Her menstruation stops and her ovaries cease to produce estrogen and progesterone, crucial female hormones involved in pregnancy and other functions. During this time, she *is* very likely to have physical symptoms, most notably the hot flashes of lore, as her vascular system adjusts to the absence of those hormones.

But the commonly held view that she'll be depressed, irrational, and devoid of sexual interest simply doesn't hold up. In a survey of more than 8,000 women, most viewed menopause as either a neutral experience or a positive one—especially when they considered that they no longer had to worry about getting pregnant or having periods.

In fact, this time of life is actually the happiest for many American women. Their incomes have often reached an all-time high, the kids are out of the house, and they've struck a nice balance between intimacy needs and the desire to be somewhat autonomous. And as you know if you share your home with a member of the fairer sex, a woman's happiness goes a long way toward ensuring her man's happiness.

There is, though, an underbelly of discontent to menopause. It is from there that the negative mutterings have spread. For about 10 percent of women, menopause is atypically harsh. They suffer with bouts of depression, lack of sexual desire, and difficulties surrounding their perceived loss of femininity. This is particularly prevalent among women who have undergone surgically induced menopause. That's when their ovaries, uterus, or both have been removed.

All is not necessarily lost for these women. Studies have shown that es-trogen replacement therapy can help. Research has also shown that testosterone replacement therapy often can boost the libidos of women who no longer have ovaries. Yes, testosterone plays an important sexual function in women too.

Also see: biological clock, empty-nest syndrome, estrogen, fertility, hysterectomy, lubrication, progesterone, progestin, sex drive, testosterone replacement therapy, young men/older women

menopause—yours

Let's admit it. Hell, let's not only admit it but praise the scrotal gods of manhood: Being a guy is a sweet deal. We don't bleed out of our crotches every month. We don't need to find someone else to open pickle jars. We're never faced with the challenge of pushing small human beings out of our bodies. And we don't go through menopause.

Or do we? Well, no, we don't go through a female-style menopause. Hers is relatively abrupt and dramatic. Ours is slower than that, more like a fungus that's been growing unnoticed between our toes for a while, but it is just as real. One day, you just start feeling vaguely uncomfortable, though it's been sowing its spores for years. Soon, you're downright ill at ease.

Blame it, in part, on your dwindling supply of testosterone. Starting in your 30s, the hormone of manhood makes itself ever more scarce. Because it happens slowly, you don't really notice. But by the time you hit your late 40s or early 50s, that sense of uneasiness is blossoming. Your energy levels are dropping. Depression may be darkening your door. Your sex drive has driven off. Combine

M

that with the psychological and social changes in an aging man's life and you've got male menopause.

Or, more accurately, andropause.

Those psychological and social changes we mentioned? They're things like realizing you're not as mentally sharp as you used to be. And finding out that it's tougher to turn a young woman's head. It's about understanding that immortality is not the birthright you thought it to be—and with that comes the desperate thought that time is running out.

That's andropause—also known as ADAM, or androgen decline in the aging male. Either way, it sucks. In part, it's the midlife crisis of lore. It's the extended dark night of the soul. It's a personal and physical reassessment that can take years to complete.

In many cases, testosterone replacement therapy can help. Not all doctors recognize andropause as a legitimate condition, so ask around for a urologist who does. He should measure your testosterone levels and ask you about other symptoms. He may even refer you to a psychologist or psychiatrist. Take his advice and go.

Also see: aging, fertility, midlife crisis, sex drive, testosterone replacement therapy, urologist, young women/ older men

More than a few women agree. When sex researcher Shere Hite asked women about it in *The Hite Report: A Nationwide Study of Female Sexuality*, of the 571 women who responded, 344 confirmed that the one time of the month when they experienced heightened sexual desire was during menstruation. The fact that pregnancy is unlikely (but, be warned, by no means impossible) during their periods leaves many women free of anxiety and ready to make love with abandon. Fluctuating hormones may also give rise to lusty feelings.

Even so, it's possible that your woman is worried about grossing you out and won't bring up period sex unless you break the ice. So let her know you're not put off by the additional mess (an old towel or two on the bed will take care of any leakage). Bear in mind that the amount of blood you'll have to contend with varies according to which day of her cycle you're in. Sometimes you'll barely notice it, other than a mild reddish tinge to the wet spot. On the middle days of her period, expect your genitals to be pretty much blood-soaked. When you're done, an immediate, shared shower can be nice afterplay.

Also see: estrogen, horny, Norplant, ovulation, period, pituitary gland, progesterone, PMS, tampon, vaginal moisture

menstruation

A woman spends a total of almost 7 years of her life menstruating (thankfully, not all at once), pounding through about 7,500 tampons along the way. That's a lot of time that, by some traditional standards, is sexually off-limits. Seems like a waste, doesn't it?

micropenis

Two words we'd never dream of putting together unless maybe we were trying to get a buddy's attention in a crowded barroom. ("Yo, Micropenis! You want another microbrew?!")

Medically speaking, *micropenis* is no laughing matter. It's the term for—and this may not shock you—an extremely small penis. By that we mean an adult length of 3½ inches or less when erect. Luckily, it's a rare condition. A "normal" penis measures 2½ to 4 inches long when flaccid, and 5 to 7 inches when erect.

Because the condition is congenital (that is, present at birth), you needn't worry that your redwood may one day suddenly shrink without warning. Boys born with the trait usually have a chromosomal defect or a hormonal deficiency and are treated at an early age with hormone supplements.

Also see: hermaphrodite, hung, hypnosis and penis enlargement, packing, penile enlargement, size—penis

microphilia

One of the rarer fetishes, microphilia is a sexual obsession with tiny women. We're talking very tiny women: 4 to 6 inches tall. Obviously, microphiles don't find real women this size, but they do collect photos doctored to portray women sitting in the palm of someone's hand. (These guys must love King Kong movies.)

There are also computer-generated images and, uh, short films along the same theme. Some of the images are reminiscent of stripped-down Barbie dolls come to life. Coincidence? Probably not.

Also see: abnormal, compulsive behavior, fetish, kinky

midlife crisis

It's as inevitable as bad coffee from a gas station: You will go through a midlife transition. But will you go through a midlife *crisis*? Will you trade in the

family sedan for a ragtop? Will you blow your savings on a hair transplant and a 20-year-old?

Good questions. Fortunately, there are some early omens that you may be on the cusp of an existential meltdown.

• One of the telltale feelings is a sense of having been cheated by life. You've scratched and clawed your way to financial and job security just to look back and say, "I worked my ass off for *this*?" You may also find yourself increasingly bored, pushing papers around on your desk, unable to decide whether to start on the task at hand or scratch your testicles for a few extra minutes. The truth is, it's not really boredom; you're losing your ability to give a damn.

• Another warning sign is your wife. Specifically, the fact that she has suddenly turned into a crone—in your mind, anyway. News flash: She's not what's really bothering you. She's just a reflection of your own worries about aging.

• Keep an eye out, too, for a tendency to take impulsive, unusual risks with money. If you're suddenly hungering to start up a chain of tattoo parlors or chuck it all to become an Outward Bound instructor, you may have trouble brewing.

• A few other precursors of problems: You hit the hooch more often. Your last child leaves home, bringing on a heavy-duty sense of emptiness. Or you lose a parent, and you realize that you're no longer somebody's kid. ("You mean *I'm* the adult now?") You make major style changes, on the order of acquiring a ponytail and an earring.

Hollywood and uncomprehending women love to make fun of men in midlife crises. For anyone in the throes of one, though, there's little reason to laugh. This is bigger than you. Get some help. Seek out a skilled therapist who has experience counseling men through this.

Also see: aging, biological clock, boredom, depression, menopause—yours, trophy wife, young women/older men

mirrors

Have you ever had sex with a full-length mirror stretched out beside you? Have you ever seen the reflection of a woman going down on you, her head bobbing in the bright, shiny glass? If not, you don't know what you're missing.

Watching yourself in a mirror is almost like starring in your own personal adult video, except without a sweaty camera operator crowding your butt. It appeals to your highly visual sense of eroticism and fulfills exhibitionist fantasies, while at the same time acting as a real turn-on for many women.

There are, unfortunately, some women who won't be very receptive. Either they're too insecure about their bodies to watch themselves or they think the mirror reduces intimacy by competing with them for your attention.

But if you share your bed with a woman who's open to the idea, you really must give the experience a whirl. If you don't want your mother to see mirrors on your ceiling, go shopping for old-fashioned upright mirrors in their own stands. Get at least two, and station them at different spots around your bed, bathtub, or '54 Chevy

flatbed. That way, you won't have to crane your neck into unnatural positions to catch a peek.

Also see: body image, exhibitionism, videos, voyeurism

missionary position

This is to sex what Wonder bread is to the sandwich: serviceable, reasonably appetizing, a little bland after repeated use. (That's not to say it can't be your favorite.) It is, of course, the traditional man-on-top-between-the-woman's-legs position.

In case Regis asks you on nationwide television someday, here's the origin of the term: European conquerors forbade their Polynesian colonial charges from having sex in any other fashion, deeming all other positions barbaric and pagan. It does have a bit of the conquering theme to it, what with the man on top, in control.

But it can also be a very intimate, loving position. It allows you to gaze into her eyes and kiss her freely. It can be very relaxing for her since you're often the one doing most of the work.

To spice things up, try placing your legs to the outsides of hers. This forces

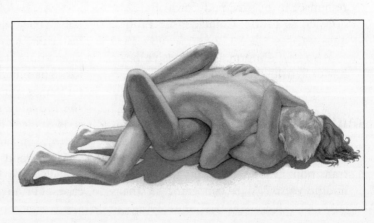

you higher up on her pelvis and puts you in greater contact with her clitoris. Or suggest that she hook her ankles over your shoulders. This variation allows you deeper inside her and stimulates the back wall of her vagina. Go easy here; it can be painful if you propel yourself like a battering ram.

The missionary position is not for all men, all the time. Especially if you've been watching your bellies burgeon over the years, having your gut pressing down on hers is far from erotic for either of you.

Also see: boredom, eye contact, routines, standing positions, water beds

moaning

There are only two good reasons for a man to moan. The first is if someone is stamping unmercifully on his left one. The second is far more enjoyable. (You'll notice, incidentally, that both instances involve the family jewels. Maybe women are right about us, after all.)

One of the many things that women can't understand about men is how we can be so quiet during sex. For them, there's an unseen connection between labia and larynx, with one necessarily engaging the other. So when we fail to emote so much as a paltry peep, they wonder and worry if we're having a good time. That's where a well-placed moan comes in. And it's a thing of beauty, really. A low, almost animalistic moan says as much in pure, unfettered sound as you could say in dozens of well-considered words.

It's also a great way to let her know she's doing what you like. For example, your moans can tell her that she's giving you head just the way you want it. Stop

when she slips into a technique that you're less fond of. And let fly another moan when she reverts to the better way of doings things. She'll remember that and make use of the knowledge next time.

Also see: communication—nonverbal, grunting, talking dirty, whispering

money

While it can't buy love, it *can* buy sex, and plenty of guys are digging into their wallets. About 18 million American men have forked out cash for sex. That number soars much higher if you count expensive dinners and presents as payment for the sex that men hoped would follow.

More than half of men who pay to poke do so on only an occasional basis, while 31 percent of middle-income men make it a habit. The greatest number of sex buyers by far are middle-age, married white guys. (All taking their new Viagra prescriptions for a spin, no doubt.) On the flip side, only about five million women have had sex for money.

Also see: escort service, gigolo, john, prostitution, sex tours and resorts, size—wallet

monilia

An old-fashioned term for *Candida*, the fungus that causes yeast infections. For more information on libidinous leavening, wander on over to the entry on *yeast infection.*

monogamy

Let us put to rest, once and for all, the endless debate over whether human beings are naturally monogamous: Yes, we are. And no, we aren't.

There. Don't you feel better?

The contradiction remains because there are two kinds of monogamy. The first, social monogamy, is when a bond forms between a social pair: husband and wife, boyfriend and girlfriend, goose and gander. To biologists, that's a lasting pair bond.

The second kind, genetic or sexual monogamy, is when a mister and his missus form a lasting pair bond *and* are sexually exclusive. For most of the animal kingdom, this kind of monogamy is rare. Even humans aren't *naturally* meant to be this way. (Think back to caveman times, when the future of the human race depended on the assumption that every man would sow his seed with as many women as possible.)

So, as a species, yes, we are socially monogamous. But we are not genetically monogamous—again, *as a species.* That's not to say that there aren't instances of both types of monogamy among couples. In fact, as if you hadn't noticed, there's a huge cultural drive to keep couples sexually monogamous, breaches of which have been the downfall of many a preacher, politician, and sportscaster.

To some degree, it's unfair to expect a man to be sexually limited to one woman. As a society, we encourage young men to go out and bag as much game as they can before they get married. Then we expect them to leave all that behind after the altar?

And we know you probably won't want to hear it, but don't think for a minute that this applies to men only. Many women have learned to enjoy the hunt and find it difficult to give up, even after bagging a fine 10-point buck such as yourself.

So we've really given you two important strategies to consider.

1. Accept the fact that we humans are biologically programmed to stray, and try to develop the emotional steel to deal with an affair (yours or hers) when it comes along. Or else think very carefully before committing to monogamy in the first place.

2. Realize that through tremendous mental discipline, people can transcend the limitations of their species. That's why we're not lunch for every large, furry carnivore out there, despite the fact that our bodies are pitifully equipped to defend us. Yes, you will come across powerful, hardwired urges to stray. But you can overcome them in ways that a horny tomcat never could. Your sense of values and honor will be your best friend in times like this.

Also see: affairs, boredom, commitment, lust, marriage, marriage—open, promiscuity, soul mates, variety

monotony

If your loins are no longer forever aflame for your long-time lover, it's not necessarily because she's let herself go or because you have a short attention span (though both of these things may be true). It's natural for warm-blooded animals to become less hot-blooded after they've been with only one sex partner for an extended time. This sexual cooldown is called the Coolidge effect, after an anecdote involving President Calvin Coolidge. One day, the commander-in-chief and his wife toured a farm. The first lady observed two chickens mating and asked how often the rooster got cock-a-doodle-dooed. More than a dozen times a day, the farmer informed her. "Please tell that to the president," she coyly replied. When the president was told, he asked, "Same hen every time?" No, a different female each time, said the farmer. "Tell that to Mrs. Coolidge," the president retorted.

The explanation behind the Coolidge effect is another example of male reproductive strategy. When a rooster, a politician, or a guy like you first becomes acquainted with a sexually responsive female, he's biologically driven to have sex with her frequently in order to make sure she's inseminated with his sperm. While your brain may not necessarily want her to get pregnant, your genes have their own agenda. They also want you to get a lot of other women pregnant so your DNA gets passed down to as many offspring as possible. Therefore, once you've been with one woman for a while and know that she's received a lot of your seed, you become less sexually interested in her and more interested in finding new sex partners. (Think your wife would buy that?)

Just remember, you are not a rooster, and we hope you're not a politician either. Your advanced, highly intelligent brain can override your genes and tell you not to knock up the hot FedEx delivery girl; it can also help you overcome the Coolidge effect with your old lady. So if you want to sustain your monogamous relationship, read the entry on *boredom* for tips on outsmarting sexual monotony.

Also see: animals, marriage, monogamy, sexual attraction, wandering eye, variety

mons pubis

The next time you're tempted to say, "Yes, Your Eminence," aim the comment at your woman's crotch. First of all, it's always a worthy target, we think. But it's also where you'll find the mons pubis, or

continued from page 194

king a bell he had worn in his penis and then removed for you. Uh, thanks but no thanks.

In Extremis

Nice pair of . . . cheeks: A jury awarded a former exotic dancer $30,000 after she sued the plastic surgeon who had used **breast implants to build up her buttocks**. The doctor testified that he charged the Florida woman $6,500 to put the implants in and $1,500 to remove them. He said there were no commercially available buttock implants at the time.

LEGAL BRIEFS

Valerie Solanas was one scary feminazi. A writer and prostitute, she penned the *SCUM Manifesto* (SCUM being an acronym for "Society to Cut Up Men") in 1967, contending therein that **men are "unfit even for stud service."** And that was one of the nicer things she said about us.

Consider: "To call a man an animal

True or Phallus?

The expression *peeping Tom* was coined because Thomas Jefferson was caught looking at a woman through the window of her home near the White House.

continued on page 208

"pubic eminence," a plush cushion of tissue beneath her upper pubic hair. If you're lucky enough to need it, the plural of the Latin form is *montes pubis.*

The mound makes a great resting spot for your cheek if you need a break from a heavy cunnilingus session. Also, your woman may enjoy it if you massage her mons pubis gently with the palm of your hand while you kiss her. Such kneading provides a nice, indirect clitoral sensation. A lot of guys don't realize that the love button itself takes a while to warm up, so stampeding directly there before she's ready may just feel irritating to her.

Also see: reproductive system—hers

mood

It's easy enough to tell when a woman is in the mood. She starts playing Sting albums.

But when she's not in the mood . . . That's the part we're interested in here. Too many men handle it poorly when a woman says she simply doesn't feel like it. And when guys react badly, they sabotage their chances for healthy sex lives in the future.

The worst way to handle your partner's sexual cold shoulder is to take it personally. After all, transient lack of sexual interest is rarely a sign that her lust for you has turned to loathing. Nor is it always a deliberate attempt to piss you off. She simply may not feel sexy, and the reason could have nothing to do with you. Maybe she forgot to shave her legs. Maybe she has a pimple on her butt. Too many guys fail to consider the pimple factor.

And guess what? You're not going to make her feel any more amorous by stomping around, getting belligerent, or—worst of all—whining about how she's "never" in the mood anymore. Acting that way will just build up resentment between the two of you. And resentment and desire are two of the most incompatible emotions in the world.

The best thing to do is accept her answer with an air of Zenlike inevitability. Hold her close, kiss her, and say something like, "I'll take a rain check then." Do it gracefully. Do it without bitterness. One night soon, you'll be glad you did.

Also see: aphrodisiac, appointments, arousal, atmosphere, begging, breast-feeding, horny, oral contraceptive, period, PMS, postpartum depression, Prozac, randy, rejection—sexual, romance, routines, seduction, sickness, variety, withholding

morning after

The morning after some horizontal recreation is a critical point in your relationship. The way you treat her after sex shows her how you'll treat her on a day-to-day basis. She knows this and, consciously or not, she's watching your every move. You already dazzled her last night (we'll give you the benefit of the doubt here). Now, it's time to do it again.

Note: Before you throw this book against the wall, we hasten to add that we're not suggesting you take the following approach with *every* woman you spend the night with. This is the way to woo a potential Ms. Right. For advice on making a clean getaway from Ms. Right-Last-Night, see *one-night stand.*

So: Start brewing up a love potion even before she wakes up. Sneak out from under the covers, and go make a

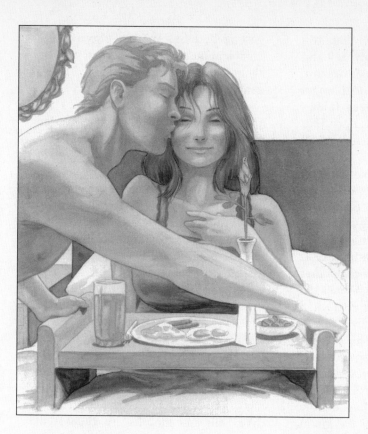

sight of a man cooking highly erotic. Indulge her.

Play footsies as you eat. Tell her how great the previous night was—trust us, she's wondering. Touch her gently every chance you get, but don't maul. After breakfast, if all goes well, you'll get a reprise of the previous night. When she finally heads home, she'll be more than ready to come back for seconds and thirds and beyond. And even years after this first special morning, these same attentive A.M. actions will be just as appreciated.

Also see: afterglow, infatuation, first time with a lover, sexual etiquette

M

pot of coffee. If there's any chocolate around, slip a piece onto the saucer. Head back to the bedroom, take a seat, and just watch her. This will probably wake her up within a few minutes. And the first thing she'll see is your baby blues gazing softly upon her. (This works just as well with brown eyes.) You have no idea how romantic it is to her that you were watching her as she slept.

Hand her the coffee, sweetened with a good-morning kiss. Tell her to relax in bed while you make breakfast. That will give her a chance to get her wits about her, freshen up, and of course, think about what a swell guy you are.

When she comes into the kitchen, make her take a seat and watch you cook. For some strange reason, women find the

morning-after pill

Before we discuss this, let's talk about the night before. You shouldn't be in this mess to start with, because part of being a man is being responsible. That means not only having some form of birth control with you but also using it. (And no, we don't mean that year-old condom you have to peel out of your wallet.) Real men do not leave contraception entirely up to their partners, especially in this day and age.

For those macho types out there who believe that it's her problem, we have three words for you: *child support payments.* And for those who have unprotected sex with a new partner who tells you she's on the Pill, we have another word, or at least an acronym: *AIDS.*

M

We'll assume, therefore, that you know your partner reasonably well and that you're in this predicament because your condom broke or her diaphragm slipped. After all, stuff happens. It happens to a lot of guys, actually: Each year in the United States, about half of all pregnancies are accidental.

You can still prevent your partner from becoming pregnant—even after the "oops"—with the emergency contraceptive known as the morning-after pill. *Morning-after* is actually a misnomer since it can be used up to 72 hours after sex.

There are three types of morning-after pills currently available. First, there's the Preven Emergency Contraceptive Kit, a regimen of pills that combines estrogen and progestin hormones. The second, known as Plan B, uses progestin-only pills. The third option involves taking a certain number of birth control pills. The dosage is different depending on the brand, so if your partner has the Pill at home, make sure that she checks with her doctor before trying this method.

All of these methods require two doses, the first within 72 hours after sex and the second 12 hours later. These pills prevent pregnancy via one or more of the following processes: keeping her ovaries from popping out an egg, preventing an existing egg from becoming fertilized, and/or stopping a fertilized egg from implanting itself in the wall of her uterus. Of the side effects reported with the morning-after pill, nausea and vomiting are the most serious, and they are far less common in women who take the progestin-only version (Plan B).

In addition to being less likely to cause adverse reactions, progestin-only pills are also better at preventing pregnancy. One study of almost 2,000 women found pro-

gestin pills to be 89 percent effective. The combination estrogen-progestin pills, on the other hand, work only about 75 percent of the time.

The sooner your partner takes the pills, the better. The effectiveness of the progestin pills, for example, jumps to 95 percent when they're taken within 24 hours of unprotected sex.

To get your hands (or your partner's) on the morning-after pill, call Planned Parenthood at (800) 230-PLAN or the national Emergency Contraception Hotline at (888) NOT-2-LATE. Or call your partner's gynecologist.

Also see: abortion, abortion pill, contraception, Pill—the

mouth

When your mother threatened to wash your mouth out with soap all those years ago, she realized two things: Soap tastes like hell, and mouths are capable of some bad, bad things. Bad in a good way, we mean.

Your mouth is one of the most supersensitive and erogenous spots on your body. A wise lover knows that the mouth of his paramour is never to be ignored. And, no, that doesn't mean you should shove your penis into it. Well, that's not the only thing it means.

Break the ice by letting her become comfortable with your own mouth. Hold her hand in yours, and kiss her fingers. Then, let her feel your teeth and tongue as you slowly draw one finger into your mouth.

Run your fingertips over her lips, parting them gently and slowly. You're testing for a reaction here. Her degree of enthusiasm about taking your finger can sometimes be a gauge of her appetite for oral sex. If she's not interested, she'll turn away or busy her mouth with kissing you.

Incidentally, even if the sucking stops with your fingers, you'll be surprised by how remarkable it feels, if you've never experienced it before.

Also see: biting, breast sucking, breath, erogenous zones, French kiss, hickey, hygiene, kiss, licking, lips, oral sex, thrush, toes, tongue, venereal disease

movies

When it comes to sexual arousal, it's been said that men respond to visual stimuli more readily than women do. For the most part, that may be true. But there's one type of visual stimulus to which women have an even *greater* response than men do: porn movies. Australian researchers found that women got a bigger adrenaline rush from watching skin flicks than did the men who were watching. (You gotta love those Aussies.)

So what will you do with that nugget of wisdom? Rent a movie, of course. But maybe not porn per se, since some women might feel obliged to prove their respectability by expressing offense at your choice of entertainment—especially if it's early in the relationship. (Besides, you don't want to risk bumping into your boss in the adult-video store. What's *he* doing there, anyway?) Since we're always thinking of your well-being, we polled top movie critics for their picks of the steamiest, sexiest mainstream flicks out there. Rent one of these classics next time you have improper thoughts on your mind.

- In *Body Heat* (1981), starring Kathleen Turner and William Hurt, watch for the ice cube scene.
- *Carnal Knowledge* (1971) stars Jack Nicholson and Ann-Margret in a tale of erotic obsession.
- *Casablanca* (1942), with Ingrid Bergman and Humphrey Bogart, is an all-time favorite study in sexual chemistry.
- *The Last Seduction* (1994) features Linda Fiorentino, Peter Berg, and a whole lot of raw, passionate sex.
- Check out *Last Tango in Paris* (1973), available in both R-rated and X-rated versions. Marlon Brando's performance is among the best work of his career.

Also see: casting couch, erotic films, lesbian, media, pornography, sex symbols, unwanted advances, videos, X-rated

multiple orgasms

You knew there had to be payback for the fact that men don't go through childbirth. Here it is: Women get to

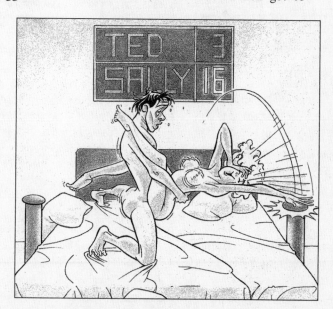

have multiple orgasms, and all we get is one—maybe two if we're lucky.

Women have this advantage because they're missing something most men have. No, not a penis—a refractory period. That's the time your body takes to recover before it can be stimulated to orgasm or ejaculation again. And as you may have noticed, that time tends to get longer as you get older. The young pup that you were may have been good for three, maybe four ejaculations on a good night. The old dog you are now is likely happy with one.

Women aren't constrained by such physical limits. Case in point: One ambitious and daring study lined up a lone willing woman with a cadre of equally willing men. The woman had intercourse with one of the men, and her orgasm was recorded by electrodes. Then she took on another guy. And then another, and another. By the time the study was all over, 50-plus men had given their best for science, and the woman had climaxed each time—and was still ready for more.

So your dilemma is this: If your woman is capable of having multiple orgasms, how do you keep up with her? You don't have to, at least not in number. There is no law that says you have to come the first time she does. Wait a while; let her enjoy herself. And if you do come, there is no law that says you have to do it again. If you're tired, let her know. If she still wants to keep going, tell her you'd enjoy watching her touch herself, or use a vibrator with her until either she's had enough or you're ready to go again.

Getting her to have more orgasms shouldn't be the goal in itself; plea-

---

Hot Dates Circa 1965 English dress designer Mary Quant popularized a new article of clothing called the miniskirt.

---

continued from page 203

Answer:

False. The term was inspired by the story of Lady Godiva, who rode naked on horseback through her town. Her husband, a local big shot, ordered citizens to stay indoors with their shutters drawn. All did except for Tom, the village voyeur.

is to flatter him; he's a machine, a walking dildo. It's often said that men use women. Use them for what? Surely not pleasure."

Solanas, who shot and nearly killed Andy Warhol, spent time in prison and mental institutions. She died in 1988, turning tricks in a seedy San Francisco hotel.

Seemed like a Good Idea at the Time

Advertisers have long linked cars and sex, of course. In the 1970s, an ad for a muffler called the SuperMuff QT showed a busty young woman wearing a bikini and standing in front of piled boxes of auto parts. The headline read STACKED AND QUIETLY WAITING JUST FOR YOU.

A second muffler ad urged readers, DO YOUR THING ON A SCATCAT COMPETITION MUFFLER. Pictured was another bikini-clad woman holding the large, phallic-shaped product.

Foreign Affairs

Some men in Borneo wear penis pins, tiny rods that are inserted though the

BAWDY BALLADS "Let's Get It On," *Marvin Gaye*

continued on page 219

suring each other and enjoying your time together should be.

Also see: afterplay, aging, female ejaculation, Kegel exercises, marathon, orgasm—delayed, refractory period, tantra

multiple partners

See: extramarital sex, group sex, monogamy, promiscuity

muscles

Stand bare-chested in front of a mirror. Now, in your mind, morph your body to the level of muscularity that you think most women prefer. Guess what? You're probably overestimating by about 20 solid pounds.

In one study, researchers recruited 200 college-age men from the United States, Austria, and France. From a stack of photos of different male body types, each man picked one photo that he thought would most appeal to women. The researchers later showed the stack to a group of young American women. Their choices overwhelmingly favored men of average build. The body that the American men thought their country-women would prefer was 15 to 20 pounds more muscular than the women's actual choices.

Does that give you a license to swill? Of course not. The body that the women preferred was still nicely in shape, just not a muscle-bound hulk. Think Mel Gibson, not Arnold Schwarzenegger. There's a reason you sat next to a bunch of sweaty guys at all those Conan movies.

Also see: abs, beefcake, bimbo, body fitness, body image, body odor as an at-tractant, body shapes, exercise, male body, PC muscle, sexual attraction, sexy, steroids, weight loss

music

When we set out to write this book, we made a conscious effort to refrain from quoting Shakespeare. But sometimes the raunchy old bard just nails it. And so it is here: "If music be the food of love," he wrote, "play on." Indeed.

Music, like coffee, comes in many flavors. The robust, hearty kind has a different effect than the tender, delicate kind. For example, researchers found that playing music louder than 90 decibels—the typical blast of sound at a rock concert or dance club—generated sensual feelings among listeners. The astute among you will realize that this is news you can use: If you want to get her in the mood, take her dancing. And of course, the dividends of dancing go way beyond the mere music; the physical contact and suggestive body moves don't hurt either.

If you want to set a more sedate, romantic mood, the opposite end of the volume dial is your best friend. Other researchers have found that soft music is much better for lowering your heart rate and kick-starting the relaxation response. So it's perfect for a leisurely meal at home, followed by a massage . . . and more.

Besides setting a mood, music also creates memories. How many times has a song or album taken you back to fond moments? Try playing her favorite music during your lovemaking. Whenever she hears those strains in the future, she'll think of you and—better yet—sex with you. If you've been in a relationship for a while, consider making a mix tape of the songs that have been the background music for your unfolding love. That kind of soundtrack, played during love-making, is sure to intensify the experience for her. And for you.

By the way, the Web site Music.com did a month-long survey near the end of 2000 on favorite music for making love. Tops on the list? The freaky-sex facilitator himself, Marvin Gaye.

Also see: atmosphere, courtship, food, mood, pornography, rave, rituals, strip-tease, underage, voice

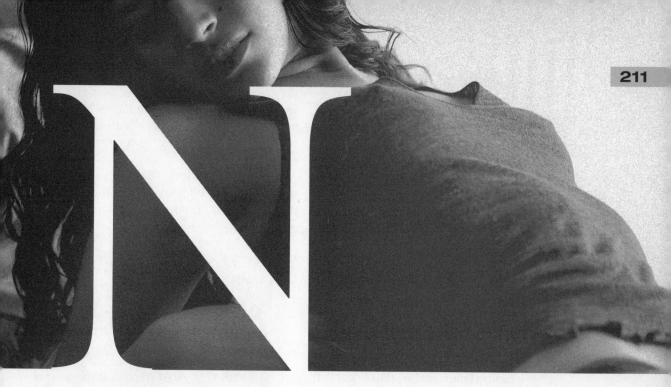

necrophilia

A sexual and emotional attraction to corpses. (Real ones. This is not the place for snide jokes about your wife's level of enthusiasm in bed.) As grim as that may sound, it's been around for a long time.

The father of written history, Herodotus, described it in the times of ancient Egypt. He told of how the bodies of noble ladies were not given to the embalmers for at least 2 days after death so that the corpses would not be violated; one presumes that the smell of a days-old corpse is enough to keep away even the most committed necrophile.

Even more troubling, on many levels, is what some soldiers did in wars of years gone by. In the book *Perverse Crimes in History*, R. E. L. Masters tells of how conquering soldiers had anal intercourse with dead and dying men on the battlefield in order to experience the rectal spasms that come with death.

As you might imagine, necrophiles tend to choose professions that allow close contact with dead bodies. That's not to say that every mortician, medical examiner, or coffin maker is some sort of perv—true necrophilia is very rare. Interestingly, necrophiles often see corpses as pure and kind, incapable of rejection and other cruel acts.

And in case you were wondering, yes, necrophilia is illegal.

Also see: compulsive behavior, fantasies, paraphilias, perversions, sex offenders, sex therapy

nipple clamps

These metal jumper-cable-like devices are sadomasochism staples (in every sense of the term). They make a powerful statement about who's in charge and who's not. For some people, that kind of head game is a major turn-on.

For those who get into this sort of thing, the arousal of being dominated combines with the clamp-induced "pain" to superheat a stimulation pot that eventually boils over into orgasm. The whole experience is short-lived, though, because after a brief time the nipples become numb and the stimulatory effects are lost. Not to mention that clamps can cause injury if they pinch too hard, are left on for too long, or pierce the skin.

As is true of most sex toys and appliances, the watchword with nipple clamps is: Never just whip 'em out and expect her to happily clamp 'em on. Talk to her first, and don't be surprised by a stern, emphatic "No thank you." After all, how much talking would it take before you agreed to let somebody put your johnson in a vise?

Also see: bondage and discipline, dominance and submission, safeword

nipples

Let's start with the question you may have asked yourself from time to time: Why the hell do *you* have them?

They happen to be leftovers from when you were a girl. Seriously. Early on in pregnancy, every fetus is female. Then, if testosterone kicks in, the wee one morphs into a boy. But the nipples have already started to take shape, so you get stuck with them.

In women, of course, nipples' most important function is to provide us with an accurate gauge of room temperature. Their vast practicality does not end there. Because of the physiological link

between her nipples and her genitals, they're a great indicator of sexual arousal. If her beams are on high while you're kissing or caressing, it's usually a sign that you've got her motor thrumming.

That physiological link we mentioned? It goes both ways. This means that time spent playing with her nipples

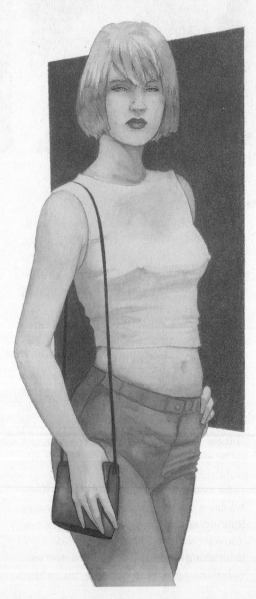

may get her even hotter down below. Some women can even have an orgasm simply from nipple stimulation.

Meanwhile, don't give up entirely on your own set. They do contain erectile tissue, after all. If you haven't already, ask your partner to spend a few moments licking, sucking, and gently tweaking them. It can be surprisingly hot. You can even try stroking them yourself during sex or while going it solo.

By the way, did we mention that women's nipples are also useful for suckling babies?

Also see: breastfeeding, breasts, piercing, size—breasts, vagina, witch's milk

no

It's doubtful that any other combination of two letters ever caused so much misery. Men are well familiar with the word *no*. We hear it when we curiously grab our penises as children. We hear it when we awkwardly ask girls to dance in junior high. We hear it when we bring up oral sex, anal sex, group sex, or sometimes even plain old missionary sex. It gets tiresome, doesn't it?

Unfortunately, we hear it so often that we tend to get a tad bitter about it. And then we act badly. We wheedle, whine, and even try to browbeat our women into changing their minds. Some guys go around stamping their feet and kicking things.

Stop stomping around long enough to put the shoe on the other foot. Let's suppose your wife asks you to tighten the washing machine hose that's been leaking for the past month. You say no, you just want to take it easy today. So then she proceeds to harangue you for being lazy. Now how willing are you to

get out that wrench? You're resentful and irritated, and the whole issue has become a battle. That's exactly how she'll feel if you continue to nag her when she doesn't feel like having sex.

One measure of a man can be found in how he handles adversity. Do you respond with pettiness or grace? When your partner says no to sex (in any of its various permutations) do you allow her to be her own person, complete with whatever boundaries and shortcomings she may have, or do you try to force your own wants on her?

It's an odd thing—the more you accept someone, the more obliging they strive to be in the future, simply because they don't feel flawed and lacking around you.

Also see: arguing, begging, date rape, marriage—lack of sex in, rejection—sexual, withholding

nocturnal emissions

See: wet dreams

nonoxynol-9

Think of this as napalm in the war against unwanted pregnancies. Also called N-9, it's a spermicide, meaning that it's designed to kill sperm on contact. The gooey foams, creams, jellies, or suppositories also make things especially slippery (lubrication being one of our favorite four-syllable words).

By itself, N-9 is not a reliable form of birth control. To significantly boost its anti-pregnancy punch, use it with other forms of contraception such as a diaphragm, cervical cap, or condom. (Bonus: If the rubber would happen to break, at least you have some kind of backup protection.)

Just don't rely on N-9 to protect you against HIV. While the spermicide had been shown to kill the virus in test tubes, a more recent study found that it may actually *increase* the risk of HIV infection in actual humans.

Also see: AIDS, cervical cap, condom, contraception, diaphragm, Pap test

Norplant

This brand-name implant contraceptive device is 99 percent effective in preventing pregnancy for up to 5 years. Within that period, it's more effective than even the Pill or sterilization.

Norplant's history has been marred by lawsuits and safety controversies. The gynecologists we spoke to deemed Norplant quite safe, the most common side effects being weight gain and occasional bleeding between a woman's periods. Our experts blame the controversy on some shoddy research from a few years back.

Norplant works like so: In a 10-minute procedure using a local anesthetic, a doctor surgically implants six matchstick-size silicone tubes under the skin of a woman's upper arm. The tubes are filled with progestin, a hormone that prevents pregnancy in three ways. First, it keeps her ovaries from pumping out eggs. Second, it thickens the cervical mucus, making it harder for your sperm to hook up with an egg. Third, researchers now think progestin may prevent a fertilized egg from taking up shop in the uterine wall.

The doctor removes the tubes after 5 years (or sooner if the patient hopes to get pregnant). Removal sometimes proves tricky, so suggest to your partner that she choose a doctor who's had some experience with the procedure.

The way we see it, Norplant works a lot like a car battery: You just put it in, and you're good for another 5 years. No pills for your girlfriend to forget to take, no messy foams or creams to deal with, and no late-night trips to the drugstore for ribbed rubbers. Just lots of great spontaneous sex. Anytime. Anywhere.

Isn't technology great?

Also see: contraception, progestin

NSU

If you're an alumnus of Louisiana's Nicholls State University, we suggest that you retire your old NSU letter jacket. Or at least wear something else when trying to pick up chicks. Why? Because no guy should walk around with the name of a sexually transmitted disease printed on his coat.

NSU stands for *nonspecific urethritis.* That's medicalese for an infection of the urethra, the tube that siphons urine from your bladder. NSU is sometimes called nongonococcal urethritis because your doctor first rules out gonorrhea as the cause of the infection. Other sexually transmitted bugs, such as the one that causes chlamydia, are to blame for NSU. Though this may be the first you've heard of it, NSU is more common than you may think. About 240,000 men saw their doctors for such an infection in 1999.

Telltale signs of NSU resemble those of other STDs. They include a watery, clear, or mucous discharge; sores on your penis; burning or itching around its opening; a foul odor; and a burning feeling when you take a whiz, especially first thing in the morning. If you have any of these symptoms, you'd better hightail it to your doc for some antibiotics. Leave NSU untreated, and it could leave you infertile.

The infection can also wreak havoc on your partner's plumbing—even though she's likely to experience no symptoms at all. So be a man, and tell her that you may have given her more than stellar sex the other night.

Our advice here is the same as what we tell you in many other places, and it's advice you probably already know: You can avoid picking up NSU by slipping on a rubber before having sex.

Also see: pee—painful, safe sex, scratching, STDs, urethritis, urologist

nudism

A term used pretty much interchangeably with *naturism*, nudism is a lifestyle as much as it is a shedding of clothes. Nudists and naturists will tell you that it's all about being able to relax in nature, to be rid of normal societal constraints, to be totally free to relate to one another without the facades we normally have in place.

If you think about it, you can see the attraction. We spend so much time covering ourselves up, even metaphorically, that it must be liberating to just dump all that for a while and not worry about it.

Not all nudists care to risk attracting the eye of law enforcement by going to public beaches: Occasional crackdowns leave the unfortunate with public-indecency charges. So they form private clubs where they're immune from prying politicians and police chiefs. These can be either landed or nonlanded clubs, meaning they either own their own land or they don't. The nonlanded clubs tend to meet indoors or travel to other clubs and resorts that permit nudity.

When you join a club, it's a whole different world than innocently skinny-dipping in a remote water hole. The social aspect becomes paramount. That's not to say that orgies are rampant; in fact, overt sexuality is normally forbidden because these groups cater to families, kids and all.

They may also refuse you if you're a single male. The ratio of men to women tends to fall heavily on the male side, so many clubs restrict the number of new single men who are permitted to join. You can pretty much forget about using this avenue as a convenient way to scout out potential mates.

Still interested? Talk to your girlfriend or wife about giving it a try. Clubs are usually very low pressure and often offer some kind of introductory tour. They realize that you're likely to be shy and uncomfortable the first time out, and they try to accommodate that. You can easily find a club near you simply by searching the Internet for nudist clubs.

Oh, and you can put aside your worries about getting a hard-on. It's really not a sexual experience. You'll see every shape and age imaginable, and it's just too casual to be erotic. Think back to skinny-dipping in high school. You were more worried about shrinkage than sudden expansion. Same here.

Also see: exhibitionism, ogling, outdoors, topless

nymphomania

Excessive sexual desire in a female. That's the official *Webster's* definition. To which we might reply, "Define *excessive.*" Or, "Yeah, so what's the problem?"

Seriously, who decides these things? Nymphomania is a concept that has con-

N

N

founded us through the ages, probably because female sexual desire has so long been suppressed, cloaked in shame, or otherwise misunderstood.

The ancient Greeks called it uterine fury (they said this in ancient Greek, of course). In the 19th century, some American doctors were not above removing the clitorises of women they considered nymphomaniacs; some foreign cultures still do this as a matter of course. The famed sex researcher Alfred Kinsey is reported to have flippantly remarked that a nympho is a woman who "wants sex more than you do." Today, we use the word with equal parts reverence and condescension.

The thing is, our feelings about it are pretty hard to pin down. It's a cultural archetype representing both our fear of and fascination with female sexuality. We want a woman who shudders with desire for us, but we don't want her to overwhelm us sexually. We want to be the object of her passion, but we don't want that passion to spill over to other men.

That said, there are those (of both sexes) who *are* out of control sexually. If a woman engages in compulsive sexual activity without regard to consequences and without satisfaction, she's got a problem. It's like eating compulsively or washing your hands compulsively. She's just using sex as her compulsive vehicle.

Also see: compulsive behavior, frigidity, promiscuity, satyriasis, sex addiction, wild women

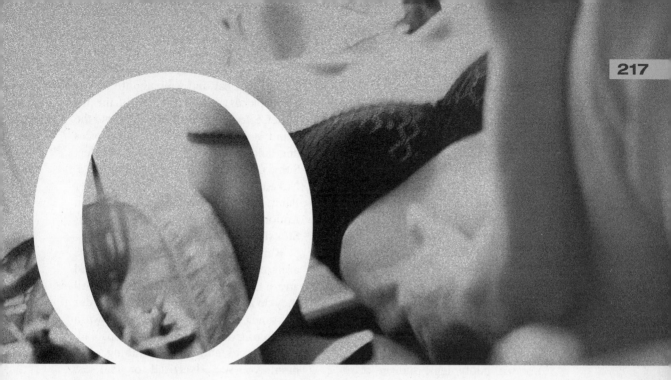

oculophilia

Break it down to its root words, and you'll see that this refers to people who are sexually aroused by eyes—which doesn't leave out a whole lot of us, we suspect. Even the great rationalist philosopher René Descartes wasn't immune. He was attracted to women who squinted.

Some guys take this a little further, all the way to oculolinctus. That's where you lick your partner's eyeball as a means of getting yourself horny. Hey, our philosophy is live and let live. Just be warned that bugs in your mouth can infect your mate's eye.

In our eyes, though, sometimes oculophilia does go overboard. To wit, there's a report of a prostitute in the Philippines who made a name for herself by removing her glass eye and encouraging her clients to have their way with her eye socket.

Also see: size—eyes

ogling

There are two constants about ogling. One, men like to do it. Two, women don't like men to do it.

Sometimes, women complain about it loudly enough that something silly happens. Like the time in 1989 when a chemistry professor got charged because he was staring too much at women while swimming in a campus pool at the University of Toronto. And the time when the city of Minneapolis declared a no-ogling policy after the gaze of city workers dwelled too long on the Midwest's fairer sex. There's even a report of a video store in Japan that barred men so that women could enjoy ogle-free browsing.

There's no question that irresponsible, lecherous eyeballing is boorish. Besides, it makes walking, driving, and piloting low-flying aircraft so much more hazardous. But that doesn't mean for a second that you have to give up the visual pleasures of womankind.

Checking her out and ogling are two different things. Many women relish an appreciative glance or two—just not a slack-jawed stare. (And be prepared; she may smile back at you.)

Also, when you find yourself in a situation where temptation is too great—say, the beaches at spring break—buy yourself a cheap pair of mirrored sunglasses. Why do you think cops wear them all the time? People can't tell if they're being watched or not.

Finally, remember that your eyes swivel all on their own. Your head doesn't have to follow them until after she's passed by. Attached men take note.

Also see: booty, legs, nudism, third-degree cleavage, topless, topless bar, va-va-voom, voyeurism, wandering eye

ointments

Consider, if you will, a simple bowl of ice cream. It's a thing of wonder all by itself. But add toppings, and it becomes a whole new thing: a sundae. Sex is kind of like that. Add ointments, and you have an entirely different sort of confection before you.

The unguents we're talking about are more than lubricants. They either add or change sexual sensations, usually by way of a warming or cooling action. Some are even edible, which leads us to our next point of interest: You can slather them on nipples and genitals, taking advantage of the very sensitive nature of those spots. But they're too sticky for wider-ranging body massage.

Besides being easy to incorporate into your lovemaking, ointments are easy to find. They're as close as your neighbor-hood adult shop. If you don't feel like hiding your car and walking into one of those places, take advantage of the Internet. Sites like Good Vibrations and the Xandria Collection have tons of choices and deliver them right to your doorstep. Some of our favorites are Lickable Love, Naked & Naughty Chocolate Finger Paint, Kama Sutra Pleasure Balm, Motion Lotion, and Xandria's Lube-a-Licious Strawberry and Watermelon Lubricants.

Remember, too, that not all ointments are created equal. We *don't* recommend any of the so-called stay-hard creams. All they do is numb your penis so it's harder to come. They will also break down a condom. Consider a cock ring instead. Also, forget about the numbing ointments you see advertised for anal sex. They're supposed to make it more comfortable for her. News flash: If it hurts her, you're supposed to stop, not anesthetize her. Any pain implies tearing tissue or other damage. Don't mask that warning sign. See our entry on *anal sex* to make it more pleasurable for her.

There are two potential problems that may constitute the proverbial fly in the ointment: These products can cause irritation, and they can be hard to strip off. Fortunately, we have solutions to both problems.

To test for bad reactions, apply a dab of your chosen ointment to the inside of your lower lip, which is the spot most like your penis or her labia. (First, make sure the lotion is edible.) Wait a couple of minutes. If it irritates you, don't use it anywhere else. Alternately, you can swab it on the inside of your wrist. This takes longer—give it 15 to 20 minutes to see if it rubs you the wrong way.

To wash it off, take a crack at it with simple soap and hot water. If that doesn't cut through, spread on some olive oil, then tackle it again with more soap and water.

A final caution: Unless the ointment is specifically labeled as a sexual lubricant, don't use it for vaginal or anal intercourse. Sexual orifices aren't very tolerant of foreign substances.

Also see: aromatherapy, body oils, cock ring, food, licking, lubricants, oysters, sexual aids, whipped cream

onanism

In the Book of Genesis, chapter 38, you'll come across the story of Onan, son of Judah. Onan was tasked with impregnating his brother's widow, but when it came down to the moment of truth, he pulled out and cast his seed upon the ground.

This didn't thrill the Lord too much, so He slew Onan. The reverberations of that moment are still with us today in the form of the word *onanism*. It means, alternately, masturbation or coitus interruptus—the old pull-and-pray technique.

Since you're busy learning new words for your old habits, here's another: *sacofricosis.* That's the practice of cutting a hole in the bottom of your pants pocket so that you can masturbate in public with less risk of detection. Pee-Wee Herman, take note.

Also see: abnormal, masturbation, taboos

one-night stand

Falling into bed with a woman you just met is great . . . until you wake up the next morning. It's not only that your standards tend to drop considerably as last call approaches—hence the phrase *any port in a storm* (and its less flattering morning-after bookend, *coyote ugly*). It's that many people find it pretty tough to have sex with no strings attached. And if you're one of those people who thinks one-night stands are totally depersonalized sex, you may want to think again. By its very nature, can sexual intercourse truly be depersonalized?

So now you have two choices: creep out like, well, a creep or handle it like a

Hot Dates 1966 A California inventor named Jon Tavel patented a torpedo-shaped, battery-operated vibrator.

continued from page 208

glans of the penis and secured on each end with a small round ball. Women in Borneo are partial to these adornments—**apparently the balls provide extra vaginal friction**.

In Extremis
Men troubled by their small penises can join **a club of like-minded guys**

named Small, Etc. The group publishes a quarterly magazine, *Small Gazette: The Smaller Man's Forum*, bulging with articles and personal ads from bisexual and gay men.

LEGAL BRIEFS
A jury awarded a San Francisco woman $500,000 after she claimed

True or Phallus
Sweden is the world's leading producer of skin flicks.

BAWDY BALLADS *"You Got to Give Me Some of It,"* Buddy Moss

continued on page 230

decent guy. Your first task come daybreak is to listen closely to what she says. She may well think that the two of you made an awful mistake. Don't be defensive.

Second, it's important to leave nothing behind—make sure you take your wallet, your tie, and so forth. Make it clear that you enjoyed meeting her but that there's no future beyond the past. If you knew going in that this was a one-time gig, don't tell her you'll call her, and don't say you'll see her around. False hopes lead to hurt feelings.

Finally, don't be surprised if you end up feeling a bit more attached to her than you expected to. (It's a myth that women are the only ones who want sex to lead somewhere.) This brings us to another don't: Don't, under any circumstances, be surprised if she's the one who wants a clean break. Essentially, the two of you went into this looking for a form of mutual masturbation. Be prepared to leave it at that. You have no right to force the issue just because you woke up smitten.

Also see: date rape, discretion, infatuation, lust, morning after, partner, travel—loneliness during, sexual etiquette, wild women, zipless sex

opening line

There's only one opening line that amounts to a hill of beans. And it's not, "Wow! Great job, God." Or "I was wondering, do you have any [insert your own nationality here] in you? Well then, would you like some?"

No. The preferred salutation is, amazingly enough, "Hi, my name is [insert your name here]; may I ask yours?" It's a simple, straightforward expression of interest. If she's older than 16, she's heard all the pickup lines; the slobbering, drunk proposals of marriage; and all those other embarrassing things men insist on saying to women. You can assume, quite safely, that she's also heard the one you were about to use.

So surprise and delight her with something she's not used to: honesty. From there, it gets even easier. Your main job is to listen. Don't feel obliged to fill the air with witty banter. Let her talk for a while, and she'll walk away thinking that you're the best conversationalist ever.

And please, please don't tell her about your car, your mother, or anything to do with stock options. (Dogs are okay, because it shows that you know how to care for something beyond a single-celled organism.) When you do pipe up, try to make it something funny. Women consistently rate a good sense of humor as a major turn-on. Hey, how else could Gilbert Gottfried get any?

Also see: eye contact, flirtation, meeting women, pickup lines, smiling, Your place or mine?

oral contraceptive

Don't get us wrong. We totally dig the oral contraceptive known as the Pill. After all, it makes our sex lives so spontaneous (provided, of course, you're with a woman whom you know to be disease-free). We don't need condoms or messy foams to prevent knocking her up, because in typical use, the Pill by itself is 95 percent effective at preventing pregnancy.

We just have one question: How come our honeys never seem to be in the mood once they go on the Pill?

It could be the hand vacs we gave them for their birthdays. Either that or the Pill may be tapping their testosterone levels. While a woman's levels of this manly hormone are significantly lower than a man's (except on Olympic teams from Belarus), the small amount that her ovaries do produce has a profound effect on her libido. And for complex biochemical reasons, the Pill can take a bite out of a woman's testosterone stores.

The Pill could be to blame if your woman has had low libido for several months after switching to this form of birth control. Just to be clear, her saying no to doing it five times a day doesn't quite qualify as low libido. We're talking about a sex drive that's lower than normal *for her*. Guys' standards don't apply.

Suggest that she visit her doctor again; a change to a brand of the Pill that provides a different balance of hormones may put some life back into her libido. And while she's at that appointment, we suggest that you run out and trade in that hand vac for something a bit more romantic. Or at least for one with all the attachments.

Also see: contraception, male pill, Pill—the, safe sex, sex drive, testosterone, witch's milk

oral sex

We always knew we were ahead of our time. Way back before the sexual revolution, when oral sex was still listed in medical and psychiatric books as a deviant act, we knew better. We can thank the feminist movement, however, for bringing a positive change in attitudes about fellatio and cunnilingus.

Today, almost as many women as men view oral sex as a normal part of lovemaking. Younger women, in particular,

have an even more casual attitude about oral sex than men their own age. A survey of 600 college students found that only 37 percent of the female respondents would say that they had "had sex" with someone to whom they'd given a blow job, while 44 percent of male respondents said they would define giving or receiving such favors as "having sex."

All this means that you're much more likely than your grandfather was to find a partner who's willing to give head—*and* to expect you to return the favor. Here's what you need to know to improve the odds still further.

• When she's going down on you, always warn her before you come. Whether she spits or swallows, she'll appreciate the, uh, heads-up. It'll give her a second to prepare, so she'll be less likely to gag and more likely to want to come back for more.

• Keep in mind that being on the receiving end of oral sex is the only way some women can reach orgasm. (Let's face it, we'd say that too, if it meant getting more head.) So try to hang in there until her moans turn into all-out screams and she begins digging her fingernails into your skin. Oh, and follow the same rule you hope she does: no biting.

• As for that post-cunnilingus kiss, not every woman likes the taste of her own secretions. (You're not wild about yours, are you?) Your best bet is to slowly work your way back up. If she turns her head when you zero in, nibble her neck instead. Then go brush your teeth and give your face a quick once-over with soap and water.

• One last thing: At this writing, it's still illegal in nine states for a man and a woman to give each other oral pleasure—even if they're married. So never engage in oral sex with a cop you don't know awfully well.

Also see: AIDS, biting, couch, cunnilingus, eat, fellatio, genital warts, give head, glory hole, herpes, lips, mouth, rimming, safe sex, sixty-nine (69), sodomy, thrush, tongue

orgasm

To too many of us, an orgasm can be as simple as a *National Geographic* article on seminude tribal peoples and a couple tosses of the hand.

That's ejaculation. And while no one is disparaging the pleasant feeling of ejaculation, it pales mightily compared to orgasm. What's the difference? In the case of orgasm, we encourage you to think globally and act locally. Orgasm begins with the same sort of activity that brings on ejaculation. It just doesn't stop there.

Unlike ejaculation, orgasm is an all-over feeling. It swallows your entire body and soul, not just your groin. Your breathing rate, heartbeat, and blood pressure rise. Let it build even more, and your whole body can spasm and thrash, from your toes to your lips. You doubt us? Ever see the full-body rapture a woman often goes through during orgasm? Yours can be just as powerful if you expect more than mere ejaculation during lovemaking.

One of the easiest ways to experience true orgasm is to put off ejaculation for a while when you're in the midst of passion. Each time you feel yourself nearing the brink, back off. Stop thrusting for a bit and slow things down. If you're too close, you may even want to pull out and concentrate just on kissing for a few min-

utes. Each time you relax and let the momentum build, your orgasmic threshold gets a tad higher. When you're finally ready to unleash, waves of oceanic pleasure will carry both of you to new lands. Or at least make the old land seem a little bit brighter.

Also see: afterglow, anal beads, chakras, clitoral orgasm, come, depression, disability—overcoming, ejaculation, get off, Janus Report, Kegel exercises, lovemaking, phalloplasty, poppers, Prozac, sensate focus, spiritual sex, time, yogi

orgasm—delayed

We can feel your eyebrows rising. Why on Earth would you want to delay an orgasm? Isn't getting to the high point the whole point?

It's that kind of thinking that earns men a bad rap among those who lie next to us in bed. One of women's most common complaints is that we're in a rush to get off, roll off, and drop off to sleep. Sure, sometimes your partner may want a quickie or a public tryst that must be fast if you're not to get caught. But usually, she wants you to hurry it up only if she's dead tired, late for a beauty appointment, or having an awful time.

Besides pleasing her, taking your time benefits you, too, bud. It nets you a chance to experience more relaxation, closeness, and pleasure with your partner, and ultimately gives you the thrill of experimenting with new sexual techniques.

The key to consistently containing coital eruptions is mastering techniques that are also used for premature ejaculation. Meander on over to the entry by that name.

You're also lucky that you have no choice but to get older: As you age, your arousal time lengthens, and delaying orgasm is no longer as difficult. So you're better able to take your time, relax, and savor sex a little bit more.

See also: aging, cock ring, Kegel exercises, marathon, public places, quickies, rear entry, tantra, time, yogi

outdoors

Men will throw back the warm covers at 4:00 A.M. to sit out on a frozen lake and do some ice fishing. Why? Because we thrive outside.

Take our favorite place to be and toss in our favorite thing to do, and you have that incredible thing known as outdoor sex. Fortunately, a sizable number of women also hear the call of the wild: In one survey, 39 percent of them named the great outdoors as a great alternative to the bedroom.

One thing to be wary of is that nature can be a mother. Shedding your clothes in the out-of-doors leaves you with only thin skin to combat the elements. Many a rural roll in the hay has been spoiled by ant bites, poison ivy, and sand in the crack. So take a blanket with you, or spread your clothes out beneath you. Also scout for anthills, beehives, and game wardens.

When mosquitoes are chewing on your hindquarters, it's hard to concentrate on the way your lover is nibbling your frontquarters. To avoid being eaten in a bad way, slather on insect repellant. Don't use it on your genitals, though, and avoid getting it in your eyes or mouth.

Old Sol is also no friend of pastoral companionship. The sun can, quite literally, burn the asses off you both. Exposing flesh that almost never sees light is a recipe for sunburn within minutes. And let us tell you, from first-hand experience, that penises do not tan so much as sauté. Keep your exposure to the sun to a bare minimum by either going for a quickie or finding a shady love nest. If you just have to do it on the beach, remember the obvious: Wear sunscreen with an SPF of at least 15 and full UVA and UVB protection.

Also see: exhibitionism, fig leaf, public places, quickies, risky sex, variety

outing

This is a term that's rapidly falling victim to its own success. Outing is what happens when someone—often a gay activist—widely announces the homosexuality of a public figure without his or her approval. It's forcing someone out of the closet, kicking and screaming.

Why do gays do this to their own? Either they feel that the public figure is acting in ways that are hypocritical or damaging to other gays, or they believe that it's for the betterment of society—that homosexuality shouldn't be something to hide. From Pentagon officials to high-profile magazine publishers to the late actor Rock Hudson, many have found themselves the objects of outing.

These days, it doesn't happen nearly as often—a reflection of society's increasing nonchalance about sexual orientation.

Also see: Don't ask, don't tell; heterosexuality; homophobia; homosexuality; politicians

ovaries

If there's a physical center to woman-hood, it's the ovaries. Either that or the television studio where Oprah's audience sits.

Almond-shaped glands the size of large walnuts, a woman's two ovaries sit sheltered in her lower abdomen, one on either side of her uterus. (Speaking of nuts: If manhood had been her destiny, the tissue that became her ovaries would've formed testicles instead.)

Ovaries do three important things: They produce the hormones estrogen and progesterone, which shape a woman's sexual characteristics (quite nicely, we might add). They cause the walls of her uterus to thicken with blood-rich cells and create a hospitable spot for a fertilized egg. And they produce eggs like those from which we all sprang.

A woman is born with about one million undeveloped egg cells, or follicles, but her body absorbs more than half of those during childhood. When she reaches puberty, 300 to 400 of the remaining follicles begin to mature into eggs at the usual rate of one a month. Her two ovaries generally alternate the egg-laying duties monthly. Unlike those of her counterparts in the henhouse, though, a woman's eggs are nowhere near large enough to scramble. Each of the little tykes is only one-tenth of a millimeter in diameter.

Every menstrual cycle, that month's mature, fertile egg floats out of its ovary and into the corresponding fallopian tube. If it hooks up with a healthy, hardy sperm, the result is a tax deduction. If it doesn't, it's expelled from the woman's body during her period.

Also see: estrogen, gonad, hysterectomy, menopause—hers, pregnancy, progesterone, rhythm method

ovulation

This is her other "time of the month." It's when her ovaries release an egg that's ready and waiting to be fertilized. Depending on your present intentions, it's either a time of dread or a chance to give her a—ahem—standing ovulation.

Yes, the only time she can get pregnant is during ovulation. But that's not a guarantee that she *will* conceive. Even under ideal circumstances, the chance of conception tops out at around 20 percent in any given month.

There are kits you can buy at many drugstores that will tell you if she's in those fertile few days. If you're trying to put a bun in her oven, having sex several times within that window of opportunity will boost your chances.

If, on the other hand, you're trying to evade ovulation, let us wish you the best of luck. First off, you'd do well to take leave of the misconception that ovulation occurs only in the middle of her cycle. It can—and does—take place at any point in the month, even rarely *during* menstruation.

Also see: contraception, fertility, marijuana, menstruation, morning-after pill, Norplant, pheromones, Pill—the, pituitary gland, progestin, rhythm method, sex drive, sperm count, sympto-thermal method

oysters

Aphrodisiacs. Oysters. Aphrodisiacs. Oysters. The two have been linked so long in the annals of aphrodisia that it's hard to say one without thinking the other. Right?

Sorry to disappoint, but there's no evidence that oysters will add any kind of magical boost to tonight's rocket ride. That's not to discount their erotic appeal, for oysters are a very sexy food. They're often part of a romantic evening filled with candles, dusky whispers, and lingering glances. Their charm lies in their mystique, their relative rarity, their shape that's oddly reminiscent of a woman's labia. Our very expectations for them can have a placebo effect on our sex drives.

Oh, by the way, oysters are good for you. They contain a truckload of zinc, a mineral that your body needs to produce sperm and utilize testosterone. So, bottom line, forget what you just read a few paragraphs ago. Pick up some oysters, expect the best, and enjoy!

Also see: aphrodisiac, food, zinc

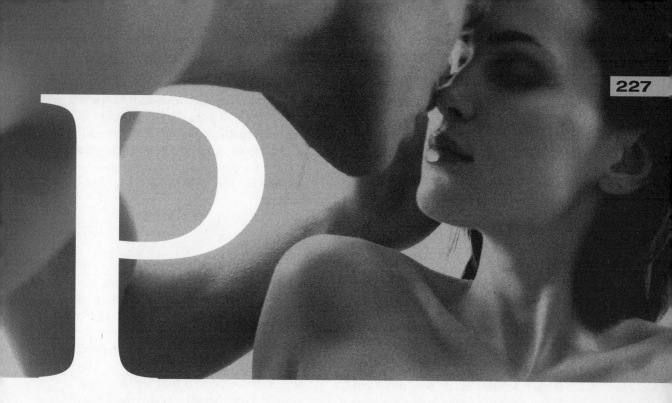

P

packing

If a female who isn't a cop tells you you're packing, say thank you and hitch up your drawers. That's because, to everyone outside the world of law enforcement, packing means your briefs are at maximum occupancy.

Packing can also refer to what your package is principally used for: intercourse, either vaginal or anal. If anal sex is on the menu, the word is usually modified to *fudge packing*. Use your imagination.

Also see: anal sex, boxers or briefs, hung, micropenis, size—penis

paddle

Man, it seemed like you could never get far enough away from the paddle in elementary school. Later, if you went to a military school or pledged at a fraternity, you stood a good chance of seeing the paddle come out again—this time in the even crueler hands of your peers.

So given that background, you'd think paddles would be the last thing any of us would want to see when we climb into bed. And you'd be wrong. For paddling, of course, is a key sadomasochistic delicacy.

Several types of paddles can be used to spank willing partners. First is the plain and simple leather paddle. Some like this type for the heavy, commanding thud it makes upon contact. A variation thereon is the slapper, made of two pieces of leather that make a loud slapping noise when the paddle encounters buttocks.

A tawse is a paddle usually made of leather strapping cut into strips at the ends. It generally makes a slapping sound as well. Last is the wooden paddle, which ranges in heft from the very light to the very heavy. Know this: A heavy paddle, no matter the material, can do real damage and is better left on the wall solely for its visual impact.

In a jam, the frantic paddler can also turn to the kitchen drawers. Wooden spoons and spatulas make for handy substitutes. But because they concentrate the force over a very small area, they also tend to leave welts and bruises. Be careful.

Also see: bondage and discipline, booty, dominance and submission, leather, safeword, sexual aids, spanking

P

papaverine

Before Viagra, there was papaverine. This prescription drug, which has helped guys get it up for some 17 years, works much the same way as the little blue pill. Papaverine is usually used in combination with two other prescription drugs, phentolamine and prostaglandin E_1. Together, they increase bloodflow to Sergeant Pecker and then trap it so that he's able to stand at attention and perform his patriotic duties.

The downside to this drug trio is that it must be injected into . . . we'd rather not say where. Luckily, all three drugs are part of the same injection, so you don't have to stick yourself three times. Plus, the needle used is the tiniest made, and the injection site on your penis has relatively few nerve endings. We know, we know; we're wincing right along with you anyway. If it's any consolation, we're told that it hurts more to think about than to actually do.

Along with a couple of unpleasant side effects (possible scarring or prolonged erections), the presence of Viagra (silde-nafil) on the market renders papaverine the less likely choice. But it does have one major upside: It gives you results in 5 to 10 minutes. That's a far cry from Viagra's 30- to 60-minute wait, and it's why some guys still opt for the injection over Viagra.

Also see: erection difficulties, impotence

papilloma

If you happen to find yourself in the company of a highly literate witch, you might tell her what a fine collection of papillomas she has on her nose. That's because *papilloma* is the 10-cent term for a wart: a benign growth on the surface, caused by a virus below the skin. But watch those warts: If they are asymmetrical, if they increase in size, or if they change color, you should have them checked out by a doctor. They might have turned into a carcinoma, which is a kind of cancer.

Also see: genital warts, STDs, warts

Pap test

Why should a big, burly fellow like yourself want to know what goes on inside a gynecologist's office? Well, for one, it lends you an air of distinguished authority the next time you play doctor. For another, it's very important if you want your partner to hang around on the planet for a while yet. Finally, your own sexual health is closely linked to hers. And aside from telling her whether she's at risk for cervical cancer, Pap tests, also known as Pap smears, can sometimes do wonderful things such as diagnose whether she's infected with the virus that causes genital warts. That's something *you* need to know.

Here's how it works. When she goes in for her yearly smear, she reclines on a table and puts her legs in stirrups. The doc inserts a speculum—a cold, hard gizmo designed to spread her vagina open. Then a sampling of cells gets scraped off and stuck on a glass slide. Yes, it's as unpleasant as it sounds, so be nice to her when she gets home.

A couple of technical points: She shouldn't douche or have intercourse for 3 days before the test. Nor should she use birth control jellies or foams for 5 days before her appointment. The reason for these precautions is simple: Anything that could cause inflammation around her cervix may result in a false-positive reading. Spare her that anxiety by laying low for 3 days. She'll thank you when it's all over.

Also see: cervix, genital warts, vagina

paraphilias

From the Greek, *paraphilias* translates roughly to "love outside the boundaries." If you're in a judgmental mood, they're also known as perversions.

In diagnosing a sexual practice as a paraphilia, therapists generally look for a pattern of one or more of the following behaviors that persists for more than 6 months: recurrent, intense, sexually arousing fantasies and actions involving nonhuman objects; or humiliation or suffering of yourself or your partner; or nonconsenting partners (obviously including children). Because these behaviors smack societal sensibilities in the face, most of them are against the law.

Pedophilia, voyeurism, and exhibitionism are the top three paraphilias for which sex offenders are arrested. Others include fetishism, klismaphilia, and necro-

philia. Some therapists include sadomasochistic practices among paraphilias; others don't.

Paraphiliacs may experience tremendous guilt over their behavior. Others object only to society's objections. Some of the behaviors and fantasies associated with paraphilias take root in childhood but really begin to blossom in adolescence. They're usually lifelong orientations, even though their sexual drawing power may wax and wane.

One thing to note: *Fantasizing* about some of these things is not, in and of itself, something you should worry too much about. When fantasy becomes reality, it's a different story.

Only a psychologist or psychiatrist specializing in paraphilias should make a diagnosis, so if you're in the "guilt-plagued" category noted above, or if you're worried about impulses that may cause you to run afoul of certain laws, book yourself an appointment to talk things out.

Also see: abnormal, bestiality, compulsive behavior, cross-dressing, date rape, exhibitionism, fantasies, fetish, guilt, incest, kinky, masher, necrophilia, pedophilia, perversions, rape, risky sex, Sade—Marquis de, sex therapy, taboos, transvestism, violence, voyeurism, water sports, zoophilia

partner

You figure it's just about sex. She thinks otherwise. Or, conversely, maybe it's you who wants to hang out awhile with this one—but she has different plans. It all comes down to that moment in time when one of you looks across the bed and, instead of a sex partner, sees . . . a partner.

P

You know what partner means. It means exclusivity. It means the person you share a toothbrush holder with. It's the person who feels pangs of jealousy when another feline in heat starts sniffing around you.

There are warning signs that a woman is getting really sweet on you. For instance, there's the classic Hallmark moment known as "I'd like you to meet my family." She doesn't want her dad to shake hands with some guy she's just banging. If she suggests a weekend at the family farm, she hopes to turn things up a major notch.

The moment doesn't have to be as blatant as that. It may be the first time she calls you at work just to see how your meeting went. Or if she's a single mom, it's when you meet the kids. Or maybe she just starts hinting around that she's, you know, not seeing anyone else. . . .

On the flip side, there are also signals that reveal that she's not interested in you for anything other than an occasional erection. She never calls you just to talk—only to schedule a date. She doesn't make eye contact unless you're talking about sex. Conversations seem to wane quickly, followed by a sudden suggestion to fool around. She has little interest in your interests. She doesn't want to know your future plans, your favorite color, your middle name.

Whichever situation you're in, you have a decision to make. If it's you who has little interest in becoming partners, you owe it to her to tell her that. A man who strings a woman along and feigns affection just to have sex is doing his part to uphold the classic female view of man as dog. Do the honorable thing.

If she's the one who wants nothing beyond pillow talk, you need honor again—as well as a certain amount of balls. Walk away with your head (the one you think with—excuse us, you're *supposed* to think with) held high. Sure, it

---

Hot Dates | **1967** Scientists found that herpes, which had been around for centuries, was transmitted sexually.

continued from page 219

Answer:
Way false. The United States is easily the world leader, churning out some 150 titles per week. Power to the people!

that a cable car accident **transformed her from a "proper young lady" into a voracious nymphomaniac.** Gloria Sykes said that after the accident, she had sex with more than 100 men—episodes that she had the presence of mind to document carefully.

Seemed like a Good Idea at the Time. . .
At one time in Europe, "massage therapy" was the genteel-sounding

prescription for female "hysteria." **A doctor feel-good would massage a woman's vulva** and bring her to orgasm to alleviate such symptoms as weepiness and frequent fainting.

Foreign Affairs
And you thought Long Dong Silver was big: In Japan, there's an annual festival during which a dozen men carry a 7-foot, 700-pound phallus carved from

---

BAWDY BALLADS | "Wipe It Off," *Lonnie Johnson*

continued on page 235

stings. But what's the alternative? If you want more than sex, you have to find someone who's ready to offer that. Otherwise, you're just spinning your wheels while the good ones pair off with some other lucky guys.

Also see: breaking up, commitment, companionship, infatuation, intimacy, morning after, one-night stand, wild women

passion

Can you imagine sex so powerful that you lose track of where your body ends and hers begins? A kiss that lasts eternities after your lips have ceased to touch? If not, friend, then you have yet to dally in the depths of passion.

You may think you simply haven't met the right person with whom to feel these atomic butterflies in your gut. Maybe. But maybe you simply haven't *been* the right person. Passion isn't something that strikes only the lucky. It's a decision you make. It's about letting loose.

Here is passion's recipe: Suspend all judgment (at least temporarily). Look at every aspect of your partner's mannerisms, beliefs, actions, lovemaking skills, whatever. Revel in them instead of grading them. And be bold. When you feel like rolling down a hill with her in your arms, don't be deterred by thoughts of how silly you'll look. That's the whole point: Passion *is* silly, frivolous, impetuous, unrestrained. It doesn't care who sees.

What's that you say? "That's just not me?" Why not? What's holding you back? We'll hazard a guess: fear. Fear is a big-time passion quasher. Fear of the unknown. Fear of looking ridiculous. Fear of being a fool. Fear of losing your dignity. Or, maybe worst of all, fear that she won't return your passion with equal intensity.

You can't experience true passion without facing such fears and taking the plunge anyway. Because passion is a lot like . . . well, like investing. Sure, the safest course is never to invest anything, not even a dollar. Then you're assured of always having at least the same dollar you started with. But the only way to watch that dollar grow to $5 and then $10 and then hundreds of dollars is to take a chance—to make an investment. Thus, investing's basic catch-22: In order to gain the biggest rewards, you have to be willing to risk what you started with.

So it is with passion. Make the investment. With luck, you'll "buy" yourself the kinds of experiences we described at the outset.

Also see: ahhh, emotions, infatuation, intimacy, lovemaking, lust, romance, rituals, soul mates, spiritual sex

past partners—dealing with

It's over, done with, kaput. You and she have gone your separate ways. That's the end of it, right? If only that were true.

A Roper poll asked more than 1,000 people whether a previous relationship had ever caused a subsequent relationship to end. Nine percent said it had happened very frequently, 23 percent said frequently, and 37 percent said occasionally. That's 69 percent or, no matter how you slice it, a lot of people whose pasts catch up with them.

If the past relationship was a marriage that produced children, that has its own special set of headaches. You and your ex are forced into each other's lives by logistics: You have to drop the kids off at her place and vice versa. And you may

P

have to deal with her telling your kids what a rotten husband you were and what a lousy father you continue to be. That resentment and hostility carries over into your present relationship. Your new woman gets mighty tired of hearing your gripes—or even just having to see her new partner always pissed off about something that happened long before she came on the scene.

There's no easy solution here, but you need to take a hard look at your own actions. For starters, you need to learn to switch off around your ex, especially when there are kids involved. She may no longer matter; they do. Don't cancel out on evenings and weekends with your kids because you can't bear to enter the hornet's nest. They won't understand *why* you don't show up; they'll just know that you don't—which only sets in motion a whole new round of blame, guilt, and bad feelings.

It's tempting, too, to come back home and gripe to your present sweetheart. Watch out. This may be a cross you must bear on your own—or with the guys over a beer. As patient as your new love may be, as nurturing as she may seem about "your problems" at the outset, it just may get under her skin that you expend so much emotional energy on your ex. Especially once you start having legitimate couplehood issues of your own to deal with. She may expect you to focus the bulk of your emotional and intellectual capacity on her. Wouldn't you ask the same for yourself?

Also see: arguing, breaking up, jealousy, remarriage

past partners—longing for

It comes to you upon the strains of an old song, the scent of a forgotten perfume, the glance of a woman with similar eyes. You say her name softly to yourself, as memories of a lover gone away come flooding back.

Welcome to the world of sweet nostalgia. It's a rite of aging as inevitable as graying hair and growing patience. You can thank the incredible powers of your long-term memory. The recollections of pleasurable times and delightful women simply cannot be excised from your mind.

But memory is selective and not infallible. In an interesting bit of revisionism, your mind allows bad memories to fade more quickly than good. That's why your grandpa was always so convinced that things were better way back when. And why you'll argue with your younger brother or your kids about how Ripken, in his day, could play rings around Jeter at shortstop.

Our point: There's a difference between loitering in your recollections for a moment (which is probably not unhealthy) and thinking that your life will be better if you track her down and give it one more try for the Gipper (which almost surely *is*). That relationship ran its course and ended, and there were reasons why it ended, and chances are, they'd just crop up again—in spades. (Can you say Liz Taylor and Richard Burton? Pamela Anderson and Tommy Lee?)

No, we're not contending that all refound relationships are doomed. Sometimes, in the intervening years, you've both learned better ways of dealing with others' shortcomings. There's that increased ability to be patient that we mentioned before. And you have a sense of comfort with each other that can take years to build in a new relationship.

So if you both find yourselves single again at the same time, what the hell . . .

go for it. But the finding-yourselves-single part is the key. You don't throw away a current relationship simply because of the memory of something that already had its day in the sun. Every relationship has its issues. Work through them. It's unlikely that you'll find your future by escaping into your past. And your wistful musings over the past may be one of the very things that prevent you from giving yourself fully to the present.

Also see: best friend's wife, breaking up, death of a partner, perfume, remarriage, single—suddenly

past partners—running into

It's only a matter of time before you run into an ex. If you're alone, you have only one person's reaction to worry about: yours. No matter how tempting it may be to fire a shot across her bow for old time's sake, don't do it. You don't have to be her friend, but there really isn't any point in being an enemy. Smile pleasantly, even if she doesn't, and act the gentleman.

If you're with your current wife or girlfriend when the past catches up with you, you've got twice as much to worry about (or maybe three times, depending on your ex's reaction to your new love interest). It's especially important not to be a goof now, because your woman is watching you closely. The mark of a keeper, in her eyes, is how a man deals with unpleasantness. The way you act with an ex gives some clue to the way you'll act with her when times get tough, and she knows that.

You can also bet that the woman on your arm is checking out your ex from top to bottom and thinking all kinds of nasty—or possibly jealous—thoughts. Once the ex has moved on, immediately put your woman's mind at ease. Say something like "Man, now that I see old what's-her-name, I feel luckier than ever to be with you." (It helps if you mean it.)

If the situation is reversed—that is, if you have an encounter with her ex—your task is simple. Don't say anything snide about the guy. Women have a protective, nurturing side and you'll be forcing her to jump to his defense. She may even feel that by criticizing him, you are, in effect, criticizing her, since she's the one who picked him. We know, it makes no sense—since she also picked you—but you ignore such quirkiness at your own peril.

Just ask her whether the situation was uncomfortable for her, and let it drop. If she wants to talk more, you'll know about it.

Also see: jealousy, remarriage

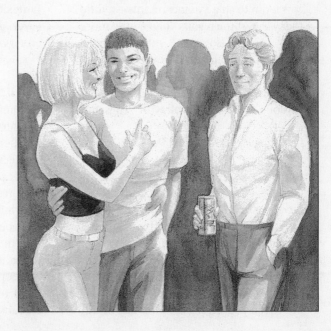

past partners—talking about

There's an odd, stomach-wrenching fascination in delving into your partner's sexual past. It's like picking at a scab: It hurts, it's grisly, but you just can't help yourself.

Some men simply aren't willing to put themselves through that. For them, whether or not their lover ever did the high school lacrosse team is best left in the past. But most people want to know at least something about the sexual histories of their bedfellows. So you need to know the rules, lest this exercise become an exorcism.

Here are some general guidelines you both can follow if you're planning a mutual information swap.

• First, establish why it's important to share these details. Does it have to do with health risks? What either of you prefer in bed? Adequacy issues? Knowing this will help each of you frame the truth in a way that will have the most positive outcome.

• Aim to share in increments—a little today, digest the results, then a little more next week. Also, make sure you have plenty of time and privacy when you discuss these issues. You need your best judgment here; talking about prior sexual exploits doesn't mix well with drugs and alcohol.

• If she lets you into Pandora's box, it's because she trusts you. Never, ever use anything she tells you in a future argument—even if she costarred in *The Satisfiers of Alpha Blue*. If you do, she'll greet your future inquiries by clamming up tighter than, well, a clam.

• Ask for the bad too. If you ask her only about positive sexual experiences, you'll get a skewed view of her past. Get her to tell you what she didn't like about

a particular experience or person. It'll do your ego good.

• It's probable that you'll end up struggling over some of the things she tells you. You'll see images in your mind of things she's done, and it'll bug the hell out of you. Some guys find it helpful to force themselves to dwell on those thoughts (preferably when she's not around, so you're not tempted to be snotty to her) so that eventually, the emotional sting drains out of those images.

• Above all, avoid the illogical (but seductive) temptation to superimpose your visceral feelings about her past relationships over your present relationship—in other words, to interpret her past exploits almost as if she were cheating on you today. She isn't. The past is past.

There's a reason why she's with you now, and a reason why she stays. She's happy with your couplehood. You're really best off leaving it at that.

Also see: communication, discretion, fantasies, first lover, first time with a lover, guilt, jealousy, lover, safe sex, secrets, virginity—hers

PC muscle

In Canada, *PC* refers to the Progressive Conservative party. In the United States, *PC* means "politically correct." But to all English-speaking men, *PC should* mean "pubococcygeus." It's the muscle behind your testicles that helps shut off the flow of urine and eject ejaculate.

A properly upgraded PC can lead you into the land of sexual mystics. For one thing, by using Kegel exercises to learn to keep that gate shut tight at the moment of truth, you can orgasm without ejaculating. This leaves you hard and ready to go again. Therein lies the secret of multiorgasmic men.

Also see: chakras, Kegel exercises, refractory period

pederast

Someone who takes part in anal intercourse. The term is usually meant to describe a man who does so with boys. It's a more clinical word for buggery.

Ancient eunuch priests used a form of pederasty to continue their sex lives after their genitals were lopped off. Even without gear, these men were able to have pleasurable sensations by having the region around their prostates stimulated.

Also see: eunuch, prostate

pedophilia

Few words evoke more bile and fury than this one. Because people have such

a potent instinctive urge to protect their offspring, pedophiles are at grave risk of losing many of their future freedoms for life when they get caught.

We bring up this highly charged topic because we have to. Consider: In 1997, of the one million child victims of physical abuse in the United States, 13 percent were abused sexually. And because of the shame it causes victims, experts believe that that number may have been vastly underreported.

In the scientific and academic world, it's important to first do one thing when you're examining an issue: Define terms. Let's do that now. A true pedophile is someone who is sexually attracted to children. The key word there is *children*—people who haven't yet entered puberty.

This is the one area where fantasy isn't so safe. If you have these feelings, you should consider seeking help, even if you haven't yet acted on your thoughts. Find

235

P

Hot Dates **September 7, 1968** Women's libbers protested the Miss America Pageant, tossing dishcloths, high-heeled shoes, hair curlers, and bras into trash cans.

continued from page 230

Japanese cypress from one shrine to another—a distance of a mile. The phallus is so big and heavy that several teams of 12 are needed. After the ceremonies, **the prior year's giant wooden organ is sold**. The festival promotes fertility and prosperity and protects against evil.

In Extremis

Small-town Iowa cops arrested a colleague found driving around

with scores of sex videos in his car and a "sexual device inserted into his body, . . . connected to a battery pack." Interestingly enough, **he was arrested not on sex charges but on drug-related offenses.**

Legal Briefs

The Oklahoma Supreme Court ruled that truck driver Elmer O. Dulen was entitled to workers' compensation benefits after he was injured and a

True or Phallus?

Georgina Spelvin was but a high school senior when she starred in the landmark porno film *The Devil in Miss Jones.*

BAWDY BALLADS "Banana Man Blues," *Memphis Minnie*

continued on page 240

a psychiatrist or sex therapist who specializes in such matters.

If your concern is keeping your daughter or son safe from pedophiles, learn to recognize the danger signs. Pedophiles often prey on kids who are loners. Be very wary of any adults befriending them, particularly if expensive gifts start showing up without common-sense explanations. Likewise, be suspicious of adults who offer to babysit for free or take your child on camping trips and such. Every grown-up in your child's life should have a defined role, be it teacher, coach, or Scout leader. It's a red flag when an adult tries to go beyond that role and create a special, private relationship with your child. As for strangers, teach your children a code word, and instruct them to ask for it if someone unusual offers them a ride home from school. If you sent that person, he or she will know the word. Talk to your kids about pedophiles and tell them to be on the lookout for adults who try to get them alone or lure them by saying, "Let's make this our special secret." Above all, encourage them to always discuss their discomfort with you whenever they think an adult is going out of his way to be physically or emotionally close, even if they think they may be overreacting. And tell them that if they're ever approached, they should immediately go to a safe place where there are other adults, such as a neighbor's house, their school, a restaurant, or a store.

Finally, give your kids some context for all this. You need to remember, and they need to know, that the world is generally safe and dependable. You don't want to instill in them a level of fear that's greater than the danger of being molested. Their concerns should be focused on specific "bad people," not the mere idea of leaving the house.

Now let's turn to the more casual use of the word pedophilia. For better or worse, it's often bandied about to describe any man who's interested in young women—say, over 15 but under the legal age of 18. (The so-called age of consent varies from place to place.) Such usage is less a medical description than a social taboo meant to keep adult men away from adolescent women (or adolescent men, in some cases).

Unfortunately, our bodies don't recognize that having sex with a girl in her teens is socially unacceptable. The attraction to a sexually maturing young woman registers in our bodies well before the taboo hits our brains. Realize, too, that not all that long ago it was commonplace to court and marry *very* young women— a phenomenon stretching back millennia. The evolution of legal limits has little or no bearing on our biological urges.

All of this leaves men in a tight spot. Act on those urges, and you go to jail. Or a very angry father neuters you. Or you lose your job, wife, and house. It's really not a good trade for a few moments of sex.

You may think that societal boundaries are unfair, but society isn't interested in fairness when it comes to sheltering its youth. Though you're not a freak for discreetly looking, you are a fool if you do more than that. Recognize the seriousness with which our culture approaches this topic and respect it. Enough said.

Also see: fantasies, incest, innocence, *Lolita*, paraphilias, perversions, sex offenders, underage, young women/older men

pee—bloody

Boxers know what it is to see blood in the urinal. Ten rounds of pugilistic pummeling to the kidneys are enough to darken the urine of even the most hardened of heavyweights.

Unless you've just gone toe-to-toe with George Foreman or any of his children, you've likely got a different sort of problem. The causes of bloody urine, or hematuria, number over a dozen. They range from the relatively benign, such as side effects of certain medications, to the truly scary, including bladder or kidney tumors. Other common causes are kidney stones, cystitis, some sexually transmitted diseases, and prostate problems. That last one may even cause you to have bloody ejaculations.

Blood in your urine or semen is never something on which to turn your back. Make an appointment with your doctor immediately. Be sure to tell the receptionist about your specific complaint so she doesn't pencil you in for a month from Sunday. "I have blood in my urine" is a line that even the most penny-pinching HMOs usually take to heart.

Also see: cystitis, prostate enlargement, STDs, urethritis, urinary problems, urologist

pee difficulties

We put this entry here because we figured that it's a good place for men to look if they're having trouble going with the flow. The most common causes of difficult urination include things like cystitis, prostatitis, other prostate problems, and some sexually transmitted diseases. Go see our related entries.

But if by pee difficulties you mean that you have trouble hitting the toilet's bull's-eye, save yourself some cleaning and your wife some nagging by sitting down to tinkle—especially for those dim, dark midnight trips. Taking a seat can hide the sound of your splashing too, especially if you aim for the upper inside portion of the bowl. That is, if you care about things like that.

Also see: finasteride, urinary problems

pee—her—during orgasm

If you've turned to this entry, it's likely because you've just had a strange experience. Perhaps you were having sex and, all of a sudden, your partner just soaked the bed sheets.

Did you just take part in your first golden shower? Probably not. What just happened is known as female ejaculation, and it's a bit freaky to a guy who's never heard of it, let alone seen it before. Be glad of one thing: It takes a hell of an orgasm for this to happen, so count yourself among the talented in bed.

For a more detailed description of what's going on, take a look at our entry on *female ejaculation*.

Also see: G-spot, urinary problems, water sports

pee—painful

Eddie Murphy used to do a riff about flames shooting out of his dick. Not just a painful, burning sensation but actual flames. It was pretty funny, sitting on this side of Eddie's penis.

It's a whole different story, though, if you're the one with dysuria, that sensation of burning or pain when you urinate.

P

You usually feel it in the part of the urethra that runs through your penis, and the pain generally subsides moments after you've finished your business. Sometimes, the pain rocks up into the area under your pubic hair. That's probably a bladder infection. The other kind of discomfort usually comes from a urethral infection. If you're younger than 35, it could mean you have a sexually transmitted disease, possibly chlamydia. In older guys, the source of infection is often coliform bacteria—that's the bug most often found in butts. You have something you want to confess?

Actually, in men over 35, an enlarged or inflamed prostate often causes urine to sit around longer than it should. The fluid stagnates, causing a burning sensation when you pee.

Whether you're on the low side of 35 or not, only a doctor can determine the reason for your particular problem. Go see one because in some cases it might be cancer that's causing the pain. Or it could just be one of the 200-some medications that list dysuria as a side effect.

Also see: anal sex, chlamydia, cystitis, NSU, penile cancer, prostate cancer, prostate enlargement, prostatitis, STDs, urethra, urethritis, urologist

pee after sex

There's a story, probably apocryphal, about a woman who always knew when her husband was cheating on her. It wasn't because she found lipstick stains, hickeys, or credit card receipts. It was because of the way he peed.

Normally, he would gush forth moments after he unzipped. But when he returned home from a dalliance, he would stand fruitlessly in front of the bowl for a minute or two before the flow started. And then she knew.

So why is it that it takes so long to urinate after you ejaculate? Blame it on the structure of your penis. When you have an erection, the spongy tissue in your penis swells, constricting your urethra. That's no problem for the high-powered pressure of an orgasm, but it forms a roadblock for the relatively relaxed mechanics of urination. Even after your woody subsides, it takes a while for your urethra to be released from the pinch. If this causes you grief, make sure you hit the head before sex next time.

One other thing: Don't be concerned if you notice that your postorgasmic urine looks awfully cloudy or seems to contain a lot of tiny particles. That's just leftover seminal fluid, possibly containing a few of the little fellas who didn't make the cut. Say a quick prayer of mourning as you flush, and get back to bed.

Also see: erection, ejaculation, penis, urethra, water sports

pelvic inflammatory disease

An umbrella term for infections that invade the female reproductive system. Pelvic inflammatory disease (PID) can lead to such serious problems as infertility or ectopic pregnancies. Sexually transmitted diseases, postabortion infections, and others fall under this dark mantle. And unfortunately, early symptoms of PID are hard to detect. By the time a woman realizes that she has a problem, she may already have developed a serious infection.

Women who use IUDs for contraception are at increased risk for pelvic inflammatory disease if they contract an

STD. Chlamydia, the fastest-spreading STD in the United States, poses an especially grave danger because 85 percent of infected women experience no symptoms.

One study suggests that douching once a week or more can nearly quadruple her chances of catching chlamydia from an infected partner. It's thought that douching disrupts the normal balance of bacteria in her vagina and allows the more dangerous organisms to take root.

Besides, there's vinegar in many douches. What's with that? She's a woman, not a salad.

Also see: abortion, chlamydia, douche, ectopic pregnancy, hysterectomy, IUD, STDs

penile cancer

Could there possibly be a scarier combination of words?

The good news is the odds: Penile cancer affects only 1,000 men a year in the United States. The two leading risk factors are unprotected sex with multiple partners—increasing the likelihood of human papillomavirus, or HPV, infection—and cigarette smoking. (So if you're going to be with multiple partners, forget the cigarette afterward.) At one time it was also believed that uncircumcised men faced a greater chance of developing penile cancer, but more recent studies have all but erased that connection. One remaining link is poor hygiene: Uncircumcised guys who don't wash themselves thoroughly tend to build up an oily substance called smegma under their foreskins, and that buildup has been linked to a higher risk of penile cancer. You'll also want to be wary if you've ever

contracted genital warts; they could be caused by a risky type of HPV.

As with most cancers, early detection means you're much more likely to survive. So put the time you spend grabbing yourself to good use: Roll your penis around between your fingertips on a regular basis (preferably not at a crowded line of urinals). Look and feel for bumps or scaly patches that last for more than a few weeks. Chances are, they're innocuous, but you should have them checked by a doctor all the same. Of course, pay attention to any blood or other discharge from under the foreskin or around the tip.

Treatment ranges from local excision of the affected area to topical chemotherapy (for slightly more advanced cases) to the option you didn't want to hear or even think about: amputation. That grimmest of outcomes aside, most men return to fairly normal function within a month of treatment, depending on the amount of tissue that had to be removed.

Also see: circumcision, genital warts, pee—painful, phalloplasty, prostate cancer, sickness, smoking, testicular cancer, urologist

penile enlargement

If you're reading this entry with anything other than casual interest, buddy, we've got to talk. First, let's take a look at what happens in penile enlargement surgery.

To lengthen it, a doctor cuts the tendons that attach your manhood to the pubic bone, then pulls the shaft away from your body—so it's not unlike exposing the foundation of a building and saying it's taller. Yes, you might gain up to an inch. But you might also end up with erections that bob straight out or even droop downward. And the more wobbly your wood, the more apt it is to fracture when things get freaky.

Well, how 'bout girth, you ask? Can't the surgery at least give you a wider pipe? Yes and no. To accomplish this, fat from another part of your body is pumped below the penile skin, like reverse liposuction. You'll look huge and chubby for a while, but your body will likely reabsorb most of this fat, leaving you with a lumpy, deformed, and possibly painful unit.

And for these "enhancements," you'll shell out $6,000 or so.

It's true that newer, more expensive, supposedly safer techniques are being developed. Some doctors swear by them. Too often, though, they're the ones who are pocketing the money.

The plain truth is, unless the size of your penis interferes with urination or insemination, you're fine just the way you are. Okay? We're tired of telling you that. Studies have shown that the average length of an erect penis is 5½ inches. That's *average*. And that spans all ages and races in our country. Also, erect penis length is the only number that counts, because flaccid length can vary widely, depending on the time of day, how you're feeling, or even how hot or cold the weather is.

Women, for their part, almost universally say that size doesn't matter. That old quip "It ain't the size of the hammer, it's how you swing it" seems to be the bottom line for them. Indeed, some women have told us they actually prefer smaller penises because they're less painful upon first entry and their owners tend to be more creative in their approach to sex.

This leads us to suggest an alternative to letting somebody hack away at your crotch: *Become a better lover.* If your woman comes so hard she nearly passes out, if she dwells on fantasies of you while she's at work, if she speaks of you to her girlfriends in giggly whispers . . . well, do you really think she'll begrudge you a measly inch?

Also see: hypnosis and penis enlargement, micropenis, penis pump, phalloplasty, size—penis, urologist

Hot Dates 1969 A half-million hippies attended the music festival Woodstock, making it the largest public display of sex, drugs, and rock 'n' roll in history.

continued from page 235

Answer:
False. Spelvin was the relatively ripe old age of 36.

female co-driver was killed in a collision with a train.

This, despite the fact that a witness quoted Dulen as saying that he and the co-driver were having sex at the time of the crash. Dulen denied that, but conceded that **his pants were pulled down a bit** and that his co-driver wore only a T-shirt.

Seemed like a Good Idea at the Time. . .
In 1908, U.S. Army doctor Joseph Richard Parke wrote about the case of a 15-year-old boy who took solo sex to a lewd and limber level. The boy's mother brought him to Parke, asking that the doc **cure her son of fellating himself**.

BAWDY BALLADS "You Put It In, I'll Take It Out," *Papa Charlie Jackson*

continued on page 249

penis

Ah, yes. The tallywhacker. The master of ceremonies. Old Blind Bob. The upstanding citizen. Big Jim and his twins. He who is exactly, gloriously, one arm's length away.

How much do you really know about your penis? Sure, you know his name, likes, dislikes, and favorite foods, but there's a lot more to him than that. Your penis is anything but the simple device it seems like from the outside. Consider first that it performs two seemingly contradictory functions: urination and fertilization. Thus it's involved in both the elimination of life's waste products and the very production of life itself. How it does this is a marvel of nature.

The penis comprises one long tube—the urethra—surrounded by three inflatable cylinders, all wrapped up in a surprisingly tough sheath of elastic tissue. Capping it off is what's known as the glans, or head. Sensitive nerve endings abound in this nut-shaped tip. In uncircumcised guys, a fold of skin called the foreskin covers the glans.

Extending from the bladder to the tip of the penis, the urethra carries urine or ejaculate, depending on your most pressing need at the moment. The urethra is surrounded by the corpus spongiosum, one of the three inflatable cylinders. The other, larger cylinders are called the corpora cavernosa. All three cylinders are made of a spongelike material filled with blood vessels and tiny chambers. When you have sexy thoughts, your brain sends signals to these cylinders, which begin filling with blood, making your penis stand at attention.

Your brain also signals the prostate, a walnut-size organ located beneath the bladder. This little guy releases the bulk of the fluid in which your sperm swim. The bladder neck squeezes shut the part of the urethra connected to the bladder, so only semen gets through to the target (this also explains why it's so difficult to get a good urine stream going right after sex). When you're done, the valves that drain the cylinders relax, allowing the blood to flow out of the penis, returning it to its floppy state.

Also see: circumcision, cock ring, condom, dildo, ejaculation, erection, fellatio, foreskin, frenulum, glans, hung, impotence, injuries, micropenis, packing, papaverine, pee after sex, phallic, phalloplasty, piercing, *Playgirl*, prepuce, reproductive system—yours, short-arm inspection, size—penis, STDs, talking dirty, urethra, urologist

penis pump

In the dark years before Viagra and other impotence busters, erectile dysfunction was often treated with this mechanical number. Also known as the vacuum constriction device, it was easy to use and had no dangerous side effects. The process also was reversible—unlike surgical implants that leave the patient with the proverbial cigar permanently ensconced in his pocket.

Here's how the pump works: An airtight cylinder is placed on your penis, then a vacuum pump—either electrical or hand-powered—draws blood into your hitherto flaccid member. A rubber ring on the base of the penis prevents blood from flowing back out too quickly.

Although the penis pump performs the job it was designed for, the resulting erection usually isn't as stiff as a natural one, nor does it last as long. The big problem with the penis pump? Stopping

P

in the middle of lovemaking to firm up your erection with the humming, squeaking device (which answers the age-old question "What's the opposite of an aphrodisiac?")

Also see: cock ring, erection difficulties, erection—firmer, impotence, medications, papaverine, sexual aids, vacuum devices

Penthouse

Think of Bob Guccione's cornerstone magazine as Jayne Mansfield to Hugh Hefner's Marilyn Monroe. Mansfield, of course, was the B-movie bombshell with a body that might make a monk question his vows. But she could never equal Monroe as the quintessential American sex symbol. So it is with *Penthouse*—always lurking hopefully in the voluptuous, more upstanding shadow of *Playboy*.

Guccione started *Penthouse* in 1969. The first, 75-cent issue sold its entire 225,000-copy press run in days, using a formula that has served the magazine well ever since: If *Playboy*'s Playmates were wholesome girls next door, *Penthouse* Pets were their raunchier sisters. *Penthouse* was the first mainstream men's magazine to publish nude photographs that included pubic hair.

Penthouse has also had journalistic high points. After publishing an article linking California's La Costa resort to the mob, the magazine became the defendant in the largest libel suit in magazine history—and won. *Penthouse* also has championed First Amendment rights and the causes of Vietnam War veterans.

Still, the magazine has always made its biggest splashes by publishing nude photos of the famous or near famous. Its 1984 pictorial of Miss America Vanessa Williams ended up costing Williams her crown. *Penthouse* has also featured nude or seminude photos of two women linked to President Bill Clinton: Gennifer Flowers and Paula Jones.

Though *Penthouse* came close to matching *Playboy*'s circulation in the late 1970s, by 2001 it had fallen well behind again.

Also see: erotica, erotic literature, fantasies, media, *Playboy*, *Playgirl*, pornography, sex symbols

performance anxiety

You've shown up for the big game but left your bat at home. Trust us, it's happened to a lot of guys—almost everybody at some point, in fact, whether we admit it or not. That's the price we pay for having a penis that's required to stand tall in order to complete the sex act.

Some therapists call this spectatoring, and for good reason. Essentially, an anxious fellow is watching himself perform (or trying to perform) rather than being fully involved in the moment. He's so worried about not being able to get the job done that, as an ironic result, he removes himself from the very sensations that *would* shiver his timber.

Try to take a fatalistic approach to it all. Simply assume that, at one time or another, you won't be able to get it up. The only question then is, What do you do when that happens?

Fortunately, we have an answer: Immediately stop the stampede toward penetration. Focus instead on pleasing one another in alternate ways. Dwell over her breasts, or parts farther south,

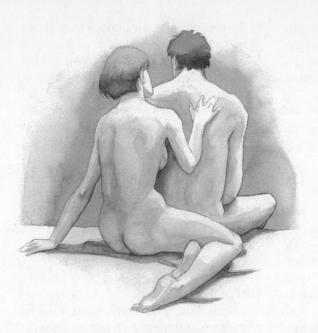

with your tongue. Give her a massage. Let her massage you. Take a break and just talk for a while. Make a concerted decision *not* to have intercourse.

You know something? You'll actually come out of this a better lover. If you expand your repertoire of skills beyond mere intercourse, you'll have one very devoted fan in bed next to you.

Also see: anticipatory anxiety, clumsiness, cunnilingus, emotions, erection difficulties, erection—firmer, faking orgasm, first time with a lover, hypnosis and performance anxiety, impotence, job loss, laughter, massage, medications, phallic, premature ejaculation, relaxation, self-esteem, sensate focus, sex therapy, spectatoring, stress

perfume

Because women are more acutely aware of smell than we are, it matters more to them how *they* smell. Ergo, their passion for perfume.

This isn't a bad thing. How many times have you caught a whiff of a woman wearing Eau de Old Girlfriend? Chances are, you were transported right back to those exciting times with the one that got away.

However, here's an interesting bit of trivia: The same perfume can produce a whole variety of slightly different aromas depending on who's wearing it. The blend of oils in a perfume mixes with the natural odor of a woman to create a totally new, individualized scent. That's why Shalimar may have smelled great on your prom date but not so hot on your mom. It's also why your woman's natural scent can send you into a hot-blooded frenzy.

Also see: aromatherapy, body odor as an attractant, body odor—controlling, breath, farting, fragrances, hygiene, past partners—longing for, pheromones, scents, sweating

perineum

In some parts of the South, this area is known as the taint. That's because t'ain't one and t'ain't the other. It's the part of your anatomy between your anus and your scrotum—the chunk that contacts a bicycle seat. It's the same area in women, except, of course, they don't have scrotums. Unless you're at a stage show in Thailand.

Like the genitals and anus, the perineum is loaded with extra-sensitive nerve endings. In women, this area is very responsive to rubbing and massaging. That could explain why they love horseback riding so much. It also means that you now have new frontiers to explore in your next lovemaking session.

We men like it a lot too. If the area is massaged deeply, it stimulates the prostate and can up the intensity of our orgasms.

Also see: priapism, prostate

period

Common slang for menstruation (other popular terms include *friend, curse, on the rag, that time of the month*). It's when she changes into her lackluster "period panties" so she doesn't wreck the tiger-striped thong you bought her last Valentine's Day.

Let's face it, not menstruating is one of the great things about being a man. Imagine if you bled out of the end of your peter every month. Imagine having to stock cotton condoms in your desk drawer. Imagine having to suddenly excuse yourself in the midst of an important meeting to rush to the john and wash out the scarlet stain that's started to leak across the crotch of your pants. There's a good reason women begrudge us for not having to go through this a dozen times a year.

Add to that the fact that a woman's period has been surrounded by myth and misinformation since the dawn of history. Some cultures—ancient and not so ancient—felt that women were unclean during this time and forbade any sort of contact with a menstruating woman.

Though we're a bit more enlightened these days, some men and women are still wary of getting it on during menstruation. Too bad, because aside from the added cleanup, it's a great time to have sex. In fact, some women are

hornier during their periods than at any other time of the month.

If you decide to take advantage of her increased interest in you, realize that even though she may be really randy, her natural lubrication may be limited, especially if she uses tampons (they *are* superabsorbent, after all). Spend extra time kissing and caressing, and use a good lubricant. It's also a good idea to wear a condom, especially if you don't know her HIV status.

Also see: estrogen, horny, menstruation, Norplant, progesterone, PMS, tampon, vaginal moisture

personal ads

Maybe you think only losers run the ever-present personal ads you see in your local newspaper or free weekly—and oh yeah, we hear they're also on the Internet these days. If that's the case, you obviously haven't taken a good hard look at the bar scene (with its increasing craziness) or the office romance scene (with its increasing legal complexity).

Some pretty classy women are mighty tired of those very same scenes. That's why they place ads. Think of it as a bonus for you: You definitely know that a woman who tries such an approach is available and looking. It saves you from hitting on, say, that cute chick on the bar stool whose husband, the linebacker, is on his way back from the john.

If you do spy someone who fills the bill, spend a few minutes thinking about what you want to say to her voice mail. You have mere seconds to convince her to call you back. Practice your message aloud a few times. Just don't write it out and read it into the phone. Scripted messages sound just like what they are. You sound lame or insincere or both.

Don't bother placing your own ad, either. The guys we know who have placed ads generally report disappointment over the number and quality of responses.

If you do end up with a date, arrange to meet her in a public place for the first few times. It protects her and it protects you. Plus, it's easier to make a hasty exit if she seems like the kind of woman who might cook your pet if you end the relationship.

Also see: blind date, date rape, dating, desperate, first date, hypnosis and seduction, Internet dating, matchmaking services, mail-order brides, meeting women, one-night stand, pickup lines, romance, singles scene, soul mates, Your place or mine?

perversions

Generally speaking, perversions are sexual expressions outside the range of what's considered normal. Of course, that raises the question of what's normal. For some people, the only allowable, normal sexual act is straight old intercourse between a husband and wife for the purpose of procreation.

Perversions are defined by society. Experts in the field think of acceptable sexual expression as a bell curve, where the large middle is made up of the most common sexual practices—kissing, touching your partner, intercourse. Group sex, anal sex, urophilia (the use of urine for sexual pleasure), and sadomasochism are among the acts that fall on the outer edges of that bell curve. Healthy sexual expression, then, covers a wide range of sexual acts, all of them reasonable as long as they occur between consenting adults.

That's why, when something happens in private between consenting adults and it helps them learn about themselves, it isn't perverse, no matter how disgusting it may seem to outsiders. But it's also why rape, and sex with children, are rightly considered perverse as well as illegal.

If consent cannot be given, you shouldn't be doing it.

Also see: abnormal, compulsive behavior, danger, fantasies, guilt, hang-ups, paraphilias, risky sex, sex therapy, taboos, violence

pets

The latest statistics from the American Veterinary Medical Association show that nearly 60 percent of American households have pets. Whether it's a dog, cat, turtle, or snake, it's not hard to see why. With their unconditional love and wacky antics, pets allow humans to express feelings of warmth, concern, tenderness, and affection without fear of rejection. This ability to be physically affectionate can carry over into our relationships with other humans, if we allow it.

This is also why pets are a good way for single people to meet. Like the clothes you wear, your hairstyle, your job, or the type of car you drive, the pet you choose to own sends a strong message to women about the kind of guy you are. A single man taking care of a dog or cat can be seen as responsible, warmhearted, and affectionate by single women. In other words, somebody a woman may want to spend some quality time with.

Use a little decorum when she comes over for her own tummy rub, though.

P

P

Lock your 150-pound mastiff in the hallway when the two of you are hard at it in the bedroom.

Also see: animals, bestiality, love, zoophilia

Peyronie's disease

Your penis can take a lot of wear and tear. How else could it survive what you did to it as a teenager? But for up to 5 percent of us, mostly between ages 40 and 60, that manhandling can lead to a condition called Peyronie's (pronounced "pay-rone-EEZ") disease. While it's not life-threatening, Peyronie's can put a definite kink in your love life. Literally: You end up with a bent erection—a right angle, in the very worst cases.

Although the exact cause of the disease isn't known, many men report either a major trauma to the penis during vigorous love-making or a number of small traumas over time. The blood pressure medication Inderal (propranolol hydrochloride) has also been implicated. Whatever the cause, scar tissue builds up in the elastic tissue surrounding the chambers in your penis that fill with blood during an erection. That scar tissue prevents the chamber from expanding completely in concert with the others. Hence the angled erections.

Treatment ranges from simply waiting for the condition to heal itself to surgical procedures to smooth away the scar tissue. A promising new option is injection with the calcium blocker Verelan (verapamil hydrochloride), which inhibits the uptake of calcium in the scar tissue. This keeps the tissue pliable.

Because Peyronie's develops gradually, it's possible to detect it early. Any hard spots or changes in curvature—not including the normal left or right slant you've had since birth—should be checked out by a urologist.

Also see: athletic sex, erection difficulties, injuries, penis, urologist

phallic

Derived from *phallikos,* the Greek word for "pertaining to the penis." In everyday usage, *phallic* is the word used to describe something that looks or acts like a penis. Speeding trains, towering sky-

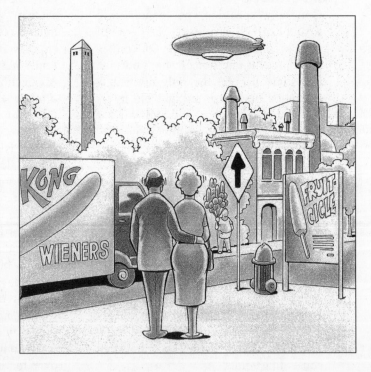

scrapers, huge cigars, Geraldo Rivera—all can be said to be phallic symbols. Many ancient agrarian cultures worshipped phallic statues and symbols in hopes of harnessing this generative power.

Some more history for you: The phallic stage was the third of five stages of human sexual development outlined by famed psychiatrist Sigmund Freud—the others being oral, anal, latency, and finally, genital.

According to Freud, during the phallic stage—between ages 3 and 6—a child's libido is fixated on sensations derived from the genitals. (Because he based his theory on a study of boys, Freud chose the term *phallic* to describe this stage, even though it affects girls as well.) Freud said that if this phallic fixation is somehow blocked by, say, prudish parents or militant nuns, the resulting adult will exhibit psychosexual distress such as anxiety or obsessive masturbation. Although this theory sometimes has been replaced, especially in America, by other behavioral models, Freud's basic idea that childhood trauma can affect sexual function in adulthood had a profound effect on the growing science of psychiatry.

Also see: anima and animus, compulsive behavior, dildo, dreams, fears/phobias, Freud, guilt, libido, penis, religion, sex therapy

phalloplasty

A general term used to describe the surgical enhancement or reconstruction of the penis. Enhancement is done by choice, as in enlargement surgery. Reconstruction is done to repair congenital deformities, injuries from accidents, or an advanced case of penile cancer—usually using skin from the underside of the forearm, near the wrist.

The organ can be rebuilt, but unlike Steve Austin, it may not be stronger, faster, or better. Though the reconstructed penis will function perfectly well for urination, sex may be difficult. To help overcome this, inflatable implants may be surgically inserted during the reconstruction process.

Reconstruction—or rather, construction—can also be done during gender-reassignment surgery. That's a sex change from female to male. The female genitals are transformed into male external genitals in an operation resembling reconstruction, but with a major difference: The nerves involved in clitoral stimulation are preserved and hooked up to the newly constructed penis. Although purveyors of this surgical technique strive to ensure that their clients maintain the ability to orgasm after surgery, it doesn't always work out that way.

Also see: hermaphrodite, penile cancer, penile enlargement, transvestism, urologist

pheromones

In the classified ads found in lowbrow magazines, pheromones are some sort of magic potion that causes perfectly rational people to fall suddenly in love with you. You wish.

Not that the theory is entirely unfounded. Pheromones—chemicals that regulate behavior ranging from sexual arousal to territorial defense—do exist throughout the animal and insect kingdoms, so there's no reason to suppose

P

that we humans evolved without them. Indeed, scientists at Yale and Rockefeller Universities recently isolated the first gene believed to be linked to special mucous membranes in the nose that may be designed to receive pheromone signals.

We're also known to have special glands in our armpits and genitals called apocrine glands. These secrete two chemicals—androsterone and androstenol—that are present in saliva as well. So what? So, they're present in the saliva of hogs, too, and hog breeders have known for years that they induce arousal in females of the species.

Researchers also have found that these two substances can influence subconscious male and female behavior. In one study, men avoided a restroom stall treated with the chemicals. Women, on the other hand, tended to *choose* a similarly doused chair. Interestingly, nearly twice as many women as men can detect the odor of both chemicals, which they deem to have a pleasant, musky smell. Researchers tell us that women are much more sensitive to the smell of musk than men are, especially during ovulation. Not surprisingly, then, most perfumes and colognes used to be made from a chemical derived from the musk glands of the musk deer.

Androsterone and androstenol don't just show up in our pits, spit, and pants. They're found naturally in celery, caviar, parsnips, and the mushrooms known as truffles, which explains why hogs are used to unearth them in the forests of France. So, theoretically, these veggies might be a good thing to have on the menu next time you're cooking dinner for a hot date. All that said, the precise mechanism by which pheromones work—and how to harness their power in humans—remains largely a mystery.

Also see: aphrodisiac, aromatherapy, body odor as an attractant, body odor—controlling, breath, fragrances, perfume, pubic hair, scents, sweating

phimosis

An abnormally tight foreskin, a condition afflicting about 2 percent of uncircumcised males. In adults, phimosis results in incredibly painful erections that make sex all but impossible while increasing one's risk of contracting sexually transmitted diseases.

The pro-circumcision camp uses phimosis as one main reason—along with general hygiene and reducing the risk of penile cancer—for circumcision in newborns. The anti-circumcision camp claims that tight foreskins are normal in prepubescent boys, and that puberty itself, or nonsurgical methods such as stretching and steroid creams, will solve the problem.

When phimosis does persist into adulthood and the discomfort is extreme, circumcision becomes the only recourse. We doubt that you need to be reminded of this, but if you suffer from any unexplainable pain or discomfort of the penis, contact your doctor.

Also see: circumcision, foreskin, penile cancer, smegma, urologist

phone sex

Like deepwater fishing and competitive farting, talking on the phone while masturbating is a primarily male activity: Nearly 99 percent of the workers in the phone sex business are women. There are two reasons why. First, it's a safe, quick way of exploring sexual activity outside a monogamous relationship. Second, because phone sex often involves role-playing, it's a way for men to act out fantasies they may be uncomfortable discussing with their partners. Therein can lie the problem, say sex therapists.

Communication is the key to a good relationship. If playing serving wench and stable hand gets you hot and bothered, imagine how much better it would be if your partner took one of those roles instead of some apathetic sex worker who's in it only for the money? (An apathetic worker who, by the way, may be 4 feet 8, 242 pounds, and covered with lesions. You have no idea who's on the other end, after all.)

Speaking of money, phone sex is an easy way to blow tons of it. At 3 bucks a minute, it doesn't take long to max out your plastic. So if phone sex is what you crave, why not try it with your partner? Dial her up from a hotel room and see where things go. She'll probably be willing to play along—and without your credit card number.

Also see: communication, dial-a-porn, fantasies, hypnosis and seduction, play-acting, talking dirty, time-saving tips, travel—loneliness during, unwanted advances, voice

pickup lines

The good news: Lines really can work. The bad news: Yours don't. That's because you're probably using a *stereotypical* pickup line, which women smell as quickly as they do another gal's perfume. And then you're toast.

It may go against conventional guy wisdom, but studies show that honesty—about who you are and why you want to talk to a given woman—is more than twice as likely to be successful at starting a conversation than some corny, canned line. And getting a conversation started is half the battle, isn't it?

P

Hot Dates 1970 The President's Commission on Obscenity and Pornography concluded that erotica does not cause sexual deviance. Most sex offenders, in fact, had less exposure to erotica than other Americans.

continued from page 240

The skeptical physician asked the lithesome lad for a demonstration. Parke later wrote: "He lay on a couch; and as the climax of the orgasm approached, apparently forgetting my presence, and every other consideration, he resigned himself with utmost abandonment to the delirium of his pleasure, rolling, gasping, writhing, and resembling nothing so much as some sort of animal, curled up in a ball, enduring its death agony.

"He was afterward committed to a sanitarium for the treatment of such cases."

Foreign Affairs
In the 8th century, Japanese Shinto priests devised the art of penis packaging to enhance sexual pleasure. The technique, called Kokigami or the Nippon slip-on, still is practiced by

True or Phallus?
The rock band 10 cc named itself in homage to the amount of sperm that a man reputedly ejaculates.

BAWDY BALLADS "I Touch Myself," *the Divinyls*

continued on page 256

Instead of using a pickup line, try an opening line. The latter is a sincere, fairly spontaneous expression of interest in the woman at hand. The former is a rehearsed script that you trot out (usually with accompanying lounge lizard persona) for every last woman. A pickup line like "Hey, baby, buy a drunken idiot a drink?" leaves her only two possible answers: No, and hell no.

Also see: bars, courtship, dating, first date, first time with a lover, meeting women, opening line, rejection—romantic, sexual innuendo, sexy, shyness, singles scene, slick, unwanted advances, va-va-voom

P

piercing

We've all seen people with pierced ears, noses, or navels, but piercings also are done in less visible, more sexually overt areas of the body, such as the nipples, labia, and penis. Ouch.

Men and women may get pierced to make a statement about their sexuality or to enhance sadomasochistic activities, among other reasons. In Europe, many couples use genital piercings as symbols of the marriage bond, having rings attached to their sex organs instead of their fingers.

This is nothing new. Roman centurions wore nipple rings as symbols of courage. Victorian women wore them to make their nipples bigger.

There are at least a half-dozen types of penis piercings available. Perhaps most popular is the Prince Albert, which goes through the urethra at the base of the head, on the underside. It derives its name from the legend that Prince Albert reputedly wore one to pull the foreskin back from the head of his uncircumcised organ.

Some penis piercings are said to enhance sex. The ampallang is one. Done as part of a puberty rite in the areas surrounding the Indian Ocean, it consists of a horizontal cut through the center of the head, above the urethra and the erectile tissue. A man may then insert through the holes a metal bar retained by discs. With the discs protruding on each side of the penis, the device is supposed to enhance intercourse for both partners, but could pose problems with anal penetration. Similar is the apadravya, described in the ancient Hindu treatise on love and social conduct, the *Kama Sutra*. This is a vertical piercing through the penis head. A protruding bar is supposed to create a vibrating sensation for the woman during intercourse.

A piercing can take up to several months to heal, and there are risks. Piercing a penis through the shaft destroys erectile tissue. And if sterile instruments aren't used, you could get a bacterial infection, such as hepatitis B or C. There's even a slight risk of transmitting HIV. Some guys also have allergic reactions to the metal used in the jewelry.

If you're still set on getting your dong pierced, ask about sanitary practices at the piercing studio. It should have an autoclave to sterilize instruments, and sterilization should take place after each use. Disposable items such as needles and latex gloves should be used once and tossed. An aftercare sheet should be made available to explain how to take care of your piercing. Avoid studios that use piercing guns; they can't be sterilized adequately. Ask whether the studio is certified by the Association of Professional Piercers.

Also ask yourself this: "Why, exactly, am I having this done?"

Also see: Kama Sutra, tattoos

Pill—the

Female oral contraceptives, collectively referred to as the Pill, were first approved for use in the United States in 1960. Advancements since then have made the Pill safer and cut down on side effects—such that it is currently the number one choice for birth control among young women.

The Pill works by using a combination of the hormones estrogen and progestin to fool a woman's body into thinking that she has just conceived, which makes her stop ovulating. It's 95 percent effective in typical use.

The obvious upside: There's no need to interrupt foreplay to put on a condom, nor, of course, are there certain days when you need to refrain from sex. It's also muss- and fuss-free. All of which spells *spontaneity* with a capital *S*. Taken to its extreme, yet logical, conclusion, the Pill allows for nonstop sex.

The obvious downside is that the Pill doesn't do a thing to protect against sexually transmitted diseases, for you or her. And because it's a form of hormone therapy, some women don't tolerate it well: They cramp, become bloated, and feel generally crappy.

The laundry list of horrifying side effects linked to the original Pill have abated amid new formulas and new studies, some of which even suggest a salutary effect on some cancers. The verdict is still out on whether the Pill helps reduce a woman's risk of developing breast cancer. But there is evidence that the Pill decreases her risk of developing ovarian cancer by up to 50 percent, compared with women who have never relied on this method of birth control. Moreover, one study found that a woman may reap these benefits by taking the Pill for as little as 3 to 6 months, with the cancer-prevention benefits lasting up to 15 years after she stops taking it. On the flip side, there is evidence of cardiovascular problems in women over age 35 who take the Pill—especially if they smoke, are overweight, or have a history of heart disease.

Also see: breast cancer, contraception, cramps—menstrual, estrogen, hormones, male pill, menstruation, morning-after pill, oral contraceptive, progestin, STDs

pituitary gland

This pea-sized lump of tissue at the base of the brain is the human body's mighty mite. It releases growth hormone that promotes the growth of bones and several organs during childhood and adolescence and that improves muscle strength in adults. When there's a deficiency of growth hormone, dwarfism results.

The pituitary also is vital to sex and procreation. For guys, it triggers the release of testosterone—the adrenal hormone that fuels most of our sex drive—and the production of sperm. In women, the pituitary gland regulates menstrual cycles, causes the maturation and release of eggs, releases estrogens, stimulates the contraction of the uterus during childbirth, and prompts the production of breast milk during lactation.

Also see: hormones, witch's milk

pity sex

You're a great guy, the salt of the earth. Everybody thinks so: your friends, your co-workers, the ladies. Throw in the fact that you're also considered pretty cute, and you could probably have any woman you want. So how come you went home with that plain-Jane chick from shipping and receiving, the one with the personality of a dandelion, after the office party last week?

Welcome to the world of pity sex.

Know this: You're not doing a woman any favors if you sleep with her once and never call again. Though your "good deed" may have given her a temporary jolt of excitement or self-worth, eventually, when you don't follow up, she's going to feel rejected or used or both. And if she's someone you work with, she may very well seek to make your life miserable forever after.

Just so you're aware, don't think that because you're in a relationship, you're exempt from this kind of situation. Pity sex is common toward the end of a relationship, when a guy throws his soon-to-be-ex-girlfriend a bone, so to speak. Try to avoid this. If you really want out, it only complicates matters.

Oh, by the way, women do this pity-oriented stuff too. Kind of gives you a new perspective on some of the gals who've slept with you, eh?

planes

The novelty . . . the thrilling risk of getting caught . . . and the oxygen deprivation from the stale, recycled air: All these things can combine to create some pretty mind-blowing sex. Too bad airborne antics are such a logistical challenge.

For the determined, we offer the following.

Start by booking a red-eye flight, which is apt to have fewer passengers. In coach, most seats have only 35 to 36 inches of legroom, which doesn't allow for much more than some petting under a blanket. You probably don't want to

get any wilder than that in the cabin anyway. Airline crews and pilots—not to mention less adventurous passengers—have been complaining about the increasing incidence of overt sexual behavior on flights.

The lavatory isn't much more spacious than the legroom in economy class, but it offers two distinct advantages. One, you're less likely to be interrupted by the drink cart or other travelers. And two—a very interesting piece of news indeed—the Federal Aviation Administration's official, uh, position is that what you do in the lavatory is your own business.

So, your partner should head to the little-pilots' room shortly after the seat belt sign has been turned off and the initial rush of passengers to the lavatories has abated. Once your lover has been safely ensconced in the restroom for a minute or two, you can nonchalantly join her. Create a little turbulence in the rear-entry position. Return to your seats separately but with matching grins. Don't forget to wash your hands.

Oh, and if you're looking for official admittance to the Mile High Club, pay careful attention to the pilot's announcements about your altitude: Sticklers insist that you be literally at least a mile, or 5,280 feet, above Earth.

Also see: rear entry, standing positions, travel as an aphrodisiac

playacting

Be grateful if you're a closet thespian. Sex therapists say that playacting, role-playing, or whatever you choose to call it, can leave bed partners begging each other for encores.

Problem is, you may get stage fright when it comes to asking your partner to pretend she's Little Bo Peep or a bawdy babe in a brothel. And she may be just as hesitant to ask you to pretend you're a domineering school principal administering a stern lecture and a few swats on the butt.

Nobody wants his partner to be offended by the fantasy he wants acted out—or to dismiss it as absurd. The key is to have a relationship built on trust. Only then can a couple completely reveal what they want and need in bed. One way to build trust is to have a relationship contract in which each of you agrees that the other is free to ask for anything. That doesn't mean you'll get it . . . but there should be no penalties for merely raising the subject.

If you've never discussed playacting with your partner, you may want to bring it up in an intimate but calm setting, such as over a romantic dinner. Don't pressure or coerce her. If she's agreeable, make the whole bedroom your stage. Then once you've played and enjoyed a few such games, you can try new ones spontaneously.

Also see: anal sex, bondage and discipline, cross-dressing, dominance and submission, drag queen, fantasies, games, john, *Lolita*, phone sex, role reversal, rough sex, zipless sex

Playboy

In 1953, using $6,600 of other people's money, Hugh Hefner launched a magazine and an empire that forever changed the American sexual landscape. That first issue of *Playboy* was thin—44 pages. But for a paltry $500, Hefner purchased color-separation plates and a photograph that ensured the inaugural issue's success. The voluptuous, naked blonde pictured in the photo: a young Marilyn Monroe. (Almost fittingly, *Playboy* also would publish the last known nude photo of Monroe, taken a mere month before she died.)

Aimed at an audience that Hefner described as interested in "good food, drink, proper dress, and the pleasure of female company," *Playboy* embraced and mainstreamed topics and pictures once deemed too risqué for public consumption. Critics complained that the publication was hedonistic and objectified women. At least one psychiatrist opined that Playmates would cause men to be frustrated and angry by setting them up for disappointment in their relationships with real women.

In 1962, Hefner began publishing a feature entitled "The Playboy Philosophy." It ran in 25 installments of the magazine, espousing a society in which sexual conduct between consenting adults was something to rejoice in, not be ashamed of. Sample insight: "If a man has a right to find God in his own way, he has a right to go to the Devil in his own way also." Putting his money where his mouth was, Hefner created the Playboy Foundation, which has contributed money to causes that include sex education programs and anti–death penalty and pro-choice organizations.

Notwithstanding jokes about picking up *Playboy* for its articles, the magazine has in fact showcased many of America's top writers—and created its share of controversy with its lengthy interviews. Jimmy Carter confessed to *Playboy* that he had lusted in his heart, while Minnesota governor Jesse Ventura said that religion was for "weak-minded people."

Playboy's circulation is less than half what it was during its pinnacle in the early 1970s. And gone are its glitzy

Playboy Clubs, where cotton-tailed waitresses did the "bunny dip" as they served drinks. Striving to remain relevant—and profitable—Playboy Enterprises nowadays has a cable TV channel, home videos, and an Internet club. Hefner's daughter, Christie, is chairperson and CEO of the company.

Of course, *Playboy* spawned a series of more sexually explicit men's magazines, including *Penthouse*, *Hustler*, and *Chic*.

Also see: erotica, erotic literature, fantasies, media, *Penthouse*, pornography, sex symbols

Playgirl

In 1974, *Playgirl* magazine leveled the pornographic playing field by featuring buff stuff for women. By its third issue, *Playgirl* was selling its show-all centerfolds to a million women—maybe. Some speculate that gay men compose a sizable portion of the magazine's readership.

Though the magazine mimics some of the features of its men's counterparts, there isn't even a pretense of the serious journalism found in the likes of *Playboy* or even *Penthouse*: "12 Buff Hunks Strip Down" is about as probing as things get here. Actors Brad Pitt and Leonardo DiCaprio have sued *Playgirl* over its planned or actual use of unauthorized, nude photos of them.

Also see: beefcake, erotica, erotic literature, homosexuality, hung, fantasies, male body, packing, *Penthouse*, pornography, sex symbols, size—penis

PMS

Common shorthand for a jumble of disturbing symptoms lumped under the term *premenstrual syndrome*. This dis-

order—known scientifically as *aggravatus regularus*—is thought to be caused by hormonal shifts linked to a woman's menstrual cycle. It usually starts 1 to 2 weeks before the onset of her period and ends with the start of her menstrual flow.

Researchers estimate that 40 percent of women in their reproductive years experience symptoms, which may include depression, anxiety, anger, breast tenderness, headaches, insomnia, hot flashes, and joint and muscle pain. At its outer limits, PMS can wreak havoc on her mood to the point where she can't function normally. In extreme cases, it has been a contributing factor in broken marriages, child abuse, even homicide.

The malady's effect on sex drive is unpredictable. Some women want less sex. Others more. Bearing in mind what we said above about homicide, men whose partners have PMS should broach the subject of sex carefully. In addition, it may help to know her cycle so you can be forewarned and ready to deal with her. Try not to argue or pick a fight; and if she picks a fight, sidestep it. Be kind and understanding.

Much remains unknown about PMS. Genetic history and stress may contribute to the severity of a woman's symptoms. Oddly, women in different cultures report different symptoms.

Also see: breast pain, cramps—menstrual, hormones, manual stimulation, menstruation, mood, postpartum depression, sex drive

politicians

Cigar aficionado Bill Clinton, Newt Gingrich, Gary Hart, and other politicos whose "peckerdilloes" have come to light don't represent a new trend in government debauchery. They're just the guys who've gotten caught.

Heck, Clinton wasn't even the first to imply that oral sex doesn't count. Virginia senator Charles Robb made that claim when his infidelities came to light in 1994.

America's tradition of political philandering dates back to the founding fathers. Ben Franklin had a common-law wife. Thomas Jefferson reputedly had a decades-long affair with a slave who also happened to be his wife's half-sister. Later, Secretary of the Treasury Alexander Hamilton explained his letters to an embezzler as proof not of corruption but of blackmail money he'd paid to cover up an affair with the embezzler's wife. Hamilton even printed a pamphlet with details of the tryst.

Rumor has it that our only bachelor president, James Buchanan, was gay and had an unusually close relationship with his married, male secretary of the treasury. President Martin Van Buren's vice president, Richard Johnson, lived for years with a slave who bore him two daughters. Grover Cleveland, like Jefferson, was believed to have fathered a child out of wedlock. Presidents Warren Harding and, of course, John F. Kennedy both had affairs while in the Oval Office.

Cabinet members have also gotten into the act. Indeed, Clinton appointee Henry Cisneros dallied with a female fund-raiser while his wife was bedridden with a difficult pregnancy.

New York City mayors have held up their end too. Long before Rudolph Giuliani stepped out with an upper–East Side woman, Jimmy Walker bedded a British showgirl half his age.

One is reminded of the old Henry Kissinger line "Power is the ultimate aphrodisiac."

Also see: adultery, casting couch, French, hypnosis and seduction, monotony, outing, *Penthouse*, *Playboy*, power, sex addiction, trophy wife, young women/older men

polygamy

Most of us would agree that it's hard enough being married to one person. Even so, some cultures practice polygamy: marriage to more than one spouse at a time. If a guy has multiple wives, it's called polygyny. If a woman has more than one husband, it's called polyandry. Sometimes, a man's wives are sisters or a woman's husbands are brothers.

Polygamy has been practiced in many countries, including Egypt, Ireland, China, and Japan. It can still be found in parts of sub-Saharan Africa and in some Muslim nations. The Muslim holy book, the Koran, permits a man to have four wives, although the practice is prohibited or discouraged in several Muslim nations.

In the United States, we tend to associate plural marriage with Mormons. Up until the late-19th century, the Church of Jesus Christ of Latter-day Saints permitted men to have several wives. In 1890, the fourth president of the Mormon church, Wilford Woodruff, issued a manifesto that generally disallowed plural marriages.

Die-hard polygamists were excommunicated from the church and formed splinter Mormon groups. A number of these groups still exist and continue to practice polygamy, primarily in Utah.

Also see: jealousy, marriage, marriage—open, ménage à trois, swinging

poppers

Street name for nitrite drugs that users inhale: amyl nitrite, butyl nitrite, and isobutyl nitrite. Poppers have been around since the 19th century and were initially used as a heart attack medicine. They've been abused as a recreational drug since the 1930s and are particularly popular with gay men. One study conducted in Los Angeles County found that gay and bisexual men were five times more likely than the general population to use amyl nitrites.

Amyl nitrite's legitimate, prescription usage is for the alleviation of angina pectoris, a heart condition that causes sharp chest pain. The drug comes in a small glass bottle or ampoule. Fluids containing butyl or isobutyl nitrite are often sold in bottles labeled *leather cleaner* or *room deodorizer*. You snap off the glass tops and inhale the fumes.

Users get a brief rush—sometimes the drug is even called rush—due to their blood vessels expanding, their heartbeat accelerating, and blood swooshing to their brains. Inhaled just before orgasm, poppers can extend and intensify the experience—or, conversely in some men, cause a sudden loss of erection.

Because they dilate blood vessels and increase the risk of tears in anal tissue, poppers also increase the chances for HIV and other sexually transmitted diseases to enter the bloodstream. Chronic use weakens your body's immune system and causes sores in your mouth and nose and even lung damage.

A word of special caution: Poppers and Viagra (sildenafil) together is an especially risky, even lethal, combination.

Also see: anal sex, drugs, heart conditions, STDs

pornography

Originally, it meant writings about prostitutes. Today, it means videos, pictures, writings, and other media intended to cause sexual arousal. While the word is

Hot Dates **1972** In his book *The Joy of Sex*, Englishman Alex Comfort showed couples how to spice up their sex lives. Some 12 million copies of the book were sold.

continued from page 249

Answer:
True. Scientists peg the normal amount of ejaculate at 9 cc, so the band was aiming to be somewhat above average.

some men today. It calls for a man to pack his pistol inside a paper sculpture of an animal. Then he imagines that his penis has the qualities of the animal, and **he and his partner act out sexual fantasies conjured up by the beast**. Scripts are available for the fantasy-impaired.

In Extremis
A woman bit off a testicle of a man whom she said forced her to perform oral sex on him. California police kept the severed testicle in a plastic bag in the police property room. The guy charged with the sexual assault said the sex was consensual and that **his accuser simply couldn't take criticism**.

LEGAL BRIEFS
An Orlando judge had a ready explanation for courthouse workers who accused him of printing out In-

continued on page 267

used interchangeably with *obscenity*, pornography is not a legal term, just a popular one.

The question of when pornography becomes obscene—and hence illegal—is an ongoing conundrum. Congress passed the first antipornography law in 1873, with the U.S. post office granting a man named Anthony Comstock enormous power to snoop through people's mail in search of smut.

Books ranging from James Joyce's *Ulysses* to Henry Miller's *Tropic of Cancer* had been banned in the United States because they were regarded as obscene. More recently, music lyrics have been the source of controversy, from the Rolling Stones' song "Let's Spend the Night Together" to 2 Live Crew's "Nasty as They Wanna Be" album.

Pornography became a truly big business with the advent of videocassettes that enabled folks to take home copies of *Debbie Does Dallas* with the same ease with which they rent *Honey, I Shrunk the Kids*. The industry shows no signs of going flaccid anytime soon. It released more than 10,000 new video titles in 1999, doing an estimated $4 billion in rentals and sales, with more than 500 million video rentals.

The overwhelming majority of skin flicks are made in the San Fernando Valley area of Los Angeles. Here's a shock: Guys are the biggest audience. It's estimated that of adult videos rented, 71 percent are by lone (and lonely?) male customers, 19 percent by women accompanied by men, 7 percent by male couples, 2 percent by women alone, and less than 1 percent by female couples.

U.S. obscenity law now states that material can be deemed obscene only if its dominant theme appeals to a "prurient interest" in sex, if the material affronts contemporary community standards relating to the depiction of sexual matters, and if the material has no serious literary, artistic, political, or scientific value. Lawmakers across the country have worked hard to find loopholes in this Supreme Court–mandated definition. They've also grappled with how to impose restrictions on the proliferation of porn on the Internet—and on children's access to it—without hampering free expression.

Defenders of the right to view porn point to countries such as Denmark, Holland, and Germany, which have repealed obscenity laws with no discernible ill effect. President Reagan's Meese Commission also found no causal link between sexually explicit materials and sexually aggressive behavior. Indeed, there are no studies showing any such connection in any American communities. However, strong conservative views in the United States continue to keep porn obscenity laws in effect for the forseeable future.

Also see: bestiality, cybersex, dial-a-porn, erotica, erotic films, erotic literature, French, hermaphrodite, lesbian, *Lolita*, mail-order sex products, media, movies, *Penthouse*, *Playboy*, *Playgirl*, Sade—Marquis de, sex symbols, third-degree cleavage, videos, violence, X-rated

postpartum depression

Though the birth of a child is a happy event, it's common for new mothers to develop "baby blues": depression, mood swings, crying jags, sleep problems, and headaches. The blues may be a result of hormonal fluctuations and changes that a woman experiences in her body shape, marital and family relationships, sexuality, finances, and self-image. For 9 out

(continued on page 262)

SPECIAL REPORT
Positions

Yet another reason to be glad you're a man and not a mouse or a moose. With the exception of the Bonobo (pygmy chimp), which indulges in numerous sexual positions and behaviors, we humans experiment far more than other animals, most of whom just revert to the same old position every time. Can you imagine Lassie ever growling to Rin Tin Tin, "Hey, big boy, wanna try people style for a change?"

Some years ago, Ted McIlvenna, Ph.D., of the Institute for Advanced Study of Human Sexuality in San Francisco, questioned approximately 200 people about the various positions and places where they had sex. The responses numbered more than 700 ways and settings: elevators, cars, and so forth. Dr. McIlvenna suspects that if he did the survey again, he'd learn about 700 new places.

Experimenting in this manner enables us to keep boredom at bay. And it's a way to learn what best increases pleasure—ours and our partners'. We don't have 700 positions for you, but the following varieties should keep you busy for a while.

Also see: anal sex, animals, athletic sex, back, boredom, couch, cramps—leg, doggie style, exercise, *Kama Sutra*, marathon, missionary position, oral sex, public places, rear entry, risky sex, sexual aids, sixty-nine (69), standing positions, variety, water beds, wrestling

P

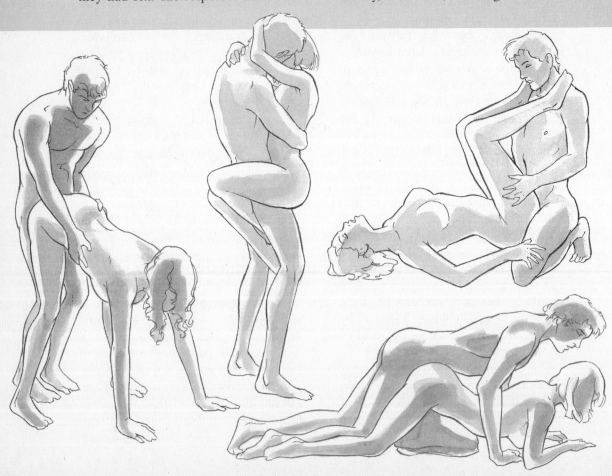

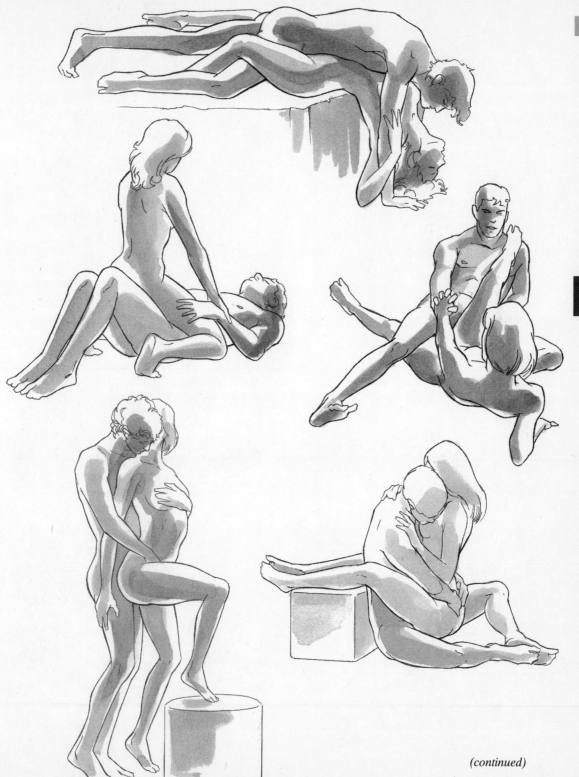

P

(continued)

P

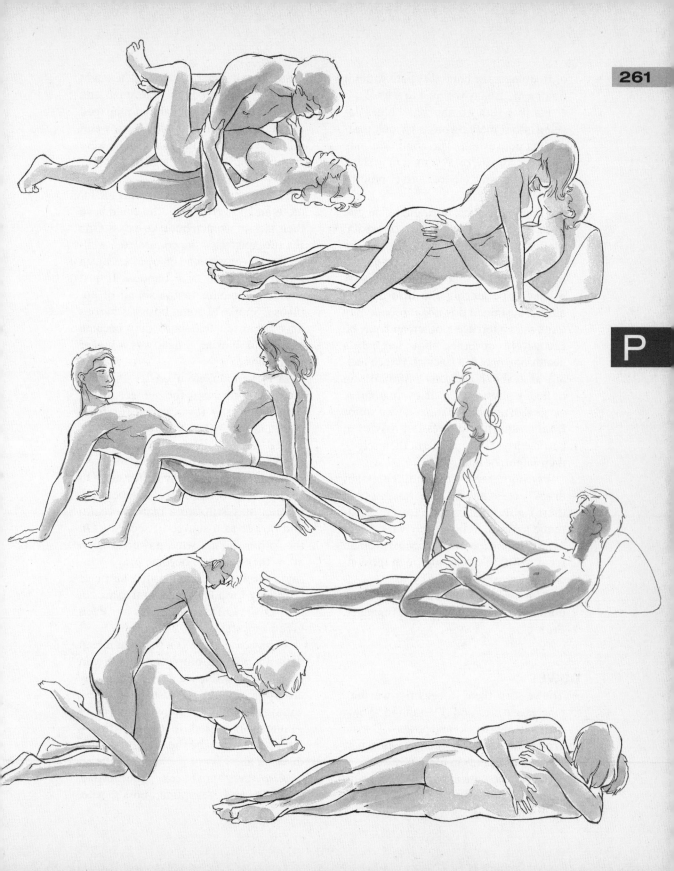

P

of 10 women, the blues dissipate without treatment, usually within 4 to 6 weeks.

For that 10th woman, baby blues develop into something more serious: postpartum depression. The condition may evolve gradually, or a woman may show no symptoms at all for 1 to 3 months after childbirth.

Though genetics, hormonal changes, psychiatric history, and a lack of marital support are among the potential causes of postpartum depression, a definitive explanation eludes researchers. A woman experiencing the disorder exhibits a sustained downbeat mood, may think she's a terrible mother, and may be excessively concerned about her baby's health. She may feel suicidal. If such feelings arise, she should call her obstetrician or family physician for an evaluation. A very small number of women who suffer from postpartum depression may even become psychotic and harm themselves, their infant, or both.

Psychotherapy and antidepressant drugs are standard treatments, but there's also no substitute for an empathetic partner. Telling your wife to get over it is not the answer. Most women recover within a year, although the condition can last as long as 3 years.

Also see: breastfeeding, depression, hormones, kids, mood, PMS, pregnancy, Prozac

power

You've seen them in celebrity-worshipping magazines and TV tabloid shows: men with megabucks and power—Donald Trump and his ilk—seemingly with a new flavor of eye candy in tow every week.

As we also note in our entry on *politicians*, Henry Kissinger once said power is the ultimate aphrodisiac, and he ought to know. The esteemed statesman and member of the Nixon cabinet managed to squire any number of actresses and other lovelies around town, as if he were an Adonis instead of a short, homely guy in Coke-bottle glasses.

(Meanwhile, there are plenty of famous and powerful men who could have their pick of women but take a pass. One sex therapist says she counseled a well-known singer who had enjoyed sex much more before he was famous. It just couldn't compare to the sound of applause. Similarly, some business barons have admitted that once they became successful, closing a deal was a bigger rush than sex.)

Why women glom on to powerful men has long been the subject of debate. Some say it's a carryover from caveman days, when the best hunter received the affections of the primitive equivalent of Elizabeth Hurley because she knew he would provide for her. On some level, even modern, independent women may still see a man of wealth and power as a source of security. On the other hand, why powerful men allow themselves to become prey—why, say, a president will jeopardize his place in history for a few quick oral exams in the Oval Office—may be an even greater mystery.

In any case, there is a way that a man with no notable power or wealth can exert sexual influence over women: Pay attention to them. Listen to them without butting in. Show them you're genuinely interested. To a woman, that—not power—may be the greatest aphrodisiac of all.

Also see: anal sex, aphrodisiac, bondage and discipline, boss's wife, casting couch, dominance and submission, dressing you to look sexy, financial difficulties, hypnosis and seduction, politicians, pussywhipped, sexual attraction, size—wallet, trophy wife, young women/older men

preference

Why one man goes gaga over willowy blondes while another's idea of perfection is voluptuous brunettes has long been the subject of debate. The latest thinking is that several factors account for the fact that we all aren't turned on by the same physical characteristics.

Many sex experts think that much of what you find attractive in a woman can be attributed to events imprinted on your tender memory before you were 3 years old. For example, when your mother, a babysitter, or a nurse hugged or caressed you in a particularly pleasurable way when you were a toddler, those good feelings are reinforced years later when you see (or even smell) somebody who reminds you of the female who made you feel good earlier.

What a society deems attractive also affects who turns your head. In some cultures, the most winsome women are those who are fat or have elongated ears or necks or other features that most of us in the West find unappealing. What was considered the norm where you grew up also can influence who you think is good-looking. Hence, the Midwestern fondness for Waspy, corn-fed

features or the preference in New York and other urban centers for more varied ethnic looks.

Also see: attraction, beauty, body shapes, fetish, interracial sex, legs, pheromones, sexual attraction, sexy, size—ass, size—breasts, size—nose, turn-ons

pregnancy

When an expectant couple's love life goes dormant, the cause is often not so much the woman's burgeoning belly as a communication breakdown. A pregnant woman has no choice but to feel her way through a bewildering array of physical, emotional, and hormonal changes—changes that can lead to lasting resentments if her man fails to either notice or sustain an open dialogue with her.

During the first trimester, for example, her interest in sex may drop precipitously, much to your alarm. Realize that it's nothing personal; it's hard for her to feel sexy when she's dividing her time between sleeping and puking.

Some women do feel renewed horniness by the second trimester, when morning sickness often abates. By the third trimester, your mate's interest in sex may drop off once more. And by

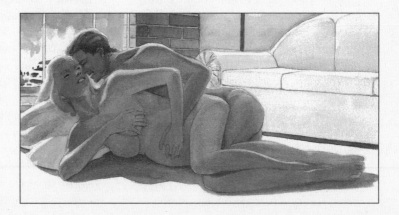

then, of course, she may be as big as some of the smaller species of orcas. Worse, she's well-aware of it. She may also experience frequent indigestion, heartburn, back pain, or other discomforts. Again, she feels more like a baby machine than like a sex machine.

Another potential impediment to lovemaking is a fear of harming the fetus. Absent medical complications, this fear usually is unfounded; most couples can have traditional intercourse throughout the woman's pregnancy because the fetus is protected by a cushion of amniotic fluid. But each case is unique, so it's best for a woman's obstetrician to advise here.

Notice that we just used the phrase *traditional intercourse*. You should not insert vibrators or other toys or foreign objects into your pregnant wife's vagina (nor should she, for that matter). Doing so could damage her cervix or prematurely break her bag of water. Also, avoid blowing into her vagina while performing oral sex. There are some isolated case reports of embolisms (sudden artery blockages) happening due to air being forced into the vagina and forming air-bubble clots. Embolisms can be fatal.

We're not likely to get much sympathy from our partners here, but we men, too, may be tired and cranky during our partners' pregnancies, particularly if we work longer hours in anticipation of those extra mouths to feed. And we may feel left out and forgotten as everybody makes a fuss over the mothers-to-be (as if we had nothing to do with it).

All these factors underscore why communication is so vital during pregnancy. And you have to engage in *good* communication, not yelling or sarcasm. Talking openly and sincerely minimizes hurt feelings and may even strengthen the bonds of intimacy.

Also see: abortion, body image, biological clock, breastfeeding, communication, contraception, ectopic pregnancy, kids, postpartum depression, size—vagina, zygote

premature ejaculation

Defining what it means to "come too soon" is, shall we say, a slippery subject. The usual meaning is the inability to delay orgasm for more than a very short period after entering your partner. Then again, some women insist that any guy who comes before they do has ejaculated "prematurely." This, of course, prompts questions of its own: How long should it take for a woman to come? And how long should a guy have to wait? These questions, in turn, lead to other questions having more to do, perhaps, with sexual politics than with pleasure. In fairness to the fair sex, the bottom line is that regardless of how and when you come, you owe it to your partner to maximize your contribution to her satisfaction. How you help her get there is up to the two of you.

In any case, textbook premature ejaculation is a common problem. (For the record, it wouldn't be if we were, say, apes. Other mammals routinely ejaculate faster than you can say "ejaculate.") And several reasons are commonly cited as to why some men have quicker triggers than others. Performance anxiety. Stress. Hypersensitive penises. Even a learned response—a vestige of boyhood masturbation, wherein rapid-fire ejaculation was the norm.

How to fix this? Sex experts recommend two closely related methods:

squeeze and start-stop. In the first, your partner stimulates you until you're just about there, then one of you simply firmly squeezes the glans, or head, of your penis with a thumb and index finger (or with both hands, depending on the sizes of the available fingers and glans), thus thwarting ejaculation. This can be done several times during foreplay to prolong it without causing ejaculation. Once you get better acquainted with your body's moment-by-moment responses, you can use this tactic during intercourse as well. It works best with the woman on top, because you're stimulated less intensely in this position, so you're better able to last longer. She can lift herself off you when you're too close, too soon.

In the start-stop method, your partner stimulates you until you're near orgasm, then stops. Once your sexual tension is diminished, she resumes. This helps a man to anticipate his point of inevitability and thereby control it. Once you master this, you can also employ the technique during intercourse, again starting, ideally, with the woman on top. (Of course, you can practice either of these without a partner too. It's just not as much fun.)

Doctors don't recommend using desensitizing creams or gels. They don't help you learn new ways of responding during sex. And if you use them but don't use a condom, they may numb your partner's erogenous zones as well as yours (then you'll be right back to the coming-before-she-does problem).

Since younger men generally come quicker than their elders do, if you're under 40, consider masturbating before anticipated sexual encounter. This may reduce your excitement somewhat and give you more self-control. Plus, it ensures that you'll definitely get off, even if your date isn't in the mood to help you.

Also see: Kegel exercises, Masters and Johnson, orgasm—delaying, sex therapy, urologist

prepuce

A fancy name for the foreskin, that retractable fold of skin that partially covers the head of your penis, unless you're circumcised. If you are, this is what the doc cut. Prepuce also refers to the fold of skin over the end of a woman's clitoris.

Also see: circumcision, foreskin, piercing, smegma

priapism

An erection that just won't quit. This is a problem? Believe it. It can be painful as hell. And after a few hours, it can be harmful. And let's face it, do you really want a bulge in your pants when you go to work? To church? To the gym? ("Honest, pal, you're not my type.")

The condition melds the names of Priapus (son of Dionysus, Greek god of fertility and wine) and Aphrodite (goddess of love). Priapus, art fans may note, is depicted in statues as better-endowed and more constantly erect than a horny Clydesdale.

Priapism is caused when blood is unable to drain out of your penis. It is *not* a result of chronic sexy thoughts or actions. Trapped in your rigid rod, the blood stagnates, acidifies, and loses oxygen. That, in turn, causes the red blood cells to stiffen, making the blood even less able to escape. This leads to damage of the erectile tissue and replacement of elastic tissue with woody, nonexpansile tissue.

Certain medications and medical conditions may cause priapism. Of the former, penile injections for treating erectile dysfunction are most often the culprit. But this unfortunate side effect is unlikely unless you give yourself too big a dose. Antidepressant and antipsychotic drugs may also cause priapism. Among medical conditions, sickle-cell disease and leukemia can cause priapism, even in youngsters. Ditto for injuries to the penis, perineum, and spine.

It's crucial that priapism be treated quickly. One poor guy who waited a week to see his doctor was left, after surgery, with a penis less than an inch long.

If you get an erection that doesn't subside within 2 to 3 hours, try taking an over-the-counter decongestant. If that doesn't help, head for the emergency room and ask for a urologist. He'll probably stick a small needle in your swollen organ to drain the old blood trapped there. Not a pleasant prospect—but it sure beats having less than an inch.

Also see: erection difficulties, Spanish fly, urologist

prison

There's no shortage of sex going on inside prisons. Sometimes it's between inmates. Sometimes it's between guards and inmates. A South Carolina prison guard was fired, for example, after having sex four times with Susan Smith, the woman who drowned her two young sons in a lake. Sometimes there's no accounting for taste. Or desperation.

As you may have heard, prison sex isn't always consensual. "Long Island Lolita" Amy Fisher said she was raped by guards while imprisoned for shooting the wife of her then-boyfriend, Joey Buttafuoco.

And just as in all those prison movies, prison sex is not necessarily heterosexual, either. For a variety of fairly obvious reasons, the prevalence of such activity is tough to measure, though it's clear that there's some truth to those old jokes about not bending over to pick up the soap in prison showers. Several decades ago, Ted McIlvenna, Ph.D., of the Institute for Advanced Study of Human Sexuality in San Francisco, studied consensual sex among male prison inmates throughout Europe. He concluded that 41 percent of prisoners engaged in consensual sex behind bars. He also concluded that heterosexual inmates who had homosexual sex in the confines of prison generally returned to the warm bodies of the opposite sex once they were released from prison.

Just be aware, in case you ever find yourself on the wrong side of the law: Because of unsafe sex and the sharing of needles, prison inmates of both genders harbor the HIV virus or full-blown AIDS more than seven times more often than in the general population.

Also see: AIDS, gang rape, homophobia, homosexuality, rape, sex offenders

progesterone

This is the hormone that complements estrogen to shape a woman's sexual anatomy. And with estrogen's help, progesterone regulates her monthly period. The mix of these and other female hormones ebb and flow, and depending on the state of her menstrual tide, your woman may want to thrill you or kill you.

Progesterone also may be combined with estrogen to treat unwanted effects of menopause. It can be taken as a pill, vaginal suppository, or cream. Taking only estrogen increases a woman's chances of developing uterine cancer. Adding the correct dose of progesterone to the mix negates this risk.

Also see: abortion pill, estrogen, hormones, IUD, menopause—hers, menstruation, ovaries, period, sex drive, testosterone

progestin

A synthetic or natural compound similar to the female hormone progesterone. Progestins are combined with estrogen in some forms of hormone replacement therapy used to ease the symptoms of menopause and reduce the risk of heart disease and osteoporosis.

Progestins also are a key ingredient, along with estrogen, in several types of contraceptives, including the Pill, Norplant, Depo-Provera, and the morning-after pill. There also is a progestin-only birth control pill that a woman must take at exactly the same time every day if it is to be most effective. Progestins work by inhibiting ovulation and thickening mucus so that sperm have a swim that's as arduous as that of salmon going upstream.

Also see: estrogen, hormones, menopause—hers, morning-after pill, ovulation, Pill—the, Norplant

promiscuity

Sex therapists say that as long as you're responsible and respectful of the people who join you in bed, there is no reason to limit the number of sex partners you have. The deciding factor for each individual should be personal ethics: Hugh Hefner has a somewhat different standard than Jerry Falwell. And a young woman born in, say, 1975 proabably has a different standard than her own mother—quite possibly a more conservative standard, given that her mother came of age during the swinging '60s.

Many people, including Hef and former flower children, do enjoy cele-

P

Hot Dates **1972** The U.S. Supreme Court extended the right to privacy to include unmarried persons' access to contraception. This decision served as the basis for the 1973 ruling that granted the right to abortion.

continued from page 256

ternet porn and stockpiling adult videos and magazines in an office cabinet. He said that he kept the material at work only because **he had teenage boys at home and didn't want them to find his stash**. The judge also contended that he had surfed sex-related Web sites only as research on how to restrict them from his kids.

Seemed like a Good Idea at the Time. . .

In imperial Rome, **handsome young men were sometimes forcibly castrated** so that wealthy women could fornicate with them without fear of pregnancy.

Some guys had it even worse: Their penises were lopped off. These eunuchs became servants of the

True or Phallus?

The rock group Steely Dan took its name from the medieval nickname for a chastity belt.

BAWDY BALLADS "You Can't Tell the Difference after Dark," *Alberta Hunter*

continued on page 274

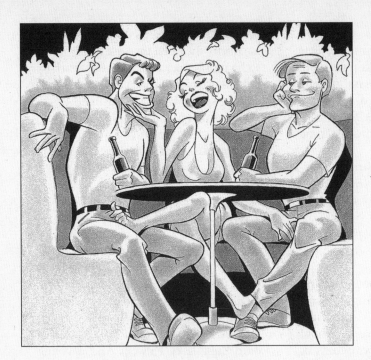

brating their sexuality with numerous partners, and feel quite happy and comfortable keeping those sexual relationships casual. This is perfectly healthy as long as both people in such a relationship are fully aware that it's casual. If one of them also has other sex partners, that should be common knowledge, too, so that everyone involved can make informed decisions about their own lives and health.

Obviously, there are bad reasons to have a lot of partners. Some men have lots of sex mostly because of peer pressure or juvenile expectations of what it means to be a man. That's no better than buying a Porsche you can't afford because you think it makes you more of a man. Women, on the other hand, may have unrelenting serial sex because they think that putting out is required to please guys. (And let's be honest here: Many of us don't do much to change that

perception.) Or they may suffer a lack of self-esteem and just not realize that they have a say in the timing and frequency of sex. Their self-images then take added batterings when they're labeled as whores: You can't deny that the studs-and-sluts double standard remains alive and well. Finally, in some cases, frequent sex can even be a symptom of obsessive-compulsive disorder, manic depression, or borderline personality disorder.

If you're genuinely concerned about someone's well-being and you feel that he or she is possibly being self-destructive or harming others, tell that person about it in a caring, nonjudgmental way. If you can't be caring and nonjudgmental, you should probably mind your own business.

Also see: compulsive behavior, extramarital sex, safe sex, sex addiction, testicles

prophylactic

A condom, a rubber, a love glove . . . you get the idea. And you know what it's for.

There's also another meaning of the word. In the broadest sense, a prophylactic is any medicine, treatment, or device that prevents or guards against a disease or other unwanted consequence. The term is applied to a condom because the sheath offers protection from sexually transmitted diseases and pregnancy. So if it could be proven, for example, that drinking beer prevented prostate cancer, even beer could be said to be a prophylactic. A crack team of our editors is working on that one.

Also see: condom, condom—polyurethane, rubber

prostate

This encapsulated male reproductive organ, at the center of so much pain and pleasure, often is called a gland—though it doesn't produce hormones. What it does produce is a thick, white liquid that becomes part of semen. The mineral-rich prostatic fluid (which gives semen its color, smell, and taste) protects, nourishes, and enhances the motility of sperm cells as it moves them through a woman's vagina.

The prostate's role in sexual health dramatically overshadows its physical stature: At 20 grams, it's about the size and shape of a walnut. Wrapped around the urethra and found under the bladder, in front of the rectum, it's a potential source of extreme sexual pleasure when massaged via the anus or perineum with a lubricated finger. The downside is that a man rarely gets through life without experiencing some prostate problem, whether it be enlargement, inflammation, or cancer. After age 40, you should have annual examinations and blood tests to assess prostate function.

Helpful hint: Many doctors believe that the trace mineral zinc benefits the prostate, because that is where zinc tends to concentrate in a man. Take 35 to 50 milligrams every day for prostate health. Also be sure to remind your wife or girlfriend that a healthy love life is good for the prostate, because sex keeps the

organ's circulation strong. Tough medicine, we know, but regular ejaculation keeps your prostate from getting stagnant and inflamed.

Also see: ejaculation, klismaphilia, pederast, semen

prostate cancer

This is the second most common cancer in American men, after skin cancer. It begins in the back part of the prostate, closest to the rectum, which explains why the dreaded digital-rectal exam is an important detection tool.

Men over 50 should have annual prostate exams because the cure rate is better for cancers caught early. If you're African-American or have a family incidence of prostate cancer, you're in the highest risk group. Talk to your doctor about starting screenings at age 40.

Treatment options vary. Many doctors recommend immediate prostatectomy—radical surgery—but there are alternatives. One being investigated is cryosurgery, wherein surgeons insert needles into a man's prostate through his perineum, then pump in liquid nitrogen to freeze the organ. In trials, this treatment is effective and spares nearby healthy tissue. However, doctors are still debugging this experimental procedure in an effort to minimize side effects, which are similar to those resulting from traditional treatments. These include inability to ejaculate, infertility, and, in some cases, impotence, incontinence, and bladder irritability.

Radiation therapy is making a comeback, especially among older men. Low-level prostate cancers seem to respond well to radioactive iodine seeds. This ap-

P

proach requires just 1 day in the hospital, during which numerous seeds are surgically inserted into the prostate with the guidance of ultrasound. It causes little discomfort and few side effects.

Then there's hormone deprivation, which rests on the fact that most cancer cells are hormone dependent. Indeed, deprived of male hormones, the entire prostate can shrivel up and die. Because this treatment involves removing the testicles or giving men female hormones (which can increase the risk of heart attack), it's reserved for older men and patients for whom other treatments have failed. This is not generally considered a cure, but it will control the cancer for years.

Clearly, the best option is prevention. You can help yourself avoid prostate cancer by eating healthfully. Don't wait until the critical age; start watching your diet now. Cancer-causing toxins are concentrated in fatty foods, so make the obvious adjustment in your diet. Also, therapeutic doses of vitamins and minerals, taken under the supervision of a doctor, may help protect your prostate. Taking 1,000 milligrams of vitamin C three times a day, 400 IU of vitamin E, and 200 micrograms of selenium may help reduce the risk, as can a chemical called lycopene, found in fresh tomatoes and pasta sauce. (Doses of selenium above the amount we mentioned must be taken under medical supervision.)

Also see: estrogen, prostate enlargement, prostate-specific antigen, prostatitis, sickness, supplements, testicles, urologist

prostatectomy

The surgical removal of the entire prostate. This open, radical surgery has served as the most common prostate cancer treatment for some 40 years. Surgeons usually cut into the lower abdomen to reach the organ, but sometimes they attempt a perineal approach, making an incision between the scrotum and rectum. This is a more direct route, with less loss of blood during the operation.

Worse, though, is what you may lose afterward: Up to 35 percent of prostatectomy patients suffer permanent, mild stress incontinence, which means that they leak a small amount of urine when coughing, laughing, sneezing, or exercising. And because the nerves of the penis, adjacent to the prostate, usually are severed during the surgery, many men are unable to get an erection for up to 1 year after. This side effect is somewhat less common than in the past, as surgeons try to use nerve-sparing surgical techniques to prevent permanent injury to the nerves that control erection.

Also see: impotence, perineum, prostate, prostate-specific antigen, prostatitis, urologist

prostate enlargement

For a man, one of life's few sure things, along with death and taxes, is the swelling of the prostate. It can grow from the size of a walnut to the size of an orange. Technically known as benign prostatic hyperplasia, or BPH, this condition can rear its ugly head any time after age 40, affecting 95 percent of us by the time we reach 70. Despite such prevalence, medical professionals aren't sure what causes it.

You, however, will be sure you have it when you notice how much of your time you spend urinating, especially at night.

You'll take a whiz and your bladder will still feel full. Your urine stream, meanwhile, won't be as strong as it was when you were writing your name in boldface letters in the snow. Most charming of all, your bladder may continue to dribble for up to 2 minutes after you *thought* you were finished taking a whiz. In a man under 40, these symptoms need to be investigated promptly by a doctor, as they could signal a more acute condition. If you're over 40 and these symptoms appear suddenly or become bothersome, or if you have blood in your urine, see your doctor right away.

Today, doctors prescribe dozens of treatments to shrink an enlarged prostate and ease associated urinary problems. While medications are effective for some men, others opt to have parts of their prostates lopped off. Herbal remedies such as saw palmetto are sometimes effective in cutting a recalcitrant gland down to size. Treatments performed on an outpatient basis by your urologist or surgeon (many of them are considered experimental) include heating and even microwaving the old boy.

Also see: impotence, prostate, prostatitis, urologist

prostate-specific antigen

A protein produced by cells in the prostate. A high number of these proteins in the blood usually indicates that the organ is infected, inflamed, enlarged, or cancerous.

Prostate-specific antigen (PSA) screening isn't medically diagnostic for cancer, but doctors perform the test because it's the best tool for finding a possible cancer at its early, most treatable stages. You

should have an annual PSA test starting at age 50. If you're African-American or have a family history of prostate cancer, you're considered high-risk and you should start tests at age 40. Following a suspicious PSA reading, a doctor must run other tests to confirm the existence of cancer, because high antigen levels also could be caused by the problems noted above, or even by ejaculating within the 48 hours before the test.

Other drugs, such as those for chemical castration, can substantially lower PSA levels, as can certain medical procedures such as prostate biopsy or catheterization. So it's important for you to give the doctor your full medical history before the test.

Also see: prostate, prostate cancer, urologist

prostatitis

Inflammation of the prostate. This can result from bacterial infection but more commonly is caused by a virus, stress, anxiety, prolonged sitting, or—trust us on this—too few ejaculations.

Patients with inflamed prostates compare the pain to crouching atop a golf ball. They complain of a burning sensation when they urinate—which they have to do often. Lower-back pain and anal discomfort are other symptoms.

Doctors can easily diagnose this condition if it is caused by bacterial infection by taking a sample of fluid from the prostate and counting the white blood cells: Too many, and you know the organ is infected.

Antibiotics are used to treat prostatitis caused by an infection. If it's not caused by an infection, it's often more difficult to treat. You can try zinc supplements to help cool the inflammation. Follow the dosage instructions on the label. Vitamin B_6 and riboflavin (vitamin B_2) can also play a supporting role, so take a B-complex supplement, also according to the package directions.

Also see: prostate, prostate enlargement, zinc

P

prostitution

Although frowned upon and forbidden for about as long as it has existed, the so-called oldest profession still thrives for a variety of reasons.

Some guys visit prostitutes regularly because they lack steady sex partners. Often, such men either don't have time to play the dating game or aren't very skilled at it. Men who do have partners seek out prostitutes to experience sex acts that they're too uncomfortable or ashamed to request from their partners (or, probably just as often, they've made the request and been turned down sharply). This may explain why oral sex is the number one service men seek from hookers, according to surveys.

Other guys get discouraged when women criticize the way they have sex. They turn to prostitutes, who won't judge their performances. Occasionally, a man will have a sexual compulsion that drives him to pay for play; frequent sex with hookers helps him reduce anxiety or gives him the illusion of control over women.

While the anonymity and nonjudgment of a hooker is appealing to some, the risks are far greater. For one thing, the trade is illegal in every state but Nevada. Getting caught soliciting a sex act draws a range of legal penalties from a simple fine to time in the slammer. To say nothing of the embarrassment that stems from public exposure—your name may be printed in the local newspaper for all to see. What's more, hookers and johns alike risk contracting sexually transmitted diseases or falling victim to violence.

Also see: brothels/bordellos, extramarital sex, gigolo, john, meeting women, money, oral sex, surrogate, trick

Prozac

An antidepressant medication (fluoxetine hydrochloride) that boosts your mood—and that often botches things in the sack.

Other antidepressants causing the same sexual side effects include Zoloft (sertraline) and Paxil (paroxetine). All these drugs increase the brain's absorption of the neurotransmitter serotonin. (Neurotransmitters are chemicals that help control muscle movement, heart activity, breathing, and other functions.) Researchers link low levels of serotonin with mental conditions such as depression and schizophrenia.

Though doctors often forget to alert patients, antidepressants cause sexual dysfunction in up to 30 percent of users by lowering the sex drive, giving a man erectile difficulties, or making orgasm and ejaculation almost impossible. Adjusting the dose sometimes alleviates the sexual side effects. The downside is that your depression may return. Similarly, an antihistamine called Periactin (cyproheptadine hydrochloride) can help a man with antidepressant-related sex problems, but the antihistamine's success may indicate that it's inhibiting the antidepressant functions as well.

Some encouraging news: Up to 40 percent of Prozac users report good results from the naturally derived aphrodisiac and erection-enhancer yohimbine. Even better: Yohimbine does not appear to short-circuit Prozac's beneficial properties. It's available by prescription; ask your doctor about it.

If you are currently taking an antidepressant and suffering from sexual dysfunction, you could also ask your doctor about a relatively new antidepressant called Celexa (citalopram). This new drug works like all the others but apparently has a much lower rate of sexual side effects.

Also see: depression, compulsive behavior, impotence, medications, yohimbine

puberty

You remember this frenzied stage of sexual development, which typically begins at around age 11 and can last until the mid-20s (or, in men, until the mid-50s, if you believe women). During puberty, you were bombarded with sex from all sides—even from inside. You woke up from wet dreams. You got a woody when a pretty girl's elbow brushed your butt. You looked under the beds for your missing sock and instead found your older brother's nudie magazines stuffed under his mattress.

Ironically, this tumultuous time was when you began to form your sexual self-image. You were expected to somehow weed through all those stimuli and manage, by adulthood, to develop a "normal" approach to sex. Whatever the hell that is, anyway.

Wait, it gets worse. Though far from emotionally mature, you were expected to manage major changes in your social and physical chemistry. How were you supposed to handle it when those girls in co-ed gym class snickered and pointed at your shorts? Okay, so they caught only an innocent glimpse of your jewels. But to you, their laughter carried much more weight. They were literally laughing at what makes you a man. Who could blame you for the shyness and mistrust of women that you followed into adulthood?

Body image was a bigger deal for us as teenage boys than many of us care to admit. We knew we didn't look like those beautifully tanned model types on TV. We had pimples and braces and long limbs dangling from stubby torsos. And even though most of our friends were in the same sad boat, nobody seemed to cut anybody else much slack. If there was a chance to have a good laugh at somebody else's expense, we took the bait.

A guy who had an uncommonly tough time during puberty may have ended up with all sorts of sexuality issues that continue to linger long after he has blossomed into the next Tom Cruise. If you see signs of dysfunction within yourself, think back to the sexual input you got from parents and peers when you were 12 to 15. This kind of self-analysis ain't easy, and it's necessarily subjective, but some events speak for themselves, such as the aforementioned link between a current inability to trust women and the way adolescent girls may have treated you.

If you can't seem to resolve a troubling issue that seems to have arisen in adolescence, therapy is a wise second step. We hate to lend credence to sar-

P

castic male stereotypes, but you don't want to be a 50-year-old stuck in adolescence. Fix the problem now.

Also see: first lover, flirtation, heterosexuality, kinky, masturbation, phimosis, self-esteem, sex therapy, wet dreams

pubic hair

Scientists believe its Darwinistic function is to trap sweat, which is full of the sexual scents called pheromones. When your sweat evaporates, the theory goes, your scent spreads, sparking chemical attraction between you and a nearby female of the species. Some researchers even believe that body odor plays a role in sexual development itself.

Now, we like scientists well enough. But we're betting that a lot of them don't get out much. So we urge you to keep in mind that there's a difference between scientific theory and common dating etiquette. We don't know too many women who want to remove your pants and get a whiff of what smells like a wildebeest on a hot day in the savanna. So keep your pubes (and everything else down there) clean. Your woman will thank you. Even if she's a scientist.

Also see: body odor—controlling, crabs, hygiene, labia majora and minora, mons pubis, *Penthouse*, pheromones, rashes, shaving

pubic lice

These tiny bloodsucking insects, which as a teenager you learned to call crabs, thrive in hairy places. They usually infest the genitals but can also lurk in leg hair and armpits, facial hair, and even eyebrows and eyelashes. They're most commonly spread during sexual activity, hopping cheerfully from one partner's pubes to the other's.

Hot Dates 1973 The film *Deep Throat* hit adult theaters. It was an overnight success that made porn chic and raked in more than $100 million.

continued from page 267

Answer:
False. The group swiped the name from the William S. Burroughs novel *Naked Lunch*, in which Steely Dan is the name of a dildo.

wealthy and companions of Roman emperors and prominent church leaders, including some popes.

Foreign Affairs
I'll cook you mine if you cook me yours: After boys are circumcised, **the Poro people of Liberia dry the foreskins**, which are then cooked and eaten by the girls of the tribe during their initiation. The girls then have their clitorises and labia minora removed, and these are dried, cooked, and eaten by the boys.

In Extremis
Salt Lake City police responded to a 911 call from a woman who said her husband refused to have sex with her. When cops arrived, they found the **nearly naked woman beating her husband**. He explained that his paucity of passion was due to the exciting Utah Jazz game he was watching on TV.

LEGAL BRIEFS
Now that's what we call making a bust: An on-duty Houston cop interrupted two ardent couples in a local

BAWDY BALLADS "Paradise by the Dashboard Light," *Meat Loaf*

continued on page 287

Crabs resemble, well, crabs—tiny gray ones. Adult lice are large enough to spot crawling around in coarse body hair, but usually only a few will share a host. The skin they inhabit may be red and itchy. Also examine a few of your partner's individual hairs. Female lice lay white eggs, called nits, which attach to the hair shafts.

Of course, if you feel you've been exposed, check your own pubic hair for nits. It takes about a week for the eggs to hatch and another week for the young nymphs to come into adulthood. But don't wait for the next generation to come around before you counterattack.

Over-the-counter lice shampoos, such as Rid, usually kill crabs. For resistant cases, more potent potions are available from your doctor. Unfortunately, it's no quick-and-easy rinse. You must completely lather the entire infested area and leave on the rather unpleasant medication for at least 10 minutes. But the treatment does work the first time. After you've killed the little suckers, the dead nits will still be dangling from your hairs. Use a nit comb to slide them off.

Don't use the medication on your brows or lashes. Your doctor can prescribe an eye-friendly petrolatum ointment, which suffocates the lice. Then you can remove them with a nit comb.

To prevent an encore infestation, wash all of your infested clothing, sheets, and towels in very hot water and detergent; and vacuum your floors, especially around the bed.

Bear in mind that crabs can live for up to 2 days without a host. When a louse falls off an infected partner and lands on bedsheets, couch, clothing, or towel, it will be desperate to find a fresh source of food—potentially you. So, as always, be careful where you put your naked butt, especially when you're with a new partner.

Also see: crabs, hygiene, STDs

public places
Herewith, two incompatible truths. First, some of us love to get naked with our partners in public. Second, it's illegal to perform sex acts in most public places. You'd think that the second fact would automatically put a damper on the first fact. Uh, no. Often, in practice, just the opposite is true: The risk of getting caught boosts adrenaline levels and makes the sex even more exciting than when it's tucked safely away behind closed doors.

Now, we're not in the business of advocating criminal disobedience or moral decadency. We feel obliged to tell you, however, that the consequences of such recklessness are likely to be minor. Even if you're caught, you probably won't be handcuffed and thrown in jail. (Note: This does not apply in certain areas of the Bible Belt. Always check local laws first.) The cops will probably order you to stop—yes, before you climax—and will likely issue a summons, which means you'll have to show up in court at a later date to defend your actions.

That doesn't give you license to be downright stupid. For instance, don't go at it across the street from a schoolyard in broad daylight. And have a cover story, a strategy. When you slip into a dressing room at a department store, pretend to be discussing the fashions or having an argument. In a restaurant, pull the old she-dropped-her-fork-and-went-under-the-table-to-retrieve-it ruse. This will work only in a restaurant that has tablecloths. And, of course, it will work only once per restaurant. Nobody drops her fork *that* much.

An interesting tidbit for those of you partial to public hanky panky: A cop we know in New York City tells us that a car, at least in the Big Apple, is not considered a public place. For everybody's safety, do your best to make it a *parked* car. Oh, and ideally, the vehicle should belong to you.

Also see: cars, exhibitionism, masher, outdoors, risky sex, time-saving tips, Venus butterfly

P

pudenda

A woman's visible external sex organs, such as the clitoris and the lips of the vagina. This term is usually used in its plural form, rather than the singular *pudendum*.

Though it describes territory we tend to hold in awe, *pudenda* is rooted in the Latin word *pudere,* which means "to be ashamed."

Also see: reproductive system—hers, vulva

pulling a train

Motorcycle-gang slang for a sexual scenario wherein one woman, often a prostitute, has serial sex with a group of guys.

Also see: gang bang, prostitution, sloppy seconds

pussywhipped

Something you hope never to hear yourself described as.

Pussywhipped, or just *whipped*, can describe a guy who's in complete thrall of a woman' sexuality, thus he serves her

with slavish obedience in hopes of getting into her beloved pants at every opportunity. In such an instance, the remark does not necessarily hold any negative implications about the woman herself. More commonly, though, pussywhipped refers to a guy who is dominated, manipulated, or just generally henpecked by a shrewish wife or lover.

Being pussywhipped has nothing to do, per se, with sexual domination of the sadomasochist variety. It refers more to bullying behavior out of bed.

How to tell if you've fallen prey to one of maledom's worst stigmas?

• Do you frequently turn down invites from your buddies or otherwise tell people that you can't do such and such because she wouldn't like it? Do you find yourself devoting all your leisure time to things she likes to do? When was the last time the two of you went to a movie that she didn't pick? A sporting event that she's not so crazy about?

• When you're both out among people together, do you find yourself stifling remarks you'd otherwise make, because you know she wouldn't like them?

• Does she belittle you in front of others? Seem to make a point of putting you through your paces when her girlfriends are watching? Who picked the couples you see socially?

• Has the household budget become pretty much her exclusive domain? Does she decide how much you spend and what you spend it on? Does anything in your house look the way you'd like it to look? Or is it all her?

• Overall, do you feel that your opinions and tastes don't carry much weight?

If you've given distressing answers to such questions and you do truly love her nonetheless, you need to figure out why you've let things get to this point. Identify the parts of the relationship that are good. Do they make it worth your while to stay? (Draw up a "balance sheet" for your relationship, with the pluses on one side and the minuses on the other. It can be an eye-opening experience.) Is she willing to work with you to make things more satisfying to you? You'll need to ask her directly. It may be uncomfortable, but it's the only way things will change.

Be aware that power struggles like this have to do with deep-seated personality traits. You're not going to fix everything in a 20-minute conversation over a glass of wine. See a therapist together—one that you pick, perhaps.

Also see: begging, communication, dominance and submission, vixen, withholding

P

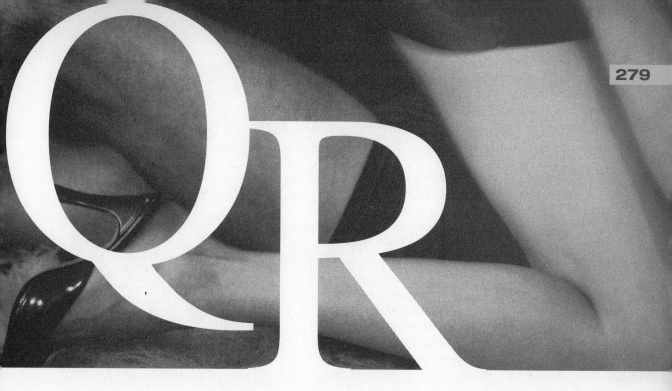

quality versus quantity

When you're young and perpetually erect, getting lucky at least several times a week is the yardstick by which you measure the health of your love life. If you're over 35, however, and you're worried that you're not having sex as often—well, you needn't worry anymore.

It's quite common for a mature man to have fewer sexual encounters than a young man. In fact, couples ages 20 to 39 have sex almost twice as often as couples over 40. An older man normally seeks a strong emotional connection with a special partner. He'd rather have occasional terrific sex with one woman than constant adequate sex with two or three women. (Note to younger readers: Stop laughing. It'll probably happen to you too.)

On the other hand, if you're getting less *and* enjoying it less, it may be because a certain staleness has stultified your love life. Try a bit more variety in positions or locations, or try watching erotic videos with your partner. Ask yourself if you're holding back sexually because of emotions such as sadness, anger, or anxiety. Qualified sex therapists also can help mature couples learn how to get the Earth moving a bit more on those less frequent encounters.

Also see: aging, arousal, boredom, frequency, marriage—lack of sex in, sex—lack of, sex therapy, variety, withholding

quickies

Your partner doesn't always want a long, slow pre-sex warmup. Before work in the morning, over her lunch hour, or during those few minutes in the evening when the kids are occupied elsewhere, she often craves a quickie—lovemaking that's fast, frenetic, and fun.

We know what you're thinking: "Wait a sec. What about all this stuff about foreplay and slow hands? What about this 'Don't rush us' mantra that women have been crooning for years?"

Don't overcomplicate the quickie experience. A quickie is a quickie. Take your cue from your partner. When she signals that she wants it *now*, she has no illusions about what she's getting into.

What signals does she give, you ask? Here's a subtle one: You walk in from work and she waltzes over and plants a hard, wet kiss on you. Or better still, she grabs you *right there*.

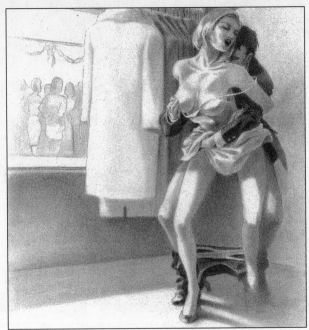

QR

Timing is vital when it comes to making a quickie work. You may have but a few precious minutes before the kids get home from soccer or the pizza-delivery guy or your mother-in-law knocks on the door. Don't waste time on preliminaries. The odds are good that a woman who has requested a quickie is already as turned on as she needs to be. (She's probably been thinking about it for a while before you got there.) In any case, all you need do to confirm this is reach down and check. No doubt the smallest amount of slithering around will ensure that she's ready to comfortably accommodate you. It's actually possible that a woman who has decided to have you right now will be frustrated by any hesitation on your part. So make her happy. (It's a tough job, yada, yada. . . .)

The key to what happens from here on in is fluency: getting the job done with as much dexterity as possible. Unzip your pants and take out your (let us hope) erection. The sight of you should only further fan her desires. If she's wearing a skirt, reach underneath it and pull off her panties. We bet she won't mind if something tears—other than her flesh, that is. Remember, you're not being rough, per se. You're being direct and forceful. There's a difference. (Think James Bond in *Goldfinger*, not Mongo in *Blazing Saddles*.)

Don't overthink the rest of it. Don't worry about technique. Half the fun is the sheer absurdity of it all. Do it standing, adjourn to a nearby couch or bed or table, whatever. Just do what comes naturally.

Once it's over, the fact that she wanted it quickly does not imply that she wants to be abandoned just as quickly. If there's time, spend a few moments holding her tight to ensure that you're both satisfied. You'll make the thrill of that quickie last a long, long time.

One caveat we feel compelled to add: We think we've been pretty clear in this entry, but this advice applies only to women with whom you have an existing relationship and some experience at reading each other's body language. A first date is not the recommended setting for a quickie.

Also see: afternoon delight, arousal, athletic sex, kids, standing positions, surprises, time-saving tips, undressing, wild women, zipless sex

randy

The origin of the word remains debatable, but the sexual connotation is believed to have evolved out of 18th-century Scotland, where originally it meant having a rude, aggressive manner. Today, it means being sexually uninhibited, lustful, lecherous, and lascivious. We know it best as a synonym for *horny*, thanks to the World Wide Web and the popularity of the *Austin Powers* movies.

Also see: arousal, horny, passion

rape

Sadly, given the pervasiveness of sexual assault, it's not unusual for a man to learn that his lover carries the emotional pain of a past rape. The legal definition of rape is forcible sexual intercourse that occurs without the consent of one of the parties (usually the woman). Rape also occurs when a woman is unable to consent because she is below the legal age (which varies by state) or because she is under the influence of drugs or alcohol, even if voluntarily, when intercourse takes place. That means that, from a legal standpoint, a woman can be raped even if she is completely cooperative.

A woman who reveals that she has been raped is generally looking to you for a secure base of trust and sensitivity. Respond with gentleness and patience, especially when it comes to sex. Certain touches can trigger horrific memories or cause her physical pain. Rough sex, even in play, may upset her. She may be leery of sexual contact altogether, so it's vitally important not to push her into having sex before she's ready. This is critical not just for the future of your relationship but also for her recovery and emotional well-being.

If your partner is raped during your relationship, you may be filled with feelings such as rage, disgust, self-criticism, and confusion. You may not want to share these with her, but if you don't share them with someone, you may unintentionally communicate the wrong tone to your partner and thereby undermine the relationship. Remember, even though you weren't the one who was assaulted, her rape is a powerful event in *your* life too.

A woman may ask you to join her in counseling as she tries to regain a healthy, positive approach to sexuality. If you are committed to the relationship, participate—although it will certainly be uncomfortable for you. Take your cue from her. Many women need some time alone with a counselor before they are ready for their partners to participate.

Sensate-focus therapy is popular for helping partners get sexually reacquainted after a woman has been raped. This technique is taught to couples who are having sexual difficulties as a result of psychological rather than physical factors. It aims to make each partner aware of what the other finds pleasurable and to reduce anxiety about sexual performance. As a woman slowly relearns how

QR

to touch and be touched, her sexual anxieties can disappear. Nonetheless, the therapy isn't a cure-all. It should never be practiced without the supervision of a therapist.

Also see: compulsive behavior, date rape, fantasies, gang rape, no, paraphilias, pedophilia, perversions, prison, rough sex, sensate focus, sex offenders, underage, violence

rashes

Red, itchy, scaly patches of skin on the groin most commonly are caused by a fungal infection called tinea cruris. Also called dermatitis or jock itch, this skin disorder resembling athlete's foot usually can be cured in a few weeks with over-the-counter antifungal creams or powders, such as Lotrimin AF.

Make sure you keep your groin clean and dry, as fungi grow well in moist places. If you're recovering from a case of jock itch, wear loose underwear for a while so your skin doesn't become excessively sweaty or chafed.

Some diseases such as syphilis and herpes cause rashes or blisters on the penis. These more serious conditions are recognizable by the oozing sores that tend to accompany the red, crusty skin. Don't mess around here. If you have blisters, ulcers, or a rash or if your itching doesn't clear up after a couple of weeks of treatment, see a doctor.

Chemical irritants and pubic parasites also will make the groin area itchy. If antifungal creams don't do the trick and you haven't recently switched to a new laundry detergent, check for the nits that indicate the presence of lice.

Also see: crabs, herpes, hygiene, pubic lice, rug burn, STDs, syphilis

rave

A spectacle of intense techno music and laser light, often flavored with the drug ecstasy. Still, contrary to the media-painted portraits, the typical rave is not a scene of rampant sex.

Based on the British tradition of all-night concerts featuring the electronic dance music and light shows that followed the decline of disco, U.S. raves began around 1988 as underground parties in abandoned Brooklyn warehouses. At that time, they were publicized only by pocket-size flyers and word of mouth. Today's raves are highly promoted affairs that fill rented stadiums and other large public spaces. Though some parties end when the venues have to close, others continue through the night.

Bad press about drug use among ardent ravers—usually teens and twentysomethings—has lately put a damper on the hottest rave sites, in New York City, San Francisco, and Florida.

Also see: alcohol, bars, drugs, group sex

rear entry

This sexual position—the most popular variation of which is the familiar doggie style—puts you behind a woman, allowing you plenty of room to move and penetrate her vagina deeply. (Rear entry does *not* usually imply sodomy, one form of which involves anal penetration.)

This is one of those sexual issues where there's little middle ground among women. Some find it fun and exciting. Others think it's unpleasant or downright degrading. Don't get irritated with a woman who says no-thanks until you consider her point of view.

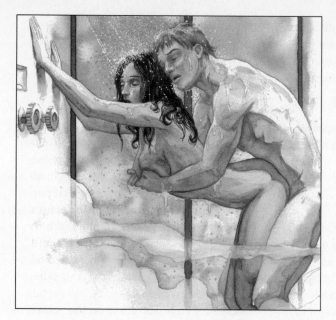

Literally. You may be getting an eyeful, but there isn't much for her to see. A lot of women like to have eye contact with their lovers, so she may feel detached when she can't see your face. You can address this problem through the strategic use of mirrors.

However, mirrors won't solve a second grievance: The position offers zero clitoral stimulation. You can remedy this by massaging her vulva while you thrust. Whatever you do, remember that the same deep penetration that feels great to you can be unexciting and uncomfortable for your partner. So adjust your thrust. And talk to her to discover what feels good for both of you.

Rear entry also makes kissing very difficult, which may be a real loss for some people. So explore more cuddly ways of taking your partner from behind. One is for both of you to lie on your sides. You won't be able to move as freely in this "spoons" position, but you'll gain a lot of intimacy. You might also lie on your back,

with her atop you, facing the ceiling.

If she lies facedown and you lie on top, you can have close rear-entry sex with more impact. Reach a hand around her pelvis to provide some added clitoral stimulation. Or, she can start with a traditional woman-on-top position, then spin around so her back is facing you. If your partner is more adventurous—or enjoys doing the work—have her sit on your lap as you both face forward in a chair or on the edge of the bed.

Finally, some men discover that the deep penetration of rear entry makes it hard to delay orgasm. If you want your partner to fully enjoy the experience, invest more time in foreplay to get her highly aroused before you enter her.

Also see: anal sex, booty, couch, doggie style, kinky, size—ass, sodomy, variety

rectum

The outer end of the digestive system, this part of the large intestine is 9 inches long, the final inch being the anus. Though it isn't a very clean place, it's usually empty. Fecal matter is stored in the rectum for only a short time, when it's ready to be expelled via bowel movement.

Contrary to what you might imagine, a rectum is not a straight 9 inches; it curves back and forth at sharp angles several times. So even though it's composed of soft, flexible tissue, when you're inserting something long and stiff—like an erect penis—into a woman's rectum, you need to be very gentle. You also want to use a water-based lubricant because the rectum produces little mucus of its own. And, of course, always wear a condom to prevent the spread of sexually transmitted diseases.

Also see: anal sex, kinky, klismaphilia, lubricants, rimming, sodomy, sphincter, suppositories

refractory period

Something we know all too well, it's a period of time following orgasm and ejaculation when a man is unable to get another erection. Generally, the younger you are, the shorter your sexual shutdown—from 10 minutes for a teenager to hours or, God forbid, days for older men.

Not all men experience this temporary impotence. For example, some men can use Tantric sex practices to learn to have an orgasm without ejaculating, thereby making it possible to experience multiple orgasms. And a 1995 study at Rutgers University found one 35-year-old guy who did not have a refractory period. Call him Old Faithful: He had six full-blown orgasms—that is, climaxes complete with ejaculation—in 36 minutes. We're doubly impressed by the fact that he did this while attached to gadgets that measured his blood pressure, pulse, and pupil size. When researchers figure out what his secret is, we'll let you in on it.

Most of us are not so lucky, which is why women, who tend to take longer than we do to reach orgasm, get ornery with guys who come too quick and then go limp and fall asleep. Remember that a flaccid penis shouldn't mean a frustrated partner. It's poor form to leave your woman all revved up with no place to go, so resort to other means of pleasing her while you're waiting for your woody to return.

Also see: afterglow, erection, multiple orgasms, sex drive, tantra

rejection—romantic

The old theory that nice guys don't get chicks sometimes holds true. Not because there's anything wrong with being nice, per se. But because a guy who's overly concerned about *not* seeming pushy isn't picking up on the cues a woman sends to indicate that she wants him to make a move. When he continues to hesitate and fumble around, she gets bored or frustrated and moves on.

Thing is, guys who come on too strong are equally likely to face rejection. Women don't sit around daydreaming of some Neanderthal who serves up one demeaning pickup line after another. Nor does today's busy career woman have time to play head games.

We know what you're thinking: It all comes down to looks, anyway. If you looked like Tom Cruise, you could walk up and fart, and they'd still go home with you. Well, before you start feeling too sorry for yourself, take a good look at the single gals *you've* been ignoring. Will you settle for nothing less than the hottest babes? That would explain your rejection ratio. Plus, you may be missing out on a great time with a woman whose looks don't quite qualify for *Playboy*.

Still, if absolutely no one seems interested in making your acquaintance, inventory your approach: Do you seem sad and desperate (that is, like you haven't had a date since you were 14)? Are you offending women with your Andrew Dice Clay–inspired humor? Do you decide what shirt to wear based on whether or not it passes the sniff test? Does your haircut say "Elvis on crack," or worse yet, does it consist of three 8-inch strands stretched futilely across an otherwise bare scalp? If you answered yes to these questions, you need to either revamp your approach or start hitting on women who are just as pathetic, crude, and/or unfashionable as you are.

We may not entirely understand women, but we do know sports, so here's a nice baseball metaphor to sum it all up for you: To get on base, you first have to figure out why you're not even getting the bat on the ball. So until you stop complaining that the calls are bad and take the time to analyze your swing, you're going to keep striking out. We hope that helps, slugger.

Also see: attraction, blind date, communication—nonverbal, dating, desperate, eye contact, masher, meeting women, opening line, pickup lines, self-esteem, sexual attraction, sexy, singles scene, turn-offs

rejection—sexual

You've spent the whole evening cozying up to a woman at the bar. You've bought her drinks, made her laugh. So you take a deep breath and invite her to your place, where, you figure, the evening will proceed to its logical conclusion. Only now she's not smiling anymore. In fact, she's fleeing, walking briskly across the club.

Shot down again.

If this sounds all too familiar, let us settle a burning question: Yes, it probably *is* you. That is, when it comes to asking a woman to bed, you're being a jerk about it. Why? In most cases, it's to compensate for your insecurities. A man who feels sexually inadequate often acts overbearing and obnoxious to disguise his fear of rejection.

On the other hand, maybe you're being a wimp. Women, much like wolves, can smell fear. And nothing is less sexy to them than a lack of confidence.

So take a good look at how you view yourself as a lover, both in and out of bed. If you're embarrassed about your sexual skills, penis size, physique, or overall appearance, you may need to do some heavy-duty self-esteem building. Do you have a female friend you trust? A sister-in-law? Ask her how you come across. You may have certain off-putting behavioral tics you're not even aware of (such as winks, head bobs, inflections, and so forth). You might also want to get some professional guidance from a sex therapist or relationship counselor who can help you identify behaviors that are turning women off.

Also see: attraction, begging, date rape, dating, desperate, first date, first time with a lover, marriage—lack of sex in, masher, no, seduction, self-esteem, sex therapy, sexual attraction, unwanted advances, withholding, Your place or mine?

relaxation

Good sex requires you to be relaxed and fully focused on giving and receiving pleasure. If you obsess over work, finances, and other daily pressures, you may well suffer erectile problems. It's not easy to stay hard when your thoughts keep wandering to that unfinished budget memo back at the office.

To purge your mind of stress, try a cognitive behavioral technique called thought stopping. Whenever your attention starts to drift away from the woman

QR

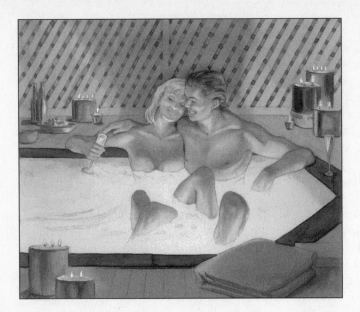

then releasing it. If your muscles are stiff, your penis probably isn't. A loose body is much more open to arousal.

Also see: anticipatory anxiety, atmosphere, biological clock, clumsiness, emotions, fatigue, frigidity, performance anxiety, stress, workaholism

religion

The clergy of many Western religions teach their flocks that sexual activity should be performed only for the purpose of reproduction. While some of these religions offer confessional sessions so that parishioners can try to reconcile their own desires with the churches' teachings, others allow no outlet for guilt and even enforce harsh penalties for "unauthorized" sex play.

Look at it this way: Whichever Creator you worship, He clearly designed sex to be pleasurable. So at minimum, if your religion makes you feel bad about your sexuality, you should delve further into what the specific tenets are and how they relate to your own sex life and conscience.

Find a member of your clergy who's open to frank discussion about sex. Tell this person that you're interested in exploring your religion's teachings on this very important subject. This is not the time to be squeamish about specifics: Ask about positions and masturbation and acts like oral sex. Yes, this will seem awkward (if not ridiculous) at first—but isn't that better than living a life of confusion and frustration?

you're inside, picture a mental stop sign. Force the distracting thoughts out of your head and concentrate on what's (literally) at hand. Notice all of the sensations you feel as you make love—not just touches but also your heart rate, breathing, and body heat. Sounds and scents too. Bothersome thoughts are less likely to break through when you stay focused on the sex.

Better still, of course, is to tackle your anxieties before you get intimate. Set aside time for problem solving. Take a sheet of paper and draw a vertical line down the center. On one side of the line, list the problems that are consuming your mental energy. On the other side, list possible solutions. Once you realize that the things causing you worry aren't so unmanageable after all, they won't get the best of you in the bedroom.

Progressive muscle relaxation is also a good way to warm up for sex. This technique involves tightening each muscle for a few seconds, starting at your feet,

If the answers you get aren't the ones you'd hoped to hear, if you're not comfortable talking to clergy, or if the cleric that you thought was open-minded turns out to be judgmental and harsh, consider some independent study. Sometimes, local religious leaders have personal biases and take much more puritanical points of view than does the official dogma. You may learn that your denomination's views aren't nearly as strict as you've been led to believe.

Realize, too, that spirituality can be pursued independent of organized religion and that different spiritual traditions may have varying attitudes about sex. Or you can practice your religion on a piecemeal basis, embracing only those precepts that reinforce the truths you know in your own heart: Adopt only nine of the Ten Commandments, or follow your faith's doctrine about charity and mercy but not about masturbation and birth control.

Also see: ahhh, abortion, abstinence, adultery, celibacy, circumcision, fig leaf, guilt, homophobia, lust, onanism, sodomy, spiritual sex, tantra, yogi

remarriage

A fresh start with a new partner should be a great second chance at romantic and sexual fulfillment. Underscore the "should be." Sadly, second marriages fail even more often than first marriages: maybe 60 percent of the time.

Speculation about the reasons could fill 10 books this size. No two self-styled experts agree on what goes wrong and which gender is more often to blame, so allow us our own theory, which is simple and unisex. It has to do with bringing the same old baggage into the brand-new marriage.

Little things that each of you do can remind the other of a soured relationship and trigger bitter feelings, dooming the relationship from the start. If you succumb to knee-jerk reactions, blowing up and telling her she's just like your ex, she's sure to get pretty bitter about it.

Rather than compare your bride to a banshee from your past, wait until you calm down—this cooling-off period is an absolute must—then explain that the specific idiosyncratic behavior really

QR

continued from page 274

park and told them **he would have to inspect the females' sex organs** to determine for sure whether they had been having sex. The officer was indicted for sexual assault.

Seemed like a Good Idea at the Time. . .

Talk about your blockbuster baseball trades! In 1973, New York Yan-

kees **pitchers Fritz Peterson and Mike Kekich swapped wives**—and families. Each divorced his original spouse and took up with the other's. Eyebrows duly raised, the Yanks dealt Kekich to the Cleveland Indians. Peterson also found his way to Cleveland, but not until Kekich was gone. Peterson later married the former Mrs. Kekich, but

True or Phallus

Playboy was the first mainstream magazine to show pubic hair.

continued on page 298

QR

bothers you. This may upset her, in which case you need to talk things out and reassure her of your love. It's the only way to put the issue behind you.

This works both ways, of course. Even though we know you're God's gift to women, she may have a nit or two to pick, and some of those nits may trace back to other men she's had the displeasure of knowing.

The key is for both of you to avoid appraising innocent, new behavior in an old, negative context. For instance, she may notice that a certain glaze creeps over your eyes as she tells you about her day. You think, "Man, the sound of her voice really turns me on." She thinks, "He's no different than my first husband. He doesn't give a damn what I'm saying. He's probably thinking about what's on ESPN. They're all alike!"

These same bugaboos also show up in the bedroom. Your playful pinch reminds her of her abusive, controlling husband. Her loud moans remind you of how your first wife faked orgasms. Don't hold in such concerns; they'll just fester and explode at the worst possible moment.

After all, you want to have one of the 40 percent of remarriages that make it, don't you?

Also see: communication, marriage, past partners—dealing with, past partners—talking about

reproductive system—hers

It's hidden mostly inside her body, and it's *way* complex compared to yours.

Here's a quick overview of the stuff that's tucked away: Lying above her vagina is her uterus, where a fertilized egg settles in and grows. The egg is fed to her uterus through a pair of fallopian tubes, where, contrary to general knowledge, conception actually happens. Above these tubes are the egg repositories known as her ovaries, which also perform a host of hormonal functions reminiscent of your testicles. See the entries on each of those anatomical parts for more detailed information.

Also see: biological clock, breastfeeding, cervix, clitoris, contraception, ectopic pregnancy, estrogen, fallopian tubes, fertility, gonad, hysterectomy, infertility, labia majora and minora, menopause—hers, menstruation, mons pubis, ovaries, ovulation, perineum, period, pituitary gland, pregnancy, PMS, prepuce, progesterone, progestin, pudenda, uterus, uterus—tipped, vagina, vulva, womb, zygote

reproductive system—yours

It's a lot simpler than hers, and in general, it causes fewer problems. Aside from those components you know oh-so-well—your penis and testicles—your reproductive system comprises the prostate, seminal vesicles, and a set of tubes called the vas deferens. For those of you who haven't seen the classic Woody Allen flick *Everything You Always Wanted to Know about Sex (But Were Afraid to Ask)*, it all works together like so:

You become aroused. Your heart rate increases; your blood pressure rises. Those 40 million or so sperm cells that your jewels produced today move out from your testicles through your vas deferens to your urethra. There, they mix with semen, the white fluid produced by your prostate and your seminal vesicles. This thick liquid waits in your ejaculatory duct, where muscles start to contract as you get increasingly stimulated by ongoing sexual activity. Finally, a series of contractions leads to the holy land of orgasm and ejaculation.

That's it. You're done. The rest is up to her.

Also see: contraception, Cowper's glands, ejaculation, fertility, gonad, hormones, infertility, orgasm, penis, pituitary gland, pregnancy, prostate, semen, sperm count, testicles, urethra, vas deferens

retrograde ejaculation

This condition occurs when the sphincter of a man's bladder opening doesn't close before he climaxes, thus allowing semen to flow back into his bladder instead of squirting out of his penis. Certain drugs, prostate surgery, neurological problems, and diabetes are its most common causes, and it rarely happens to healthy men. When it does, they're unaware of it; they just assume they've had a "dry come."

Though retrograde ejaculation isn't dangerous, it does make it unlikely you'll get your partner pregnant. Some would-be fathers with diabetes or prostate conditions have to stop taking their medications in order to conceive. There are also drugs that can reverse the condition.

Occasionally, however, the problem is permanent, and a couple wanting a baby has to undergo sperm retrieval and artificial insemination.

Also see: ejaculation, infertility

rhythm method

This supposed means of natural birth control relies on a woman's menstrual calendar to figure out when she's fertile so she can avoid having sex at that time.

The rhythm method is based on the biological fact that ovulation occurs 14 days before her period begins, plus or minus 2 days. So she need merely count back from the first day of her period to identify the day on which she ovulated. In theory, if she usually gets her period on the same day each month, that means she ovulates on a regular schedule as well.

Problem is, last month's ovulation date is not an accurate predictor of this month's. Even if your partner generally has a consistent menstrual cycle, factors such as physical activity, stress, and illness can prompt her ovaries to kick out an egg off the usual timetable now and then. And if this happens, there's no way to know about it until after the fact. If you luck out, she'll merely get her period unexpectedly (which can actually be pretty nerve-wracking if *unexpectedly* means "late"). If you're not so lucky, she won't get it at all (get ready for 18 years of wracked nerves, Dad).

Basically, the only "natural" way to guarantee that you won't have sex with her while she's ovulating is to never have sex with her. No wonder the rhythm method has a 25 percent failure rate. And anyway, who wants to abstain at the precise moment when she's apt to be juiciest and most easily aroused? If you're looking for effectiveness and convenience in a contraceptive method, try the Pill, an IUD, a diaphragm, or a condom and spermicide.

Also see: abstinence, contraception, ovulation

rimming

Stimulating the anus by licking or sucking.

If the very thought of having somebody burrowing around down there makes you want to hike up your shorts a bit tighter, no problem. It's not your gig. Be aware, though, that it suits some couples just fine. That obviously means it suits some women just fine. Some get turned on by feeling dirty and perverse. Others discover that their anuses are chock-full of sensitive, sexually provocative nerve endings.

If your partner suggests this practice and you're feeling especially playful, don't think you have to bury your tongue halfway up her large intestine to please her. As is true of the vagina, the anus has the highest concentration of nerves at its opening, so licking just around the hole will probably get the job done.

Bear in mind: You can get diseases from rimming. The anal area is loaded with bacteria, and you can also contract HIV if an infected partner has a rectal laceration. So it's best to use a latex barrier when you're in the mood for this particular meal.

Of course—file this under *common sense*—hygiene is paramount here. A nice bath or shower beforehand should improve the experience for both participants. And *never* put your tongue in her vagina or any other body opening after it's been in the anus.

Also see: anal beads, anal plug, kinky, oral sex, rear entry, sodomy

risky sex

The issue here boils down to what you're defining as "risky." Performing sexual activities at the risk of being observed or getting caught is very exciting for couples who have a touch of exhibitionism in them. If it doesn't harm anyone physically or emotionally and it doesn't force a chagrined friend to post bond for you on a regular basis, it's probably okay to keep right on doing what you're doing. (Just pull the blinds when there are kids around.)

Problem is, many other risky behaviors do cause harm. A guy who likes to have sex with strangers may easily catch diseases or cause unwanted pregnancies he never knows about, till the paternity suits arrive. A husband who enjoys extramarital one-nighters puts his marriage in jeopardy and may expose his wife to sexually transmitted diseases. A self-styled Don Juan who gets a kick out of persuading unwilling women to give in after they've already said no several times may end up explaining his particular slant on seduction to judge and jury. Partners who like to have sex while driving may close their eyes during orgasm and lose control of

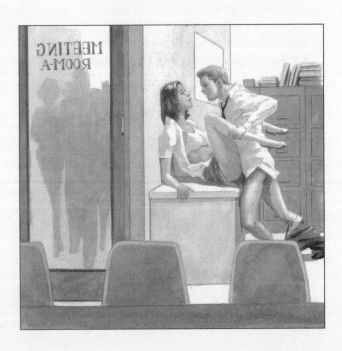

their cars—or distract passing motorists and make them lose control of theirs.

Even some exhibitionists run the risk of one day discovering that they can't get aroused *without* the element of danger. Other couples find that, in order to keep getting that same jolt, they have to keep escalating the risk to truly outlandish levels—till one day they're doing it while skydiving. It would be a damn shame to turn sex into such a big production that you get no enjoyment at all from a good old-fashioned romp in a darkened bedroom.

Also see: affairs, atmosphere, boredom, cars, compulsive behavior, danger, exhibitionism, kinky, planes, public places, STDs, variety

rituals

You read this word and think, "Boredom." That's not how we're using it here.

Establishing practices that you perform each time you have sex or reserving a specific practice for important sexual occasions can bring you and your lover closer together by personalizing and individualizing your relationship. A sexual ritual is a special act that you evolve and perform with your partner only. We don't want to get too touchy-feely here, but like a wedding ring, a ritual symbolizes your deep commitment to each other.

Case in point: One aging couple retired together in the mountains of northern New Mexico. Their home was adjacent to the tracks of a historic train that passed by at dusk several times each week. They began to meet on the back porch whenever they heard the train's approaching whistle. There, they'd hold hands until the train passed and the sun set. Several years later, the train's mellow whistle still signals to these long-time lovers that it's time for them to drop their evening activities, meet on the porch, and prepare to make love.

Another man, an artist, has his lover describe in intricate detail a place she'd like to visit. As she talks, he paints tiny landscapes on the nails of her fingers and toes.

A musician tells us that when he wants to be intimate with his wife, he sits down at the baby grand. His spontaneous composition lets her know whether he wants lengthy, gentle lovemaking or a turbulent session of hot sex. Sometimes she joins him at the piano and reads prose that seems to complement the music—everything from excerpts of Henry Miller to romantic monologues from Shakespeare.

Okay, okay, we're not losing our grip. You don't have to go hunting for the CliffsNotes of *Hamlet*. But look, the point is to keep the sex hot and cement your bond. That's why another woman reports that about one evening a month, she makes a point of putting fresh, silky sheets on the bed. When her guy gets home from work, he finds her sprawled on the mattress, wearing a black body stocking and flipping through photo albums that document their history as a couple. He joins in the reminiscing, and as they plan future adventures, they fall into lovemaking.

That doesn't sound so bad, does it?

Also see: appointments, boredom, commitment, contraception, fetish, food, intimacy, *Kama Sutra*, passion, routines, tantra

road erection

This phenomenon, also known as highway hard-on, is a spontaneous erection that seems to pop up most often when you're behind the wheel of a car. It's common among younger men (though spontaneous erections in young men aren't exactly rare to begin with). With all that testosterone coursing through a young guy's veins, it doesn't take much pressure to provoke an erection, so a little suspension-system vibration or a few potholes here and there will definitely do it. As you age, drive-by erections decline significantly.

There's nothing wrong with enjoying a little sexual stimulation while you're cruisin' down the road. But if you're tempted to take the next step—masturbation—our advice is to pull over before you pull off.

Also see: cars, erection, masturbation, stimulation

road head

We know you've had the fantasy: getting a good blow job while cruising down the interstate at 80 mph. In fact, up to 14 percent of you have had the reality, according to one survey. So-called road head is erotic, exciting, exhilarating . . . and oh, yeah, extremely dangerous.

Oral sex is generally best when not potentially fatal, so we recommend that you quickly find a place to park when a lovely passenger offers to work your stick shift for you.

Also see: cars, fellatio, give head, kinky, oral sex

role reversal

This sexual philosophy is not for the faint of heart (or the faint of other body parts, as you'll see), but if, like us, you've wondered what it would be like

to be a woman, it may be as close as you ever get.

Role reversal concerns itself with who gets to penetrate whom. A surprising number of women nowadays are strapping on dildos while their guys are busy greasing their rumps. If you can get past the homoerotic overtones—and with a gorgeous woman in the room, that's not as difficult as you may think—you may consider this worth a try.

Make this sex play the main dish, or use it to whet your appetite for a more traditional second course. Just be sure to lube up before insertion. And wash the dildo thoroughly or slide a latex condom on it before you put it anywhere inside her later on.

Also see: anal beads, anal plug, dildo, heterosexuality, homosexuality, lubricants, rectum, rimming, sexual aids, sodomy, sphincter, variety

romance

A link between the dreamy idea of love and the reality of a sexual relationship. You may feel true love for your woman, but if you don't take romantic action now and then, she may wonder if she's just a good lay. Such action benefits you, as well, because a feeling of romance is what may fan her desire for sex.

Men and women can operate on different sexual speeds. You may not need a gourmet dinner or a nicely wrapped gift to feel like getting it on. She, on the other hand, may be slower to rouse, sexually. She may want to feel loved, fussed over, swept away. She may require more sweet talk—*heartfelt* sweet talk—and more touching.

Romance is about building a bridge across the canyon that separates the sexual styles of a man and a woman. It forces you to slow down and find out what makes her feel special and sexual. It gives you time to create an environment that makes her excited about making love.

Think of romance as an all-day activity, not just a few minutes of foreplay. Start the morning by pouring her a cup of coffee, giving her a little kiss, then taking out the trash. (Trash is romantic? Uh, no. What's romantic is the fact that you remembered what's important to *her*—and a tidy, stenchless, garbage-free home is important to her.) Call her in the middle of the afternoon to say you can't wait to see her later. Bring home flowers or a bottle of her favorite wine. Turn off the television, fold up the newspaper, and forget about the problems you had at the office.

Just focus on the woman you fell in love with.

Also see: arousal, birthdays, flowers, kiss, mood, routines, surprises, sweet talk, variety

rough sex

It's a potent female fantasy—though one that's often misinterpreted, with regrettable (and sometimes illegal) results. A woman who hints about making love more aggressively is usually not looking to have sensitive body parts sundered or her head bashed against the nearest bedpost. Rough sex for most women is a role-playing game in which you create the illusion of forcefulness. You tease; you don't draw blood.

It bears repeating that the operative word here is *illusion*. Before you engage in rough sex, you and your partner should mutually agree upon a safeword that means "Enough." No matter how

much you're enjoying yourself or how close you are to coming, if your partner utters the safeword, cease and desist immediately!

That said, you also should be alert to your partner's nonverbal cues about desiring a bolder approach to lovemaking. If you think she's in the mood, you might start by backing her up against a wall— again, not too hard at first—and holding her there tightly. Employ your fingernails and your teeth, but use them as pleasure tools, not weapons. Monitor her response as you gently scrape your nails down her back and nip her neck or breasts. If she doesn't flinch, dig a bit deeper, bite a bit harder. Be a little more forceful in removing her clothing. Again, pay attention to her reaction as you go along.

Arguably the most misunderstood concept in sex is rough intercourse itself. No woman enjoys being jabbed with a fully erect penis when she's not yet lubricated or otherwise ready. The roughness comes in more in the way you move once she's fully aroused and you're actually inside her. Try rocking her hard and fast in a setting where she won't get bruised or rug-burned; a soft mattress is ideal. Gradually increase your pace or force. Here, too, nonverbal cues play a big role. Look for wincing or an attempt on her part to disengage. Learn the difference between a pleasurable moan and a painful groan.

It's a delicate balancing act: You have to learn to push the limits without exceeding them. Further complicating things, different women have different limits. And at different times.

If you're not sure whether your woman is enjoying it or just how hard she wants it, by all means, ask. There's nothing wrong with a well-placed "Have

QR

you had enough yet?" or "Do you like this?" You may even get a breathy "No, baby, I *love* it" in return.

Also see: biting, bondage and discipline, communication, communication—nonverbal, date rape, dominance and submission, kinky, masochism, playacting, rape, rug burn, violence, wrestling

routines

A couple can't live without 'em in this fast-paced world. Somebody has to feed the dog, somebody has to scrub the toilet. (Just not you. Right?)

But the same routines that make life hum pleasantly along can also reduce your love life to ho-hum. Caught up in the daily rigmarole of writing out checks and grocery lists and taking clients to dinner and kids to soccer, partners often start taking each other for granted as well. You work late; you "forget" to have conversations. Romance becomes something you squeeze in here and there, time permitting.

If daily tasks crowd out your love life, you need to readjust your priorities. Turn off the TV, put down the remote control—it's been the downfall of many a relationship—and go press your partner's buttons instead. In fact, stop reading, right now, and get to it.

What's more, in breaking out of ruts, it's important to shake up gender traditions, even in tasks as seemingly benign as cleaning that commode. She's unlikely to feel sexy in the evening if she's spent the afternoon disinfecting the john. What will put her in the mood is seeing that you're willing to do your share of the dirty work. So grab the toilet brush once in a while. (What, you're still here, reading this? You're supposed to be se-

ducing her. *Go ahead.* She'll love it. And so will you.)

On the other hand, there are some routines that can actually enhance your love life. Like actually being the one to suggest an evening stroll. Or checking in with her every day, just to show her she's on your mind. She'll find these calls sweet and pleasing—and they may put her in the mood for pleasing you later.

Also see: appointments, boredom, financial difficulties, rituals, romance, travel as an aphrodisiac, variety

rubber

The condom came by this familiar nickname logically enough: Rubber condoms replaced lamb intestine as the most popular prophylactics in the late 1800s, shortly after the development of vulcanization—a process that transformed crude, natural rubber into a thin, strong, stretchy material that was cheaper and easier to convert into condoms than were animal skins. Also less porous, rubber condoms created a more effective barrier against viruses and bacteria.

Some forms of liquid latex, which replaced crude rubber in condom manufacturing during the 1930s, are also natural rubber substances produced by plants. Most condoms are still made of latex today. When used properly, rubbers are astonishingly effective in preventing unwanted pregnancy and disease.

Also see: condom, condom—polyurethane, contraception, prophylactic, safe sex, STDs

rug burn

Red, scabby, itchy, burning battle scars can appear on your knees, elbows, hips, shins, thighs, back—wherever your skin rubs against carpet while you and your partner spend quality time on the floor. If you want to avoid these flesh wounds, consider carpeting your home with nylon and wool, which tend to be easier on tender flesh than the commonly used synthetic fiber, olefin. Another factor to consider is the structure of the pile. Cut piles—plush, velvety carpets, the denser, the better—are much softer than loop piles like berber.

The phrase *rug burn* is also used to describe any sexual chafing. If you're one of the lucky guys who gets rug burns from bed sex (and we do mean lucky—it means you're getting lots of sack time), consider buying satin bedding or sheets with a high thread count. The higher the thread count, the less abrasive the material.

If you end up with a rug burn, cool it by holding the injured area under cold running water for 15 minutes. You can also use cold compresses. Then apply a lotion that contains aloe vera.

Also see: athletic sex, back, exercise, rashes

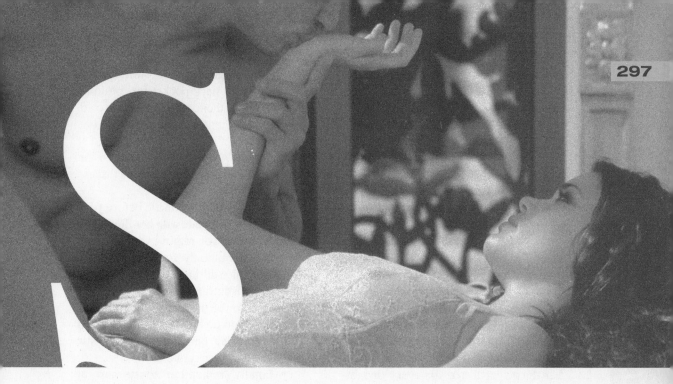

Sade—Marquis de

You know this guy, even if you haven't heard his name before. He's the fellow who gave us the terms *sadism* and *sadistic*.

Born in France in 1740, the Marquis de Sade was a nobleman whose writings and cruel sexual preferences spread his name far and wide. He spent a goodly portion of his life in prison for the sexual torture of various prostitutes and neighborhood boys and girls. During one of his prison spells, his wife, who had been his partner in crime, left him. She retired to a convent.

To combat the boredom and anger in jail and, one assumes, the lack of available sex partners, de Sade dashed off reams of material that later became books, novellas, and plays. Among them were *The 120 Days of Sodom and Other Writings* and *Justine, ou les Malheurs de la Vertu*.

His works remain banned in France to this day. Elsewhere, though, his books were (and are) read ravenously. Some people, not surprisingly, see him as the incarnation of absolute evil. Others tout his message of sexual liberation, even if it takes forms unpalatable to others.

Also see: bondage and discipline, dominance and submission, erotic literature, fetish, French, paraphilias, pornography, rough sex, violence

safe sex

You know as well as we do that to avoid a host of sexually transmitted diseases, you have to wear a condom every time you have sex with a new partner. Trouble is, too many of us consider safe sex just another ritual of early courtship that we can move beyond as a relationship progresses (kind of like leaving each other's company when we have to break wind). Once we begin to feel emotionally secure in a relationship, many of us make the mistake of assuming that our partners are disease-free and monogamous. So we say goodbye to the condoms. And, potentially, we say hello to STDs.

Here's the bottom line: You should always practice safe sex. That's because some STDs (specifically, herpes and genital warts) are difficult to detect through routine tests and can be carried relatively symptom-free, meaning if you or your partner have them, you may not even know. That said, if condom-free sex is of utmost importance to you, have it only after you're both completely monogamous and you've taken the following steps.

• First, get tested for every imaginable STD. For 6 months thereafter, even if you each get a clean bill of health, you have to remain faithful to each other and, most important, continue using condoms.

• To keep you on track during the 6-month waiting period, keep your condoms where you're most likely to use them: by the bed. Also carry a few with you when you go out. Don't store them in your wallet or back pocket for too long. Heat weakens them, as does extreme cold. Make sure you get the right fit. Too big, and it could slip off. Too small, and it could break. Avoid novelty and lambskin condoms; they don't prevent disease transmission.

• Put on the prophylactic before your penis comes in contact with her fluids, and keep it on until you remove yourself from her. Use it not only for vaginal intercourse but also during anal sex (when the risk of transmitting diseases is highest) and when you're the recipient of oral sex.

• If you go down on her, use a dental dam (available from sex shops) or plastic wrap to cover her genitals.

• Finally, remember to be careful when you take off the condom; don't be sloppy with the semen.

• When the 6-month wait is up, you each have to get another HIV test because the virus doesn't register on tests until 6 months after infection (so if you contracted it less than 6 months before the first test, it wouldn't have shown up

---

Hot Dates 1974 Students across the country staged group streaks and nude cross-campus dashes.

continued from page 287

Answer:
False. *Penthouse* pioneered in the pubic hair department; *Playboy* followed suit.

Kekich and the former Mrs. Peterson struck out.

A few years later, Cleveland had a ticklish situation of its own. Centerfielder Rick Manning began sleeping with the wife of pitcher Dennis Eckersley. The Indians, like the Yankees, felt they had to rid themselves of one of the players, so they dumped Eckersley. Wrong choice. "Eck" went on to have a long, outstanding career, while Manning fizzled.

Manning and the former Mrs. Eckersley eventually married—and divorced.

Foreign Affairs
The House of Spartacus in Johannesburg, South Africa, may be the world's first brothel for straight

BAWDY BALLADS "Jack U Off," *Prince*

continued on page 305

then anyway). Remember, if either of you carries the viruses that cause herpes or genital warts, you still may be able to transmit them.

Keep all this in mind even if you both come up clean and agree to remain monogamous. After all, safe sex is better than no sex.

Also see: abstinence, brothels/bordellos, condoms, contraception, cybersex, dial-a-porn, dry hump, fears/phobias, femoral intercourse, first time with a lover, Internet dating, past partners—talking about, phone sex, promiscuity, risky sex, sex education, STDs

safeword

Before you handcuff your mate to the headboard or engage in any other rough play during sex, you and your partner should mutually agree upon a safeword that means "I've had enough. Stop right now." Having such a code word leaves you free to scream and beg and bully and whine and threaten and plead all you want as part of your sex games, knowing that the one and only safeword is always available to put an end to things if they get too rough.

Clearly, then, *No* or *Enough* or *Stop* are not ideal safewords since you may blurt them out in the heat of the moment. The best suggestion we've heard for a safeword is . . . *safeword.*

Once she utters your code word, *immediately* stop what you're doing and untie or uncuff her. Stop no matter how much you're enjoying yourself—even if you're just about to come.

Also see: bondage and discipline, chains, dominance and submission, flogging, handcuffs, paddle, rough sex, spanking, whips, wrestling

satyriasis

A satyr is a creature from Greek mythology, part man and part goat. This handsome fellow was also overly fond of sex. Hence, satyriasis, the male counterpart to nymphomania. Dictionary-defined, it's a man's excessive, often uncontrollable craving for sex.

You can get a full accounting of the phenomenon by checking out the entry on *nymphomania.* The same basic mechanisms are at work. Just substitute *male, man,* or *he* wherever that entry reads *female, woman,* or *she.*

Also see: compulsive behavior, sex addiction

scents

Odors are essential in attraction and arousal, particularly for women, who have very keen senses of smell. Sexy scents can quickly turn on a female. Foul odors can just as quickly do the opposite.

Some odors can assist your natural sexual scents, or pheromones, in sending a sensual message. According to aromatherapists, the essential oil ylang-ylang is a turn-on to women, while sandalwood has the same effect on you. Put a few drops of oil in a diffuser to scent your bedroom, or add a touch to bathwater. Perhaps the best way to use essential oils is as aromatherapy massage oils. Both ylang-ylang and sandalwood oils can be used undiluted; just keep them away from your eyes. Oh, and some people experience less-than-sexy side effects from ylang-ylang, specifically, nausea and headaches. So use it in moderation until you're sure of its effect on your partner.

The myriad fragrances of nature can also add a new dimension to your sex

S

life. Have sex on a freshly cut lawn (not on the new mulch), on the beach (far from the dead horseshoe crab), or even in a bed covered with rose petals (unless one of you has allergies).

Also see: aromatherapy, atmosphere, body odor as an attractant, fragrances, perfume, pheromones

scratching

Most women aren't as appalled by our necessary adjustments as we may think. Hey, they understand that there's a lot of flesh dangling down there—amid all that hair, no less—so things are bound to get itchy and shift out of place now and then. Besides, many women grew up watching baseball, where scratching and adjusting are, of course, required by the rule book.

Of course, there are such notions as politeness and discretion. Accordingly, always keep some keys or loose change in your front pockets for those occasions when there's no avoiding a scratch. Jiggle the keys around, or pretend you're digging deep for a few coins. Save it for moments of true discomfort, though, because people will catch on eventually. Nobody needs to find his keys *that* often.

When the itch strikes while you're sitting down, lean back in your seat, fold your hands in your lap with one on top of the other, and slowly, surreptitiously get the job done with the pinky finger of your bottom hand. It takes a little practice to get this right, but if you're like most guys, you'll have plenty of itches with which to perfect your technique.

Also see: crabs, herpes, hygiene, NSU, rashes, yeast infection

scrotum

The loose, wrinkly, soft, sensitive pouch of skin that holds your testes. It hangs outside your body as a form of climate control, ensuring a temperature several degrees cooler than inside your body, where sperm would be scorched. That's why it swings low when you're sweating your way through a heat wave—to keep the little swimmers as cool as possible. The shrinkage that you experience when you take a dip in a cold pond happens for the same reason: The muscle inside your scrotum, called the dartos, contracts and pulls your sac closer to your body to ward off a chill.

In case you ever wondered, that line that runs up the middle of your sac actually has its own name. It's called the raphe, pronounced "ray-fee," and it's left over from where the two halves of your scrotum fused together while you were an embryo. Now that you're out of the womb, it's purely decorative—kind of like a racing stripe.

Also see: epididymitis, infertility, injuries, perineum, reproductive system—yours, testicles, testicles—undescended, testosterone replacement therapy, vasectomy

secrets

She wants to know you deeply. The darkest details of your love life may open her up to greater sexual intimacy if you open up and reveal them. Your most embarrassing sexual failures, whispered in the quiet of a darkened bedroom, may make her want to soothe your psyche with a tender, loving touch. Your most private sexual thoughts may spark her own libido and imagination.

Or, they may create a welter of problems that ultimately cause her to walk.

Secrets are sacred. They can be gifts of honesty and intimacy in a relationship. When you reveal your inner thoughts to one another, you express mutual trust. Both of you must treat those confessions as shared treasures. Never repeat them to anyone.

Just be cautious when actually discussing past sex. As we note elsewhere in this book, even the strongest relationships have been known to falter after partners opened a Pandora's box of sexual reminiscences. No matter how much she loves you, she is not immune to jealousy. And neither are you. (Did we really need to tell you that?)

For instance, we're guessing that if she's not the best lover you've ever had, she doesn't particularly want to know it. Your best bet here is to show her how to be a better lover for you, without confiding details about past mind-blowing sexual episodes that are likely to make her feel very small—and worse, very unsexy.

So protect from her scrutiny any thoughts that you think may hurt her or that you fear she may one day use to hurt you. Besides, a little mystery is, well, sexy.

And as for sharing your deep, dark sexual secrets with others besides your lover, we'll paraphrase an old quote: Three people can keep a secret . . . if two of them are dead. So don't tell friends anything "in confidence" that you don't want to hear repeated back to you (or your partner) soon after. That, folks, is the secret of keeping your secrets secret.

Also see: affairs; communication; discretion; Don't ask, don't tell; fantasies; intimacy; jealousy; past partners—talking about; trust—rebuilding

seduction

The best seducers read body language: the way a woman stands, the movements of her hands, the wideness of her eyes, the breadth of her smile. A man who can interpret those signals will have little trouble sweeping her off her feet—and into his bed.

The important thing to recognize about seduction is that it's not just you making a sales pitch; it's a negotiation. At various points along the way, an interested woman throws off certain cues that signal her mounting desire (or her desire to mount you, as the case may be). She expects you to perceive, acknowledge, and act on those cues. So ask her questions about herself, and pay very close attention to her answers—not just what she says but also how she says it. Does she seem to sway toward you for a moment as she tells you that she recently became single again? Or does she just state it matter-of-factly?

This is critical because a woman whose come-hither vibes are ignored starts to feel just as rejected as the woman who asks a man outright to sleep with her and gets turned down. Pretty soon, her pride forces her to put up a wall, to be less demonstrative about her interest. And then the seduction is over.

If the tables are turned and that Venus you met at last Friday night's dart game puts the moves on you, how should you react? If you're interested, reciprocate simply by being yourself. Smile, ask her lots of questions about herself, and let her discover who you are. Enjoy the seduction for what it is: a highly charged erotic buildup that culminates in some kind of connection, be it a phone number exchange or a romp in bed.

Also see: aphrodisiac, flirtation, communication—nonverbal, courtship, date rape, hypnosis and seduction, rejection—sexual

self-esteem

The shrinks might say it this way: Forming intimate relationships is nearly impossible in the absence of high self-esteem.

We'll say it more bluntly: It's hard to get a woman to appreciate you when you don't feel worth appreciating.

A healthy self-image means confidence in your competence in and out of the bedroom and a sense of being worthy of love. It may just be the single most important aspect of sexual attractiveness. Let's be clear here: Self-confidence is not arrogance. You don't need to be boastful to let the world know that you feel good about yourself. You only need to understand that your accomplishments are more important than your failures. And you need to have a sense of humor about those failures. That, in turn, makes you less afraid of failing in the future. Which, again in turn, makes you more likely to go after what you want.

Now, we realize that for many guys, it's not easy to follow that advice. So we won't even attempt to give you a short course in self-esteem. We'll simply urge you to go to a good bookstore and ask the clerk to point you toward the self-help aisle. We're betting that it's one of the biggest sections in the store. Browse the shelves till you find a book that seems right for you.

Or consider taking one of the many courses offered by Dale Carnegie

Training. Unlike some of the Johnny-come-lately motivational gurus, the folks at Carnegie have been at this for a long time, and many graduates swear by their approach.

Also see: anticipatory anxiety, attraction, body image, clumsiness, dressing you to look sexy, emotions, jealousy, male body, midlife crisis, performance anxiety, promiscuity, puberty, rejection—romantic, rejection—sexual, sexy, shyness, slick, soul mates, spectatoring, virginity—hers

semen

This thick, white ejaculatory fluid is produced by your testes, prostate, and seminal vesicles. But you're probably more concerned with where it goes than with where it comes from. Obviously, if it squirts into someone's vagina unhindered by a contraceptive device, you could become a daddy. If it goes into a condom, you're less likely to pass on or contract a sexually transmitted disease. And if it goes into someone's mouth, you'd better hope she was expecting it.

One survey revealed that only one woman in four is willing to swallow semen. When the other three beg off, chances are, it's because they don't like the taste, which can vary from sweet to salty to bitter. The flavor of your semen is determined largely by what you eat. Large quantities of meat and fish give semen a bitter taste. Cheap liquor turns it acidic. Dairy foods and asparagus can make it taste downright foul. But you can sweeten your semen by eating lots of fruits and drinking juices.

Some women also claim that semen smells like bleach, which makes sense since it contains chlorine. Sperm makes up only 2 to 5 percent of semen. Its other ingredients include calcium, cholesterol, citric acid, lactic acid, magnesium, nitrogen, phosphorus, potassium, sodium, urea, uric acid, vitamin B_{12}, and zinc. It's also high in proteins and sugars, and it's a regular diet beverage, with an average of only 40 calories per ejaculation.

Also see: aging, cum, ejaculation, fertility, gusher, prostate, retrograde ejaculation, sloppy sex, sperm count, tantra, urethritis, vasectomy, wet dreams, wet spot, zinc

sensate focus

A form of sex therapy invented by sex researchers William H. Masters, M.D., and Virginia E. Johnson, Ph.D., in the early 1960s and based loosely on tantric yoga practices that strive to prolong arousal and heighten the sexual experience. The treatment facilitates arousal and enjoyment by inviting each partner to learn the touches that turn the other on before they each get off. With the proper coaching of a sex therapist, sensate focus can help partners with performance anxiety get over their fears, and it can be especially successful as a form of therapy for people who've experienced sexual trauma.

For couples who just want to have better sex, taking the time to talk and touch can really heat things up. Here's one version of the technique, in case you're curious about trying some sexual self-improvement.

1. In the first two sessions, breasts and genitals are off-limits. Take turns touching each other anywhere else on your bodies, concentrating on the physical sensations of being touched without being preoccupied with sexual arousal and performance.

2. Advance to the second stage of touching, which includes breasts and genitals but prohibits intercourse and orgasm.

3. A few sessions later, you can touch each other at the same time, rather than taking turns. You can use your hands to help each other to orgasm, but you still must refrain from intercourse.

4. Begin the last stage with mutual touching. Then proceed to genital stimulation—but not intercourse—with your partner on top.

5. Finally, go ahead and have sex any way you like.

Also see: anticipatory anxiety, performance anxiety, rape, sex therapy, spectatoring

sex addiction

Like other addictions, addiction to sex is characterized by urges and behaviors that are extremely difficult to control, harmful to others, and detrimental to your career, relationships, and every other aspect of life. Sex addicts use sex as a drug that either dulls emotional pain or causes a physical and psychological high. They usually have a desperate need for love and believe that sex *is* love.

Though most sex addicts are men (lucky us), women can also be afflicted. Many women with sexual compulsions are attracted to dangerous situations such as prostitution or violent relationships. Others are terrified of being abandoned and have difficulty coping when their sexual relationships end.

For years, people have tended to laugh off sex addiction as being in the same category as, oh, addiction to pizza or long vacations in Monaco. Only, perhaps, with the travails of Bill Clinton have people begun to give serious thought to the costs of excessive, obsessive sex. Treatment is available through group-counseling organizations such as Sexaholics Anonymous and Sex Addicts Anonymous or from sex therapists.

Thankfully, getting over a sex addiction (unlike overcoming compulsive gambling or alcoholism) doesn't require forsaking sex. Recovery entails dealing with the underlying emotional issues that prompt the addiction, learning how to face anxiety and stress with responses other than sexual behavior, and improving social skills. More serious compulsions, however, such as the impulse to have sex with children or dead bodies, require more intensive therapy.

Also see: compulsive behavior, fantasies, necrophilia, nymphomania, pedophilia, promiscuity, satyriasis, sex therapy

sex appeal

See: beauty, preference, sexual attraction, sexy

sex drive

Next time you bring up sex and a woman complains, "That's all you think about!" point out that men and women have fairly equal libidos, according to studies of the subject. The difference in how the two genders perceive their respective sex drives may occur because of other dynamics that affect male-female relationships, causing us to confuse other factors with low sex drive. For instance, when you're pissed off at your partner, you probably don't want to get frisky with her. Well, okay, that's not necessarily true; if she's hot, you probably want to

nail her anyway. But we can almost guarantee that when *she's* pissed off at *you*, sex won't be uppermost in her mind.

Your woman's sex drive is also strongly influenced by her reproductive cycle. Her libido is highest during the 3 days of her ovulatory phase, which occurs about 8 days after her period ends. She's probably least lustful for the 2 weeks afterward, known as the luteal phase, when her body produces the progesterone that makes her prone to PMS. Some women, however, do feel sexually aggressive in the middle of this phase.

Libido-sapping problems affecting both sexes include diabetes, alcoholism, fatigue, anxiety, and depression. Even some remedies for depression, such as the medications Prozac (fluoxetine hydrochloride) and Zoloft (sertraline), inhibit sexual desire.

The key to keeping your sex drive strong is to stay active and healthy: Continue having sex, eat right, and exercise. Vegetables are the best foods for enhancing virility, because they're rich in vitamins, minerals, and carbohydrate. In addition, you may want to take a good multivitamin.

While your sex drive will begin to decrease after middle age, your woman's may increase postmenopause because she'll no longer have to worry about unintended pregnancy. And both of you may be more sexually motivated, because you'll tend to have fewer family and career responsibilities dampening your sexual energy.

Also see: depression, DHEA, fatigue, hormones, horny, libido, menopause—hers, menopause—yours, oral contraceptive, PMS, Prozac, randy, road erection, sex therapy, sickness, stress, supplements, testicles, testosterone, testosterone replacement therapy, zinc

sex education

The wealth of information that we use to increase our sexual know-how is ever-growing and becoming more freely available. The Internet brims with sex sites, such as that of the Society for Human Sexuality, which posts facts, news, and statistics about sex. Most bookstores have sections of erotic how-to guides that couples can share, though you should avoid trying to find useful literature in so-called adult bookstores. (Save those books for masturbation, not information.)

Sexuality workshops can be found in most major cities. Visit a local sex-toy store to find a calendar of classes. Ask store clerks for additional information about sex seminars in your area. And don't be embarrassed; there's little you could say that would shock or upset somebody who spends every day surrounded by anal plugs, nipple clamps, and foot-long dildos.

You may want to consult a sex therapist to find out how to improve your sexual style. Therapists can address individual issues more directly than any seminar or class can, by directing you to the resources that will work best for you. They also are better able to take into account your personal tastes and morals.

Oh, you were expecting us to tell you how to educate your kids, not yourself? You may get some help from your children's schools: 47 states either require or recommend sex-ed classes. But you shouldn't just wait for the high school health teacher to drag out diagrams of fallopian tubes.

It's hard to give you specific guidance about precisely when to start the instruction, but no matter the age, if questions come up, never take the attitude that your kid is too young to know. Answer honestly, in a manner that's appropriate for the child you're dealing with. Keep details to a minimum. "The baby grows inside the mommy's belly" is probably all you'll need to say to younger children. Always use correct anatomical terms in-

S

Hot Dates 1974 Strip club owner Larry Flynt turned his club newsletter into *Hustler* magazine.

continued from page 298

women. **"They are hot women, and they are looking for a hot man,"** says a gigolo who works at the club.

In Extremis

Proving once again that men don't need sweet talk to get in the mood, a Circleville, Ohio, man who woke to find his ex-wife in his house tried to get her to have sex with him—unaware that **she had just fired a bullet** into his chest. She took a pass, saying, "I just shot you." His ex added that she would have fired several more times had the gun not jammed.

LEGAL BRIEFS

During a prostitution sting in Colorado, **cops engaged in sex with hookers** rather than arresting them once the women agreed to have sex for money. A sheriff's spokesman ex-

True or Phallus?

Penthouse magazine published nude photos of Jackie Onassis when she was 41 years old.

BAWDY BALLADS "My Big 10-Inch Record," *Aerosmith*

continued on page 312

S

stead of slang or "baby" names ("Oh, that thing between your legs? Why, that's your pee-pee!")

Be sure to surround the mechanics of sex with your personal values. As far as teaching abstinence, surveys show that kids whose sexual instruction focused mainly on abstinence were just as likely to have sex as were those with different sex-ed curricula. So what? So, instruction that focuses only on abstinence is less likely to equip a child for pregnancy avoidance and safe sex. With studies showing that more than half of kids have had some sexual experience by the time they graduate high school, this is no small concern.

Also see: brothels/bordellos, erotic films; innocence; *Joy of Sex, The*; kids; kinky; sex research; sex therapy; surrogate

sex—lack of

There's a lot of this going around. One study found that one in five Americans has not had sex in at least a year. A lot of other folks simply get less action than they'd like. In fact, surveys report that at least half of women and nearly 70 percent of men want to have more sex.

Sex deprivation can cause depression and anger as well as stress that overspreads all other aspects of your life. It can even have physical effects. That line we used to give girls on dates? About blue balls? It's true, at least sometimes. A hard-on of any duration that's not followed by orgasm (especially when it's accompanied by a high level of arousal) may bring about that testicular aching of lore. This is due to blood trapped in the genitals. Women in similar circumstances can experience similar symptoms, which

raises a valid question: Why don't we all just do each other a big favor?

A dry spell in men also contributes to prostate infections resulting from poor prostate drainage. More frightening still, for guys with high cholesterol, the old adage "Use it or lose it" applies. Cholesterol-filled arteries can prevent normal nocturnal erections. If a guy with that problem doesn't get it up when he's awake either, his penis can be starved for oxygen-rich blood, leading, in extreme cases, to permanent impotence.

So ladies, if you care about us, *really* care . . .

Also see: abstinence, celibacy, horny, marriage—lack of sex in, masturbation, prostitution, quality versus quantity, rejection—sexual, withholding

sex offenders

These troubled and troubling individuals whom women fear and good men despise are not necessarily shadowy figures lurking in dark alleys. In fact, the more dangerous a sex offender is, the more likely he is to choose victims he knows. Women are four times more likely to be raped by someone they know than by a stranger. Eighty to 95 percent of molested children knew their abusers beforehand. On the other hand, guys whose gigs include peeping, exposing themselves, or surreptitiously groping usually target nonacquaintances.

Most arrested sex offenders are unmarried guys from violent, low-income environments (though they're not invariably men, contrary to popular opinion). Growing up in war-zone homes—watching adults battle and perhaps suffering abuse themselves—they learned to view sex as a form of power, not an act of love.

As adults, they commit their crimes out of fear of women, hostility, lack of empathy, or a desire to dominate.

Because such abuse is a vicious cycle, passed from generation to generation, the best thing we can do to protect the women and children we love is to vow to keep our own houses in order: Prevent today's vulnerable young boys from becoming tomorrow's sexual predators. By the time we have to resort to the common strategies for dealing with convicted offenders—prison, community-notification laws, behavioral therapy, and drugs—it's already too late.

Also see: compulsive behavior, date rape, exhibitionism, gang rape, genetics, incest, masher, necrophilia, paraphilias, pedophilia, pornography, prison, rape, sex therapy, violence, voyeurism

sex research

A lack of facts has caused the spread of much misinformation about sex, sexuality, and sexually transmitted diseases. Although unsatisfying sex is at the root of most marital problems and is a cause of great anxiety for millions of men and women, sexology is the least studied biological science. While the U.S. government does fund studies on STD treatments and birth control, only about $10 million—all private funds—are spent each year to learn more about the enhancement of erotic experiences. (Americans treasure the pursuit of happiness, but a lot of us don't want our tax dollars to pay for it.) Among the organizations that work to provide accurate information to men and women who are interested in improving their sexual functioning and pleasure is the Kinsey Institute for Research in Sex, Gender, and Reproduction. The top

group researching childhood sexuality education is the Sex Information and Education Council of the United States.

Also see: Freud, *Hite Report—The*, Janus Report, Kinsey, Masters and Johnson, promiscuity, sex education

sex symbols

From silent-film "It Girl" Clara Bow to this month's *Playboy* centerfold, beautiful celebrities have long captured our attention. Gorgeous, glamorous, and unattainable, sex symbols are perfect fodder for fantasies. An infatuation with a comely face or body on a movie screen or magazine doesn't mean you're less attracted to the real woman in your life. In fact, it's a whole lot safer than indulging your obsession with Clarice the intern. In other words, sex symbols are safe outlets for satisfying your need to ogle. Remind your partner of that the next time she karate kicks the Victoria's Secret catalog out of your sweaty hands.

Also see: casting couch, beefcake, fantasies, media, movies, *Penthouse*, *Playboy*, *Playgirl*, pornography, va-va-voom, wandering eye

sex therapy

Some people seek therapy for serious problems such as sexual trauma and compulsions. Others consult a therapist just to find out how to have better sex. About half of all married couples seek counseling: Typically, unsatisfying sex is the reason. The top three sexual complaints that bring people into the therapist's office are erectile dysfunction, premature ejaculation, and low sex drive. And sex therapists say lack of communication is often to blame.

S

Many sex therapists work closely with urologists, gynecologists, and family practitioners, so one way to find a good counselor is to ask for a referral from your doctor. The American Association for Sex Educators, Counselors, and Therapists has a Web site, www.aasect.org, that provides a list of sex therapists by city and state. Or you could also just open the phone book. Sex therapists are often listed under "Counselors"; most specify that they deal with sexual problems. If you're comfortable doing so, you can also ask people you know for recommendations. Make sure that any doctor you consider has the proper credentials: He or she should have a master's degree or a Ph.D. and should be a certified (or licensed, depending on the state) psychotherapist, psychologist, psychiatrist, family or marital counselor, or sex therapist.

The most important factor when choosing a sex therapist is whether that particular doctor is right for you—whether he or she is a person you can talk to openly about very private matters. You'll probably have to pay for a few sessions with a therapist before deciding if the two of you have a rapport.

Not all relationship problems are successfully resolved in therapy, but many sexual problems can be overcome if you commit yourself to participating in a serious course of treatment.

Also see: communication, compulsive behavior, fantasies, fears/phobias, guilt, incest, manual stimulation, marriage—lack of sex in, paraphilias, performance anxiety, perversions, phallic, premature ejaculation, puberty, quality versus quantity, rape, sensate focus, sex addiction, sex drive, sex education, sex offenders, spectatoring, surrogate, urologist, vaginal injuries, violence

sex tours and resorts

Several Internet Web sites and some travel agencies offer trips to places where prostitution is cheap, legal, and abundant. Thailand is the country most often frequented for easy sex, particularly the (disagreeably named) capital city of Bangkok. Rio de Janeiro in Brazil and Angeles City in the Philippines are also hot sex spots. Other locales include Costa Rica, Cuba, the Dominican Republic, Columbia, Cambodia, Russia, and the city of Prague in the Czech Republic.

Exotic, willing women in faraway lands where you'll be a rich, anonymous stranger . . . Sound like a dream come true? The reality is much less sexy. In many of these locations, young girls, most of them under the age of consent, are trapped in a slave-trade form of prostitution. Most of the men who take advantage of these trips do so out of a compulsion to exploit women, not a lack of sex back home.

If you're looking not to become a john but just to get some vacation jollies, there are plenty of singles resorts and cruises. Consider Club Med, Hedonism, or Breezes resorts as well as some Carnival cruises. Your travel agent can't guarantee that you'll get lucky on these trips—you can't reserve a woman as easily as a room with a view. But if nothing else, you can enjoy the sights, be they ladies or landscapes.

For those of you already hitched, resorts like Couples and Sandals offer Caribbean vacations heavy on romance. Or if you're in the mood for something a little racier, consider the Retreat for Couples (once called the Sexuality Playshop). It's a sexed-up version of the traditional marriage-encounter weekend offered by pastors, psychologists, and counselors nationwide. It preaches similar principles of love, integrity, and honesty; but it's much more sexually explicit. (Ever attend a dinner buffet where the entertainment was X-rated videos?)

Also see: brothels/bordellos, prostitution, singles scene, travel—planning

sexual aids

The most common products purchased to enhance the sexual experience are vibrators, dildos, penis pumps, cock rings, anal plugs, and lubricants (for specifics, see the entries devoted to these topics). Some people use these items—particularly vibrators and penis pumps—as true *aids*, to help them become or stay aroused. But these devices aren't only for sexual problems. They are also intended as toys, either for you alone or with a partner.

Let's dispel a myth right here: There's nothing wrong with using a vibrator during sex. We know that there's a kind of macho stigma about the idea of "not being able to get a woman off without help." But lots of women, given their druthers, go nuts over the kind of continual, buzzy stimulation that you can't possibly duplicate anyway (unless you happen to be battery-operated). So what's the problem? You're just giving her what she wants. Isn't that exactly what you want to do?

Dildos, meanwhile, can be used as part of your pump-priming routine, alongside other activities like oral sex and manual stimulation.

If you have trouble getting it up, try a penis pump (also, see our entries on *erection difficulties* and *impotence*). If you have trouble keeping it up, a cock ring might do the trick. Talk to your doctor before you experiment with these gizmos.

Under certain conditions, they can cause nerve damage and other medical problems.

Lubricants are essential during anal sex . They also make regular intercourse more comfortable for both men and women, or for women who experience now-and-then dryness even though they're turned on.

Also see: anal beads; aphrodisiac; aromatherapy; beds; ben wa balls; body oils; bondage and discipline; costumes; couch; drugs; food; French tickler; *Joy of Sex, The*; *Kama Sutra*; Kegel exercises; K-Y jelly; lingerie; mail-order sex products; medications; mirrors; music; nipple clamps; ointments; piercing; pornography; supplements; underwear; vacuum devices; vaginal injuries; Venus butterfly; vibrating sleeve; water beds; whipped cream

sexual attraction

Some stereotypes hold true: In general, guys go for looks, women go for money. That may seem shallow, but it's an evolutionary strategy that helps keep the gene pool deep. Men need females with youthful, fit bodies to bear them healthy children; women need males with the resources to support those progeny. This is true the world over, though the definitions of "good" looks and "enough" money change depending on what part of the world you're in.

Beauty and wealth are certainly not the only criteria for attraction, however (it's a good thing, too, because otherwise you'd be holding out for supermodels while Bill Gates was trying to keep his harem happy). Most people find themselves drawn to those with whom they have a lot in common. We tend to seek out partners whose jobs, incomes, educational backgrounds, religious beliefs, and other attitudes are similar to our own. This reduces the frequency of nasty disagreements that cut into the time we spend doing the nasty. It's also good for our egos: We like knowing that someone else thinks we're right.

Of course, there are those who believe that opposites attract. They just better hope they find partners who agree with them on that.

Also see: attraction, beauty, body shapes, eye contact, flirtation, horny, infatuation, legs, pheromones, preference, power, sexy, size—ass, size—breasts, size—nose

sexual etiquette

A good bedside manner calls for kindness and a sense of humor. Treat your woman with the same respect that you hope to receive from her.

Coital courtesy begins even before you get into bed. Hygiene is just as important, if not more crucial, at a slumber party as at a dinner party. If either of you is less than fresh, consider taking a shower together, and make the cleansing part of foreplay.

Remember during oral sex that there's not a woman out there who enjoys having her head forced down over your penis. And by all means, let her know when you're about to come. That's the one time when she doesn't like surprises.

In the heat of the moment, she may ask you to transform into anything from a stern master to a carnival geek to a filthy pig. Just remember that, when it's over, (a) she's not a slut for doing that and (b) you must transform back into

the gentleman we hope you were beforehand.

If you're at her place, use common sense to figure out whether she wants you to spend the night. It's a safe bet that a woman who's snoring softly and snuggling close to you doesn't want you to get up abruptly and start pulling on your chinos. Then again, if she's wide awake, staring at the clock, or pacing around the room, you should probably find those pants, give her a kiss, and go home.

Suppose she wants you to stay but you're not interested? Never just eat and run unless it's a lunch-hour quickie. Hold her for a half-hour, then explain that you have to work early in the morning, you still have a project to finish that night, whatever. (Have the excuse ready beforehand so it doesn't sound like what it is: a last-minute alibi.) Thank her. Go.

Lastly, don't tell her you'll call her later unless you really plan to. She might've just figured it the same way you did: as a moment in time. But if *you* start raising her expectations about what the evening signified, well, you can't blame her later for being angry, disappointed, and confused when you let her down.

Also see: clumsiness, farting, first date, first time with a lover, flirtation, hygiene, laughter, morning after, one-night stand

sexual innuendo

In the right hands, this is a marvelous tool for letting a woman know you're interested—and gauging her interest as well. A sly, witty double entendre not only lets a woman know that you appreciate her femininity and sexuality but also gives her the opportunity to respond in kind.

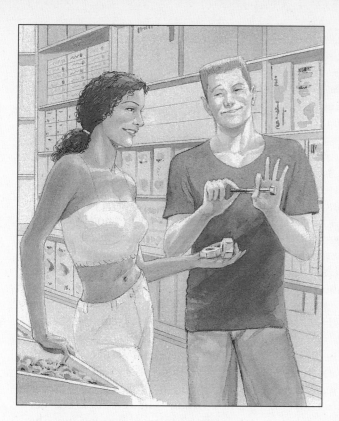

At its best, innuendo walks a fine line between suggestiveness and subtlety. It should be provocative enough that she knows you're hitting on her, yet innocuous enough that she can pretend she doesn't know, in case she's not interested. Sample situation: You're at a crowded party one night, talking to a woman you already know casually. You seem to be getting along quite well. She brushes her hair away from her neck, then says, "It's really hot in here."

To which you reply, "Yeah, you look really hot." And you smile at her and hold eye contact.

Now, tone matters here. If you sound like a dreadful parody of a porn star, just about any woman will run for cover. When the technique is handled clumsily—as is too often the case—you make yourself seem corny, cheesy, or downright crude. You look like a buffoon to *all* women, even those who may have been interested at first.

But assuming you sounded halfway normal (and you didn't overdo the emphasis on the word *hot* or follow up with the decidedly unsubtle "Why don't you take off your shirt to cool off?"), you can tell a lot by the woman's reaction. If she smiles coyly, bats her lashes, or—ideally—says something equally jocular in return ("You look pretty hot yourself"), she's letting you know that the two of you are in sync and that she's not completely averse to introducing sex into the equation. Conversely, if she acts like you're really talking about the room temperature ("Someone should open a window"), that's your cue that she's not into you. Be thankful that she's giving you the chance to make a graceful exit, instead of coldly shooting you down.

An important note: Be very careful about innuendo in the workplace. While some female co-workers may play along with a little good-natured, suggestive repartee, others may be annoyed, uncomfortable, or even intimidated. See "Special Report—Jobs and Sex" on page 156 for important pointers.

Also see: dial-a-porn, flirtation, foreplay, opening line, pickup lines, rejection—romantic, talking dirty, winking

sexual revolution

Bra burnings. Group streaks. Woodstock. *Deep Throat. Roe v. Wade.* Those of us old

S

enough to remember these historical milestones should be glad we didn't drop so much acid that we *can't* remember them. As for those of us who are too young to remember, well, we're the ones reaping the benefits of those tumultuous times.

The sexual revolution of the 1960s and '70s can be summed up in two words: *freedom* and *permission*. In 20-years' time, we tore down the prison walls that had jailed our sexual expression since the Victorian age. Sex went from shush to chic, seemingly overnight.

Historians have all sorts of theories as to what sparked this coital crusade, including the bicycle craze and Beatlemania. Most history buffs agree, however, that the first flame of the 20-year fire was the Pill. It was, essentially, sexual freedom in a dial pack. The first oral contraceptive—called Enovid—hit the market in 1960; and with it, women began uncrossing their legs and unzipping their skirts. Once the worry about

becoming pregnant was eased, women were free to have sex simply for the pleasure of it. Casual sex, premarital sex, extramarital sex. Even married women began having sex more often. One study from the mid-'60s showed that married women who were on the Pill had sex 39 percent more often than married women who used other forms of contraception. More sex *and* more spontaneity—now that's what we call sexual freedom.

The permission slip came in 1966, when two sex researchers from St. Louis named William H. Masters, M.D., and Virginia E. Johnson, Ph.D., published their findings in the book *Human Sexual Response*. It was an instant bestseller and topped the charts for 6 months. The researchers had observed more than 690 men and women having sex and masturbating to the point of orgasm. (We've already volunteered to participate in any follow-up studies.) In their book, Masters and Johnson explained the physiology of

Hot Dates 1977 The San Francisco sex-product retailer Good Vibrations was established.

continued from page 305

Answer:

False. *Hustler* published the pix of Onassis on a Greek island, taken by a photographer with a long lens, after *Penthouse* and *Playboy* nixed them.

plained that the officers "thought they needed to do what they did to make the case."

Seemed like a Good Idea at the Time. . .

If you think the concepts of free love and open marriage originated in the 1960s, you're off by at least a century. In 1848, Yale Divinity School student John Humphrey Noyes founded the Oneida community in upstate New York. The group sub-

scribed to something called complex marriage, in which **every man was married to every woman**. Complex marriage supposedly would promote social equality by overcoming selfishness and breaking down barriers between the genders at work. As Noyes himself wrote, it would "at once raise the race to new vigor and beauty, moral and physical."

Noyes also was a proponent of male continence, a practice

BAWDY BALLADS "Come Back Pussy," *Dickie Williams*

continued on page 319

sexual arousal, making an orgasm sound as natural as a heartbeat. In doing so, they dispelled the Freudian myth that mature women should skip stroking their clitorises and strive only for vaginal orgasms through intercourse. They also revealed that women were capable of having multiple orgasms. Women began to feel cheated of the pleasure they had been missing out on—and they tried to more than make up for it, setting out on what one *Esquire* magazine article termed "the Quest for the Holy Wail." Of course, we men were more than happy to help them in their crusade.

More empowerment of America's sexual coming of age arrived with Englishman Alex Comfort's book *The Joy of Sex*. Published in 1972, this erotically illustrated guide served up a menu of sex positions and games way beyond the missionary position. It permitted couples to engage in sex play, to romp in their bedrooms. (Bring on the bondage and blow jobs, baby.) Some 12 million copies of the book were sold.

Of course, the sexual revolution wasn't all fun and games. The dynamic decade has been blamed for everything from the high divorce rate to the increased incidence of sexually transmitted diseases. But we think the far-reaching positive effects of the sexual revolution far outweigh the bad points. And while the Pill and Masters and Johnson's research gave women much to thank the revolution for, we have plenty of thanking to do ourselves. It liberated men and women alike from the great sexual repression, opening doors we never knew were closed. Suddenly, sex became more mutually satisfying. We're now free to play in bed, to play out of bed, to try new things, to please her, to have her please us. And we're loving every minute of it.

Also see: clitoral orgasm; free love; flapper; *Hite Report, The*; *Joy of Sex, The*; marriage proposal; Masters and Johnson; multiple orgasms; oral contraceptive; oral sex; Pill—the

sexual thoughts

Statistically, we're told, sex thrusts itself into young men's minds about every 5 minutes. The frequency tends to decrease with age, but most 40- to 49-year-old men still think about sex at least once every half-hour.

Regardless of age—and this may surprise you—men with high sex drives and active sex lives think about sex *more* often than guys who aren't getting any. And guys who spend a lot of time in long-winded meetings or toiling on assembly lines probably spend more time thinking hot thoughts than do, say, air-traffic controllers or alligator wrestlers. That's because, as we're sure you've noticed (though hopefully not since you opened this book), you're more likely to have sexy thoughts when you're bored. Indeed, you might call it being bored stiff.

Being publishers of informative and educational books such as this one, we're forced to think about sex all day long. And we like it that way. Sadly, not everyone has that benefit built into their workday. So you'll have to find another excuse for having pleasant daydreams. Jack it up a notch, the both of you. Give your partner this book to read. Find ways to have more sex. Then, you'll each think about sex a lot more often. We'll coin a phrase: A sex thought a day keeps the blues at bay. Works for us.

Also see: dreams, fantasies

sexy

What makes a man sexy? Lucky for you, women aren't always looking for the hard, chiseled, six-pack-stomached specimens who appear on magazine covers.

Surveys show that the one trait women overwhelmingly check out first is your eyes. They peer through your portals in hopes of discerning your levels of warmth, confidence, and trustworthiness. From there, the biology of love quickly fires or falters. Literally hundreds of factors are rated, dissected, programmed, and interpreted during this initial contact.

Granted, if God didn't supply you with a set of Mel Gibson's baby blues, well, them's the breaks. But you can work at things like not seeming shifty-eyed, and you can certainly work on your eye contact—or your tendency to let your eyes glaze over when you're talking to a new woman.

To further enhance sex appeal, try smoothing out some of the rough edges. Not only is cleanliness next to godliness, but it stands a much better chance of getting you next to her. Well-groomed hands, well-kept hair, a pleasant body odor, and a gleaming smile (sans spinach between teeth) also should tilt the scale in your favor.

The voluptuous rapper Lil' Kim once said, "Sexy is anything that shows who you are." This, of course, assumes that who you are doesn't suck. That aside, women find it sexy when a man shows confidence in what he's about. Just remember that confidence isn't the same as machismo. If you're not sure where to draw that line, start by talking less and listening more. It will keep your ego in check while also exhibiting your sensitive side. Ask questions—and take genuine interest in her replies. If a woman takes a while to get to the point, don't make a habit of interrupting or otherwise coercing her to cut to the chase.

Last, in the immortal words of Mother Teresa, "Let us always meet each other with a smile, for the smile is the beginning of love." Don't let her vow of celibacy detract from this bedrock truth: A wide, genuine smile may be just what's needed to put you in a position to show off those rippling abs.

Also see: dressing you to look sexy, eye contact, hygiene, male body, power, self-esteem, sexual attraction, size—wallet, smiling, stud muffin

shaving

Some men—and yes, some women—find the clean-shaven look intensely erotic. Completely shaving pubic hair—or sculpting it into shapes such as hearts, triangles, or narrow strips—can prove arousing by affording a clearer view of the sex organs.

Visuals aside, shaving can elevate the sensation of touch to fantastic levels. Genital grooming also has an olfactory impact: Clean skin does not hold smells as a mat of wet hair does. And, of course, there are no pesky short hairs to tickle the back of your throat during oral sex (or get lodged embarrassingly in front teeth when you're rushing out to that job interview).

Maintaining baby-smooth genitals can prove taxing, however, especially for someone with sensitive skin. Here are a few tips to reduce irritations such as ingrown hairs, rashes, and chafing.

1. Wash the pubic area with soap and water, and rinse thoroughly before and after shaving.

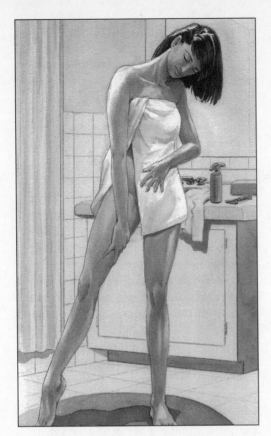

2. Use a fresh safety razor. A sharp blade will reduce nicks and cuts as well as the need to take multiple swipes. Also make sure to pull the skin taut before you pass the blade over it.

3. Apply powder, a cold washcloth, or an astringent (which may sting a bit) such as witch hazel to close the pores after shaving.

4. Apply an antibacterial cream or blemish cream to red spots to stave off rashes and ingrown hairs. Be careful not to apply creams on or in the vagina.

5. Last but certainly not least, the newly shorn should wear underwear without elastic bands, since elastic can rub directly against the shaved area.

Also see: beard burn, boredom, hair, kinky, pubic hair, variety

short-arm inspection

Military slang for the once-mandatory inspection of a private's, well, privates. The exam became protocol after World War II and was commonly conducted when soldiers returned from leave to see whether they'd picked up anything besides a souvenir. A soldier who extracted pus while milking his penis was given a shot of antibiotics. The corpsman's cursory glance would also check for lesions, spots, chancres, and crabs.

Modern inspections are voluntary and more thorough. If a soldier or sailor believes that he's infected, a doctor performs a visual inspection but also takes a culture from the urethra and draws blood to test for syphilis or HIV. As an extra precaution, the patient gets a hepatitis B vaccination series.

The comprehensive treatment is indicative of the military's dedication to keeping their arms shipshape—even the short ones.

Also see: STDs, venereal disease

shyness

All of us experience bouts of bashfulness or so-called situational shyness. During a job interview or while bedding a new lover, we blush and perspire more than we care to; yet somehow we stutter and stumble our way through. Unless we're pathologically shy—in which case a routine attempt to quell nervous butterflies is like trying to slay a squadron of demonic beasts. In the dark. Underwater. With a toothpick for a sword.

But enough with the cheesy metaphors.

Contrary to what you may think, shyness isn't always expressed visibly. Some of us do show the characteristic signs of introversion, avoiding eye contact and talking in near whispers. Others over-compensate with extroversion, assuming the role of party guy while protecting their true identities.

There's no simple strategy we can give you to get over your own shyness. Volumes have been written on the subject, and some therapists and motivational speakers make a comfortable living off others' chronic social discomfort.

What we want to call your attention to is how the subject of shyness figures in determinations you make about the opposite sex. Don't automatically assume that a woman who walks around with her nose in the air is uppity, and don't assume that the chick who won't give you the time of day thinks you're a toad. Both could be covers for a bad case of shyness that makes it all but impossible for them to relate smoothly to the opposite sex.

(One caveat: If this little intrigue is playing itself out at work, be wary. You don't want to push the issue with someone who's not receptive, lest you open yourself to claims of sexual harassment. See "Special Report—Jobs and Sex" on page 156.)

The crux here can be summed up by the adage "You can't tell a book by its cover." There could be a wonderful, caring woman concealed beneath a very off-putting exterior. And in fact, many women (and men) who "present" as being shy undergo a rather astonishing metamorphosis when they finally find someone who makes them feel comfortable.

So don't rush to judgment when somebody appears aloof and uninterested. It may be her way of saying "I'm afraid you'll hurt me" or "I don't know how to flirt" or simply "I was brought up in a house where nobody talked to each other." Maybe you'll unearth the gem that no other guy had the wits to dig for.

Also see: anticipatory anxiety, clumsiness, desperate, eye contact, first date, first time with a lover, flirtation, frigidity, masher, opening line, pickup lines, pity sex, puberty, self-esteem, signals

sickness

When you're not well, you don't feel like doing it. It's not just a question of being in a lousy mood, either. As your body's immune system mobilizes to fight illness, nonessential functions such as sex drive—which we consider pretty essential, actually—shut down so as not to distract from the task of getting you well again.

So don't make matters worse by stressing out if you can't get it up when you're sick. It's just your body saying, "Not tonight, honey." (And if your under-the-weather partner says *explicitly* that, don't make a big deal about it. If she doesn't feel up to it, she doesn't feel up to it. There's always tomorrow.)

An illness that includes a high fever takes its toll on your sperm count. In fact, a fever above 102°F not only kills sperm that you intended to use in tonight's festivities but also leaves the little guys playing catch-up for as long as 3 months. So if you've been battling some lingering ailment like the flu or chronic bronchitis at the same time you and the missus are trying to make a little tax deduction, don't worry—you're probably not sterile. Just get better and try again.

Realize, too, that sex is comparable to exercise in that it can temporarily drain the immune system. But don't get us wrong here: Overall, sex provides a host of physical and psychological benefits that cannot be discounted.

Also see: body fitness, breast cancer, compulsive behavior, cystitis, depression, ectopic pregnancy, epididymitis, fatigue, heart conditions, infertility, injuries, medications, NSU, pelvic inflammatory disease, penile cancer, prostate cancer, prostate enlargement, prostatitis, rashes, retrograde ejaculation, STDs, testicular cancer, thrush, toxic shock syndrome, urethritis, urologist, vaginal diseases/infections, venereal disease

signals

We men know what to do with a big, wet kiss. We also know what a slap in the face means. But alas, many of today's signals fall into a fuzzy gray abyss that tests our decoding skills.

Experts agree that most of the thousands of signals that women send us fall into two categories: those of interest and those of limitation. Here are a few positive signals.

Short, darting glances. A woman directs a quick gaze, singling out one man, then looks away. Luckily, she often repeats the move, figuring us for the inattentive dummies we are.

The hair flip. She raises her hand and run her fingers through her hair, smooths it with her palm, or twirls a lock around her finger. She may embellish the move by tossing her head or even by leaning toward the guy she's interested in.

The parade. You know this one: It's when she strolls by with an exaggerated erect posture—chest out, hips in full sway—that's often enough to put you in an erect posture yourself.

A woman also sends "I've had enough of you" cues long before she actually says the words. Sneers, frowns, and impatient sighs you already know about. Other signs of waning interest: crossing her arms, picking her teeth, and checking her nails—and if she actually starts clipping them, you're in really bad shape.

Also see: communication—nonverbal, courtship, flirtation, rituals

silk

Is there a sexier material in all the world? The feel of silk sheets, or silk panties—better still if they're slick with her wetness. The sight of your lover's shape shrouded by a silken veil. The subtle rustling sound the fabric makes when touched. Add all of this together and you have the recipe for a new peak of sensual arousal.

Before you go out and blow a few hundred bucks at Victoria's Secret, however, bear this in mind: Though many women love to be surprised with sexy silk underthings, some women interpret such a gesture as a gift you're really giving to yourself, and thus not really a gift at all; you don't want to make your woman feel like some kind of prop in your own sexual fetishes and fantasies. Still other women may take it as criticism of their customary choices of bedroom attire or perhaps even their inherent sex appeal. ("So, you're saying I need to wear lacy nothings to really turn you on these days?") Forgo that shopping spree until you're sure of your partner's feelings on the subject. One helpful question to ask yourself: Does she have any silk now? Have you ever seen her in silk lingerie? Does she ever drop hints that suggest she's looking for you to buy her those kinds of gifts?

The answers can make the difference between a night given over to enhanced

S

pleasure and a night spent arguing about how "selfish" or "manipulative" you are.

Oh, one other thing: If you're going to surprise her with a lingerie gift, make sure that you know her size. There's almost nothing worse for a woman's self-image than trying on stuff that's supposed to make her look sexy but that makes her look ridiculous instead.

Also see: lace, latex, leather, lingerie

singles scene

Gentlemen, it's time to log off your computers, switch off *SportsCenter*, clean behind your ears, and go meet some women.

Whaddya mean, you don't feel like it?

Wouldn't you rather have someone to share that pizza with? A hard-bodied girlfriend who could give you a run for your money mountain biking on the trails? Someone other than your stuffed Touchdown Monkey to sleep with? Well, guess what: The pizza guy ain't gonna deliver you a woman. You have to step out into the world, friend.

• Start where you feel most comfortable. Like the sports bar. Watch the game with some people. If you spot a girl who interests you, fine. If not, hey, at least you didn't miss the game. And you've taken the first step. Just realize that in such establishments, there are often more guys than girls.

• The places that offer a better male/female ratio are those with dance floors. We know; you don't dance. Well, they do. So if you can handle yourself on the dance floor, chances are, you'll spend less time handling yourself at home.

• List the activities you enjoy, and join a group that's doing them. Your dedication to the sport that ended your last relationship may be the bonding force for a new one. Load up your gear and go where fellow cyclists, rock climbers, or kayakers gather. Aside from putting you face-to-face with women, this will expand your circle of friends (which at least indirectly increases your chances of meeting a new girlfriend). Some singles organizations plan active, outdoor outings. More low-key mixers can be found at art museums, bookstores, nutrition centers, and local theaters. Check your newspaper, alternative newspaper, and local Internet sites.

• Volunteer for community projects. (Pick an activity where you can sincerely show some interest, though. Don't be the clod simply looking to get laid.) You'll meet people who are positive and caring, while doing something worthwhile.

• For the truly adventurous: Consider selling out. Join a book club or take classes in realms such as cooking or sewing. Yeah, it may be kind of uncomfortable at first, and you'll hear about it from your buddies. But the end result will put you (and probably you alone) in a room full of eligible women each week. Can you say, "Coffee or drinks after class?"

• Last, don't overlook the strong bonds of religion. In small towns, churches may be the only venues for singles events. Most people like to date and marry those with similar religious backgrounds—56 percent for dating, 72 percent for marrying. Here again, though, don't show up for the services simply looking to score. God tends to frown on that.

Also see: bars, blind date, dating, Internet dating, matchmaking services, meeting women, personal ads, rave, sex tours and resorts

single—suddenly

Regaining single status through divorce or the death of a spouse is one of the most traumatic passages of a man's life. No matter what the circumstances are, the reality is that a part of you has been taken. Physically, emotionally, sexually—sometimes financially—you feel drained.

How to recover from such a loss? The first step is to allow yourself to grieve—not easy for most of us, so drilled as we are since boyhood in a sense of "manly" stoicism. The healthy approach is to deal with your emotions first, then move on. This is important because some of us try to outrun our feelings by jumping into new relationships. If you go the route of a so-called rebound relationship, understand that your sense of loss is still there and will have to be dealt with at a later time. And in the meantime, it's bound to complicate the new relationship with another layer of feelings.

Being single again can be an opportunity to reassess your life, to recast yourself into the person you once wanted to be. Channel your energies into improving your fitness, your mind, your appearance, your self-esteem. Avoid the usual security blankets: booze, drugs, binge eating, mindless or risky sex, and the temptation of a rebound relationship. You may just create other problems that you'll need to deal with long after the immediate crisis has passed.

As for recovery timetables: There aren't any. Some men take months to heal, others take years. If you become truly reacquainted with yourself, you'll know when it's time to start dating. One good indication: If you notice that even your closest, most empathetic friends are suggesting that you step back out into the singles scene, you've probably been living a hermit's life too long

Also see: breaking up, death of a partner, depression, heartache, past partners—longing for, remarriage

S

Hot Dates **1979** A Virginia minister named Jerry Falwell launched a group called the Moral Majority. The backlash to the sexual revolution had begun.

continued from page 312

whereby a man did not ejaculate during sex. Not only did this legitimize complex marriage by eliminating those pesky unwanted pregnancies, but, in Noyes's words, it elevated intercourse to "a place among the 'fine arts.'" Unlike men, women were expected to experience orgasms during sex.

Critics dismissed Noyes as a religious charlatan and a sexual con man. Still, at its zenith, Oneida numbered 300 adherents.

Foreign Affairs

You think Nevada bordellos epitomize debauchery? **Roman brothels featured geese for sodomizing**, homosexual and heterosexual hookers—even sex with infants.

In Extremis

A medical journal reported on the case of a man with genital pain who admitted that about 12 years earlier, during foreplay, his wife had stuck a mascara brush into his urethral opening, where

True or Phallus?

Dream-team lawyer F. Lee Bailey was publisher of a skin magazine.

BAWDY BALLADS *"Grandpa Can't Fly His Kite," Clarence Carter*

continued on page 326

sixty-nine (69)

This doubly satisfying oral sex position, wherein you please your lover while simultaneously being pleased, can be a quasispiritual experience eliciting unparalleled feelings of intimacy. The downside is that it can also be overwhelming. Some of us get so hot and bothered while approaching orgasm that we forget to help our lovers—whose genitals are in or near our mouths—achieve the same. Another small hurdle is that it can be an awkward position to climb into. It may be a topic worth discussing with your lover before she wonders why you're facing her feet and trying to pull her atop you.

That particular orientation—you on bottom, her on top—is in fact the most common position for 69. Variations include man on top or each lover on his or her side. (If you're truly advanced or a gymnast or an acrobat, you may wish to attempt the standing 69 position.) Side to side works particularly well if one partner is much heavier than the other, as it lessens the "I can't breathe, dammit" feeling that tends to take the magic out of sex. It's also ideal for people who have pain in their necks, hips, backs, or shoulders, allowing maximum body contact with minimum physical stress.

Side to side also proves beneficial for beginners who want to experiment without blurting out "Hey, let's try 69!" While she lies on her side, maneuver yourself around and slowly kiss your way down her body until your tongue tickles her clitoris. At the same time, configure your body in somewhat of a fetal 69 posi-

tion. What you're trying to do here is give her some "wiggle room"—that is, put your erect penis near enough to her face so that she gets the message, without actually jamming it in her mouth in a rude or graceless manner.

If she's up for it, she'll get the hint and return the favor. If she's not, *don't* stop what you're doing. Remember, she's under no obligation to do this for you.

Also see: back, eat, oral sex

size—ass

From the buxom Venus to the featureless figures shilling for Calvin Klein, the size of the so-called perfect female ass has fluctuated more than Oprah Winfrey's dress size. Research tells us that over the years, though we seem to like our women smaller overall (at least in the United States), the preferred waist-to-hip ratio has remained relatively static. In fact, the fleshy pinups of 30 years ago

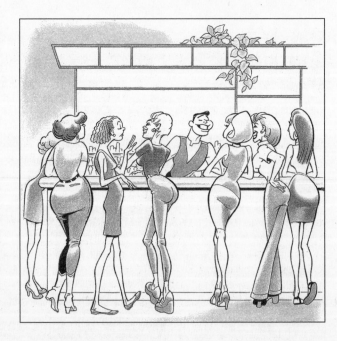

had the exact same ratio as today's slimmer *Playboy* centerfolds. In other words, no matter what size of booty we like, we seem to agree on one thing: The waist above it should be a lot smaller.

Apparently, body shape flips a Stone Age light switch in our quest to attract mates who will bear us healthy offspring. A low waist-to-hip ratio signals relatively high reproductive ability. Naturally, women in their prime reproductive years are the most desirable. A high waist-to-hip ratio can be a sign of pregnancy, old age, or illness.

But who needs research to tell us this? Maybe we just find a shapely figure dead sexy. Who would you rather watch during the Olympics: the entire lot of prepubescent gymnasts or the shapely skater Katarina Witt? Especially when her costume rides up to reveal her exquisite ass. Our baby's got some back. And we men, regardless of race, age, or occupation, like it that way.

Also see: anal sex, beauty, body shapes, booty, preference, rear entry, sexy, sexual attraction, spanking, thongs

size—breasts

There are two well-known schools of thought here. School 1: More than a mouthful is a waste. School 2: Bigger is always better. Whichever camp you fall into, keep this in mind: Breast size has nothing to do with breast sensitivity or a woman's sexual desire. Grapes, if you will, can be equally as sensitive as grapefruits. (Helpful hint: Never use such lines around women. They tend to hate fruit metaphors as applied to female body parts.)

Breast size changes when a woman becomes aroused. Nipples perk up, and the breasts and their darkened areolas swell. Sometimes, the areolas outpace the nipples and swallow them, giving an illusion of lost sexual interest until the nipples catch up. One nipple may also grow while the other doesn't. This is especially true of women who have breasts of unequal size to begin with, or women who have "innie" nipples.

Women who have breastfed may experience little breast growth during arousal, possibly because milk production increases the venous drainage of the breasts. Older women whose breasts sag due to degeneration of elastic tissue don't experience much growth, either.

It may surprise you to hear that implant surgery—properly done—can increase size without ruining sensitivity. Typically, though, the more breasts are fiddled with (surgically speaking, that is), the less feeling they have. Breast reduction surgery affects sensitivity more than enlargement because it's more invasive: The surgeon usually removes the nipple, extracts some fatty tissue and skin, then stitches the nipple back on. Aren't you glad you're not a woman?

Also see: arousal, beauty, body image, body shapes, bras, breast enlargement, breastfeeding, breast reduction, breasts, breast sensitivity, implants, media, nipples, preference, third-degree cleavage

size—eyes

Whether the size of a person's eyes can give you insight into their personality depends on how much faith you put in personology. Personologists observe the size, shape, and placement of eyes to deduce an assessment of character, thus lending their own version of credence to the expression "The eyes are the windows to the soul." In their eyes, anyway.

Many people have one eye larger than the other. Personologists tell us that the ideal distance between the eyes should measure the same as the size of one eye from corner to corner. If the space between the eyes is smaller than the largest eye itself, according to personology, the individual in question may be intolerant and picky. If it's larger, then the person could be hypertolerant, avoiding issues rather than addressing them.

You don't have to buy into personology to know that feelings are also communicated through the size and shape of the eyes. What guy hasn't felt—and instantly recognized—a woman's angry glare? Her eyes narrow and the muscles around them tense up, giving the appearance that her eyes are smaller than they really are.

When a woman gazes at her lover or something else she finds pleasurable, the opposite happens: The muscles around her eyes seem to relax, causing her eyes to open up and appear larger. Some experts believe that this so-called lover's gaze is a physiological fact (and it's different from the state of relaxation prior to sleep, when eyelids may actually close slightly). Her pupils also enlarge, or dilate, while she doesn't break eye contact with her partner once a sentence is finished (as is the norm in casual conversation). So keep your own eyes open to whether she's eyeing you up—it may be one more way for you to tell if she's in an amorous mood.

Also see: eye contact, hypnosis and seduction, makeup, oculophilia, ogling, smiling, winking

size—nose

Beauty can be as plain as the nose on her face—that is, if the nose is small, straight, and diamond-shaped instead of long,

hooked, and bulbous. So says a New Mexico State University computer program called FacePrints, which tells us that the culturally ideal female visage in America has a high forehead, full lips, a short jaw, a small chin, and the above-described nose. Researchers have found that symmetry also rules: The more centered the nose (and other facial features), the more attractive the image to the average onlooker.

The size and position of one's proboscis have something to say about health as well. Most obviously, a bent or broken nose may tell of past injury or surgery. And red and runny nostrils are a sure tip-off of someone's cold or allergies (or bad habits involving a drug that rhymes with *broke*). But did you know that a swollen and bluish beak is associated with cirrhosis? That a "saggy nose" or depressed bridge could spell syphilis? Indeed, an asymmetrical nose may serve as an indicator of poor health at the chromosomal level—signifying disturbances during embryonic development due to inadequate nutrition, genetic anomalies, or other adverse conditions.

Also see: beauty, male body, papilloma, preference, sexual attraction, sexy

size—penis

Those of us who have never used the word *hoist* to describe taking our penises from our pants—and that's most of us—find it hard to avoid feelings of inadequacy while watching porno flicks. There's a member bigger than life itself—long enough to make even a female horse bray in astonishment. The truth of the matter, though, is that Hollywood's magic played a part in creating that monster. The magnifying effect of the lens (the same lens that, they say, adds 10 pounds to one's physique) can give the illusion of added inches. Want proof? When the actor pulls out and puts his penis in his hand, take note of the penis-to-hand ratio. It doesn't look so monstrous after all. In fact, you'll be inclined to say, "Why, it looks nearly the same size as mine does when I . . . imagine what it would look like if I ever put it in my hand."

The size of a flaccid phallus can be affected by a number of factors, including time of day, temperature, and how you feel, so the measurement of an erect penis is the only one that really counts. One study involving hundreds of men determined that the average length of an erect penis—across the ages, across the races—was 5½ inches.

Certain health factors can play havoc with the heft of your hard-on. Smoking, for example, not only restricts the blood supply to the penis but can also have a damaging effect on elastin, the ingredient responsible for your skin's suppleness and flexibility. If your skin can't stretch to its full potential, neither can your erection. Body weight also affects size. If you're gaining, the fat deposits near your pubic bone increase the cushion around the base of your penis and give the illusion that your member is shrinking. The good news is that losing pounds, and thereby shedding that layer of fat, can make your penis seem that much larger.

Also see: hung, hypnosis and penis enlargement, micropenis, packing, penile enlargement, weight loss, vaginal injuries

size—vagina

We rightfully sing the vagina's praises for many reasons, yet we seldom stop to give it credit for what may be its most remarkable feature: It's one of the truly great expanding organs of all time. Far more so than a penis. How would you like to have to give birth through your pecker? And to think we complain about kidney stones. . . .

The unstimulated vagina clocks in at a modest 3 to 4 inches long. During sexual arousal and intercourse, it expands its accordion-like folds to accommodate the very largest penis. (Yes, even yours.) Before diving into a deeper-is-better mentality, remember, it's the first one-third of the vagina that's densely packed with pleasure-sensing nerve endings—and that's something even a 3-inch erection can satisfy.

But back to childbirth. That's when the vagina-cum–birth canal manages to serve as conduit for a human being whose head can be anywhere from the size of a fist to the size of a large grapefruit. Possibly upstaging even that feat is the vagina's amazing—and, to us, blessed—ability to recover. Thanks to that astonishing elasticity, it returns to almost normal size within 6 to 12 weeks of delivering a child, promising many more years of happy use. Of course, this depends on certain factors, including the size of the baby, the amount of time spent pushing, and whether there were complications.

Though childbirth causes permanent changes to most women's vaginas (yes, they're slightly looser), the changes don't usually interfere with sexual satisfaction—for you or her. If the vagina doesn't tighten up on its own, a regimen of Kegel exercises can give Mother Nature a hand. The workouts will help restore the vagina to close to its original size and muscle tone. After regular ses-

S

sions, Kegel masters boast of having tightened their love muscles to the point where they have control over the way they grip a man's penis.

Also see: Kegel exercises, vagina

size—wallet

Is that a bulging wallet in your pants, or are you just glad to see me?

More to the point: Does your wallet have to be bulging in order for women to be glad to see *you*?

Well, it depends. While few women admit to lusting after men solely for their bankrolls, many do want partners who are financially stable and who exhibit a drive for success. A survey of more than 2,000 gals for the book *What Women Want* suggests that today's women basically can't fall in love with guys who are perpetually down on their luck. They don't want to spend the rest of their lives worrying about where the mortgage payments—or more likely, in this case, the rent money—are going to come from.

Does that mean that you have to put on a lavish display every time you go out on a date? No. As you learn elsewhere in this book, both sexes evaluate literally hundreds of biological and character cues during the dating/mating process. One of them—but just one of them—is your fiscal responsibility. Let us emphasize that there's a difference between *responsibility* and *wealth* per se. You don't have to be Donald Trump to find a nice woman.

But if you exhibit one or more of the following symptoms, don't be surprised when the woman in your life starts having visions of cars and furniture being repossessed: You're constantly broke, despite a decent salary. Or you bounce checks on a semiregular basis, possibly because you can't balance your checkbook. Or you end up having to pay cash for everything because your credit is so bad. Conversely, it's also a bad sign if you use actual credit cards (that is, not debit cards) for everyday staples like food and gas. Perhaps worst of all is needing to sell (or God forbid, hock) things you already own in order to generate cash to buy new things.

That said, you want to be aware of the type of woman you attract. Sadly, there are some women out there who won't mind coming along for the ride until the party bus runs out of gas. If you suspect that your girlfriend's attention may wane as your checking account drains, ask yourself the following questions to gauge her true interest in you.

• Is the spending one-sided? The score doesn't have to even out to the penny, but we hope she's splitting the bill or picking up the tab on occasion. If it's your nature to always pay the bill, with some luck, she's reciprocating by buying you thoughtful gifts, cooking you dinner, or planning surprise getaways—on her own dime.

• Is it okay with her if you just hang out together now and then? No cash shouldn't mean no date. If she always expects dinner and a movie and turns up her nose at simply watching TV or going for a walk, you may have a gold-plated gold digger on your hands.

If your worst suspicions are confirmed, have a serious talk. If that resolves nothing, file for a breakup before she has you filing for bankruptcy.

Also see: financial difficulties, job loss, money, power, sexual attraction

skin

You may have heard it said that the skin is the body's largest organ. That also makes it the body's largest sex organ. Kissing, tickling, and gently blowing the skin give rise to thousands of mini-erections known as goose bumps. Sultry, suggestive comments cause facial skin to radiate, hot and red. Continual stimulation, from sucking the fingertips to massaging the skin with glistening oils, transforms the entire organ into a massive erogenous zone. Finally, upon orgasm, it smolders with an aura of rouge, serving as an external signal of inner serenity. (You may be wondering: Is this true for guys too? Yes, though our rougher skin and general hairiness makes it harder to notice.)

For a rewarding intimate experience, try something called the full-body caress. A session of this can last from a few minutes to an hour. Take off your clothes, and have your lover lie facedown. Warm some oil in your hands and place them on her back. Holding them there for a short time establishes a connection and helps both of you relax. Lightly caress her entire back. (Don't knead or pummel her skin as you would during massage.) Then gently stroke her arms, legs, feet, neck, and head. If the moment seems right, softly touch her breasts and genitals. When you're finished, allow your hands to linger in one spot before gently removing them.

The goal of these sessions is not to have sex per se but to take the time to enjoy the sensations of each other's touch.

Also see: beard burn, erogenous zones, hickey, massage, nudism, prepuce, rashes, rug burn, scratching, shaving, smegma, stimulation, sweating, tickling, touch

slick

To us, this word conjures breathless-making images of sexual wetness and the slippery sliding of naked bodies. To women, it has a somewhat different connotation: the smooth operator. The slimeball. The fabled lounge lizard.

It's great to be comfortable conversing with women, to know the trendiest drinks, to display the confidence of a man who knows his way around the ladies. There's a fine line, though, between the guy we've just described and the slickster, who's willing to tell any lie, dish out any line, adopt any persona in order to get laid. Picture gaudy necklaces, greased-back hair, a thin mustache, and a shirt that's open at least one button too low, as well as cheesy compliments, sly winks, and Burt Reynolds–inspired eyebrow moves (which tend to work only if you're Burt Reynolds).

We've all seen guys like this—though not, we hope, in the mirror. Slickness may get you across the threshold, but unless there's some tangible honesty behind it, you may quickly get tossed right back out the door.

Slicksters do get occasional phone numbers and one-night stands. The women involved may be equally slick, or they may be lugging some serious emotional baggage and looking to define themselves through sex. . . . But hey, who are we to judge? If both parties are looking for short-term flings, these matches may be made in heaven.

Typically, the relationships and the lifestyle forged through slickness are every bit as superficial as the moves and the lines. Realize that women who knowingly go home with smooth oper-

S

ators are the type who go home with smooth operators—meaning that you're probably not their only sexual conquest this week or this month. Realize, too, that unless a slickster evolves through the phase, he becomes the bar scene's comic relief and the butt of jokes by female comedians everywhere.

You say you're a slickster and proud of it? We grant you, you perform a valuable public service for the rest of maledom: You serve as a model for how we shouldn't act.

Also see: bars, flirtation, one-night stand, opening line, pickup lines, self-esteem, sloppy sex, sweating, winking

S

sloppy seconds

Who better to define this term than the drummer of the punk rock band Sloppy Seconds? The band's unusual name came about when Steve Sloppy and his cohorts were noodling around while the movie *Porky's* played in the background. "The characters were talking about a gang bang," he recalls. "One guy called out, 'I'm going first'; another called out, 'I've got sloppy seconds'; and another said, 'I've got slippery thirds.'" Thus, a band was christened, and a sexual euphemism rose to new heights of popularity.

Though the origin of the phrase is unknown—*Porky's* notwithstanding—it is still used to describe the second-in-line position when several guys are having sex with one woman, or, in more vulgar terms, the first car behind the locomotive when pulling a train.

You might think of it as boldly going where one man just went before.

Also see: best friend's wife, gang bang, gang rape, group sex, lubrication, ménage à trois, multiple orgasms, nymphomania, pulling a train, threesome, vaginal moisture, wet spot

Hot Dates **1980** The Equal Employment Opportunity Commission issued guidelines on sexual harassment. Six years later, the U.S. Supreme Court ruled that sexual harassment was indeed illegal.

continued from page 319

Answer:

True. Bailey was listed as the publisher of *Gallery* magazine when it debuted in 1972. In a statement to readers, Bailey said he thought "good writing is very valuable." Uh-huh.

the tip of the brush broke off. Doctors discovered that **fibrous tissue had covered the brush piece**, trapping it. It had to be surgically removed.

LEGAL BRIEFS

A man told Virginia police that he crawled into bed with three sleeping women and had sex with one of them because he suspected she was a lesbian. A sheriff's investigator said, **"He thought it would bring her back right and make her act right."** The would-be lesbian reformer was charged with sexual assault.

Seemed like a Good Idea at the Time. . .

How many naked Pentecostals can you fit in one car? Twenty. That's how many eased out of an auto that hit a tree in Louisiana: 15 adults emerged from the passenger cabin and five kids popped out of the trunk. None of the passengers—all believed to be related—was seriously hurt.

BAWDY BALLADS **"Let Me Bang Your Box,"** *the Toppers*

continued on page 337

sloppy sex

A vigorous exchange of bodily fluids. Messy, sloshing, spewing sex. Most men have fantasized about starring in their own porno flick, complete with the money shot in which they come all over a woman's body.

Some sex experts believe that the pornographic industry has conditioned not a few of us to think that's what we should do. And sure, from the actor's perspective, it does look rather enjoyable and manly. But is that joy truly shared by the actress?

As with so many other sex acts that are a matter of personal preference, the best way to find out how your lover feels about having your semen spilled over her skin is to ask her beforehand. And that's *well* beforehand—not just as you're hitting the point of no return. If you do ask and she declines, don't take it personally.

Also see: come, ejaculation, female ejaculation, gusher, lubrication, premature ejaculation, semen, slick, water sports, wet spot

smegma

Also known by the unflattering nickname *head cheese*, it's a white paste composed of the dead skin and natural lubricants that form under the foreskins of uncircumcised males. (Circumcised males don't produce smegma.) To avoid buildup of the funky-smelling stuff, retract and wash the loose skin around your penis every day while you're in the shower. This should ensure that you won't have to endure cheesehead jokes unless you're a Green Bay Packers fan.

Also see: circumcision, foreskin, hygiene, penile cancer, phimosis, prepuce

smiling

A gleaming display of your pearly whites is one of the most effective lady-killers in your arsenal. In one survey, a whopping 97 percent of women responded that a man yearning to earn their attention should smile. Few strategies can be more engaging than a smile coupled with laughter—genuine laughter, let us emphasize, not that canned routine you dredge up when Aunt Hattie tells that same asinine joke each year at the family reunion. The approach is friendly, disarming, and contagious. It not only presents you as lighthearted and humorous but also acts as bait to attract women with similar qualities. When you pull the old grin and guffaw, she'll either reciprocate or rebuff it with a blank stare or a sneer.

In gauging her response, it pays to be able to tell whether she's really smiling or just being polite. A real smile illuminates her entire face. Her forehead crinkles, her cheeks dimple, her eyes soften, her body may actually turn toward you. For an example of an artificial smile, picture the IRS auditor as he says, "Thank you for coming in today, Mr. Jones." If that's the reaction your grin garners, just walk away before things turn ugly.

Also see: communication—nonverbal, flirtation, laughter, lips, makeup, masher, opening line, seduction, sexual innuendo, sexy, signals, tickling

smoking

Not a few doctors believe that the labels on cigarettes warn of the wrong side effects. If the surgeon general really wants to curtail smoking, instead of linking smoking to death, he should probably detail how it affects sex. One major study showed that

S

smokers have lower sex drives, less sex, and less satisfying sex. While nonsmokers in the study bragged that their sex lives ranked an 8.7 out of 10, their puffing counterparts mustered a mere 5.2. This disappointing figure may be related to the negative effects that smoking has on the cardiovascular system. Since blood supply problems are not restricted to one area of the body, smoking-related conditions such as coronary heart disease often show up in the genitals first. Nicotine has an instantaneous impact down there in that it constricts bloodflow to the penis and reduces the size of erections.

The good news is that both heart disease and impotence can be reversed if you catch them early on. The bad news is that if you ignore the problem, your penis may soon resemble the limp butt dangling from your lips. And that's something that Joe Camel and the Marlboro Man never bothered telling us about.

Even if cigarettes don't kill you or Mr. Happy, they might keep you from leaving a living legacy when you die of something else. Smoking increases your risk of infertility by lowering your sperm count. And besides being less plentiful, your sperm might also be less viable: Among the smokers in that big study, there was a notable decrease in the sperm's ability to push upstream and penetrate through an egg's wall. So even if you can't kick the habit for your own sake, maybe you can do it for the kids.

Also see: drugs, heart conditions, marijuana, penile cancer, size—penis, urinary problems

sodomy

The broad definition covers homosexual and heterosexual anal sex as well as oral sex, sex with animals, and, in at least one medical dictionary, "'unnatural' sexual intercourse." The negative connotation stems from the root word *Sodom,* which was one of the Bible's twin cities of sin (kin to Gomorrah) that God destroyed with a blizzard of brimstone and fire.

Up until the early 1960s, all 50 states had laws criminalizing sodomy between consenting adults. Today, fewer than half of the states do, and even in states in which such acts are illegal, enforcement of the laws is rare.

Also see: abnormal, anal sex, bestiality, bisexuality, cunnilingus, fellatio, homosexuality, klismaphilia, oral sex, paraphilias, perversions, religion, rimming, taboos, zoophilia

soul mates

Spiritual philosophers have long written that the only path to true love is the re-union of one soul shared by two bodies. Such a soul, they expound, is separated into two halves upon exiting the astral plane and moving to Earth. Each half wanders through life satisfied but a tad unfulfilled unless it can find its mate to make it whole again. Most people who aren't philosophers take the more worldly view that good relationships are made, not born of some higher dimension. We're not going to deny that some couples seem to be linked by mystical bonds. But even for those who have such a connection and are truly devoted and committed to each other, let alone for the rest of us, maintaining a relationship can be difficult.

Those spiritual theories about severed souls actually offer some practical advice on this subject. Such scriptures say that both halves of a divided soul develop into defined, well-rounded personalities.

Each is self-sufficient, confident, and capable of living alone. Their union, therefore, is a bond of two sturdy structures standing as one and reaching a new level of fulfillment, as opposed to two needy figures leaning upon each other, unable to stand on their own.

This is a good foundation for a relationship, regardless of whether you believe in the concept of soul mates. In fact, a guy who's well-adjusted, self-reliant, and sure of himself doesn't have to wait for one perfect mate; he'll be compatible with many potential partners. Maybe finding your soul mate depends not on fate but on controlling your own destiny.

Also see: companionship, love, monogamy, partner, passion, self-esteem, spiritual sex

Spanish fly

Nearly everyone has heard the urban legend of the shy lass who was transformed into a sexual dynamo after a beau dribbled some of this stuff into her drink. Many a horndog has embarked on a search for this magic potion after hearing how ravenous it made the girlfriend of his cousin's roommate's brother—how she rode the lucky guy until he shot blanks and how she then resorted to riding the gear shift until she was satisfied.

Good story. Too bad it's not true. For one thing, despite its name, there are no flies involved in Spanish fly. It's actually a powder made from southern European beetles. And though it has earned a reputation as a killer aphrodisiac, the truth is that it can literally kill you. After ingesting the bug, early users felt a burning in their loins, which they attributed to passion. The source of the fire was actually their irritated digestive and urinary

tracts working to discharge the poisonous active ingredient, cantharidin, from their bodies. Olé!

While Spanish fly may cause short-term arousal in the genitals, that feeling is soon replaced by severe abdominal pain, vomiting, bloody diarrhea, priapism, shock, and sometimes death. So, in the mood yet?

Also see: aphrodisiac, date rape, drugs, priapism

spanking

This is one of the most basic sado-masochistic (S/M) practices. Many people who would never dream of trying hard-core S/M will toy with spanking as well as blindfolding and light bondage (such as holding or lightly tying their lovers' wrists). For expert comment on the subject, we turned to the Mistress Moth, a professional dominatrix. "It requires no real training and no accessories, and it is generally safe," says Moth. "And the ass is usually quite accessible in moments of passion when an exploratory smack might be introduced." So you'll want to think about introducing those exploratory smacks now and then. But make sure, first, that your partner herself is "accessible." As is true of all S/M play, it's best to start small here. A light tap on the butt may well elicit a purring "ooohh" from her, encouraging you to do more. But it may also elicit a stern "Watch it, buster."

The attraction of a good spanking is in part the intimacy of direct hand-to-buttocks contact. The act also provides the exhilaration of mild pain without any real consequence of agony—like many S/M practices, spanking is not so much about pain as it is about heightened sexual arousal. The sting of a slap

S

makes skin more sensitive and stimulates the nerve endings in erogenous zones.

It can also serve as a transition to harsher realms of pleasure and pain. But that probably depends on just how naughty you've been.

Also see: bondage and discipline, booty, dominance and submission, paddle, rough sex, Sade—Marquis de, safeword

spectatoring

This is a term coined by sex researchers William H. Masters, M.D., and Virginia E. Johnson, Ph.D., to describe the act of mentally observing, critiquing, and worrying about your performance (or your partner's performance) while making love. While all of us have done this at one time or another, it's a problem if you spend more time judging your performance than enjoying it. A man who takes spectatoring to the extreme by worrying about getting an erection actually reduces his chances of having one. The same can be said of a woman who ruminates on achieving orgasm.

Therapists work to solve the problem by first looking at the larger issues of the relationship's overall health. Once those have been resolved, the couple learns a therapy technique called sensate focus, which was also developed by Masters and Johnson. Sensate focus teaches the couple to concentrate on the physical sensation of every touch leading up to and during sex: the heat of each kiss, the tingle of skin against skin, the weight of one body atop another. This allows the partners to focus on their physical pleasure, to the exclusion of mental distractions that would make them spectators to their own sex lives.

Also see: anticipatory anxiety, body image, clumsiness, erection difficulties, fears/phobias, frigidity, hang-ups, hypnosis and performance enhancement, Masters and Johnson, performance anxiety, self-esteem, sensate focus, sex therapy

sperm count

"Normal" is at least 40 million of the little whippersnappers in each shot. Of those, half must be motile (a fancy word for "moving") if you hope to produce an heir.

Here's an interesting theory: In his book *Sperm Wars: The Science of Sex*, British researcher Robin Baker says that the mere thought of your wife cheating on you can send your count soaring. He argues that when a woman has sex with more than one man, the rival sperm wage deadly battle within her. The victor's sperm can then go on to fertilize her egg. So even if you only suspect your wife of cheating, that's enough to send your sperm count through the roof—up to three times higher than its normal level. You boost the ranks of your troops to increase their chances of winning the war.

Globally, the ranks of spermatazoan soldiers may be dwindling. Several studies suggest that over the past few decades, sperm counts have fallen worldwide. This phenomenon is blamed largely on pollution. So far, though, it doesn't look like the human race is in any danger of extinction: There are now more than six billion people inhabiting this Earth, with another billion expected by the year 2013.

To help keep your own count in the normal range, start by reducing stress and getting regular exercise. Simply put, a healthy, relaxed body produces healthy sperm. However, frequent exercise to the point of overexertion can harm your sperm production and sex drive, so don't overdo it.

If your exercise routine involves sports, wear a protective cup. Injuries to the testicles can have a negative long-term effect on sperm production. A postgame dip in the sauna or hot tub will cause a temporary drop in sperm count. So will celebratory drinks and smokes at the local taproom.

Finally, make sure that you get treatment for any chronic health conditions, and have your doctor monitor the medications you take to control them. Diseases such as diabetes and drugs prescribed to treat high blood pressure, gout, peptic ulcers, and Crohn's disease can lower sperm count. In addition to having regular checkups, see a urologist specializing in male-factor infertility if you suspect that your numbers are low.

Also see: boxers or briefs, ejaculation, fertility, infertility, male pill, marijuana, ovulation, reproductive system—yours, semen, sickness, smoking, supplements, testicular trauma, time, urologist, water beds, zinc

sphincter

A sphincter is like an opinion: Everybody's got one. Or more, actually. While one particular sphincter—the sphincter ani, or anal sphincter—garners most of the spotlight, other bands of circular muscles quietly open and close many of your body's orifices without fanfare. Examples of other constricting muscles are in veins connected to your heart (the hepatic sphincter) and in your bile duct (sphincter choledochus), your eyes (sphincter pupillae), and your pancreas (sphincter of Oddi).

But you're not really interested in any of those, are you? After all, who fantasizes about doing secret, naughty things to a pancreas? No, you only want to know about the one buried between the butt cheeks. And we're obliging fellows, so we'll tell you.

The anal opening actually consists of two sphincter muscles stacked one on top of the other. The lower one is the muscle you relax when you head into the bathroom with the sports page. The upper one is an involuntary muscle that is normally closed to incoming traffic. Even if you and your partner aren't uptight about anal play, your upper sphincters will be.

So here are some hints on solving the sexual riddle of the sphincter. The keys are relaxation and lots of water-based lubrication, such as K-Y jelly. You may want to start by massaging the area before moving on to gentle—we repeat, *gentle*—penetration with a finger. When the sphincter and its owner have relaxed enough to accept two fingers, they're probably also ready for whatever else you and she have in your dirty minds.

Also see: anal sex, klismaphilia, rectum, rimming, sodomy, suppositories

spiritual sex

"As the deer pants for water, so I long for you—oh, God!" While the author of Psalm 42 may not have intended the sexual connotation, he nonetheless gave us a fitting simile describing spiritual sex.

Many people's religious training unfortunately focuses on the separation between the flesh and the spirit—the first being sinful, the other sacred. But the notion of spiritual sex takes the more encompassing view that when we embrace our sexuality, we honor our spirituality. And vice versa.

S

Spiritual sex necessitates that both lovers give themselves over fully to the sexual experience. The extraordinary energy and overwhelming sensation of peace and well-being that can occur at the moment of climax are actually very similar to the feelings reported by people who have had near-death experiences. It's not without reason that the French call orgasm *la petit mort,* or the little death, and that Renaissance poets frequently used death as a metaphor for sex.

The flip side of the connection between sex and death is the fact that sex is also the vehicle for the conception of life. If you believe in the existence of the human soul, what could be more spiritual than the act that is capable of giving body to a new one? In this respect, sex is a godlike power that makes you part of the creative force of the universe.

So go ahead and tell your woman that you're a sex god—and she is your goddess. That thought should lift your spirits, even if it's not quite spiritually uplifting.

Also see: afterglow, chakras, lovemaking, orgasm, passion, religion, rituals, soul mates, succubus, tantra, yogi

sponge

For more than 1,000 years, natural sea sponges were used as contraceptives. The theory was that when inserted in a woman's vagina, the sponge would prevent pregnancy simply by soaking up sperm before they could reach a waiting egg. As late as the 1930s, fine-grained rubber sponges soaked in olive oil were prescribed by clinics as a barrier method of birth control.

The modern version of the vaginal sponge was available over the counter in the United States from 1983 to 1995 and provided both barrier and chemical protection equivalent to that of other barrier methods, such as the diaphragm. The man-made sponge infused with spermicide was inserted in the vagina up to 24 hours prior to intercourse and disposed of some 6 hours after sex.

The sponge was taken off the market when the manufacturer chose to stop production rather than spend the money to bring its plant up to FDA standards. (Interestingly enough, the device itself never lost its FDA-approved status.) In 1999, another company snapped up the right to manufacture it, and the product was expected to be available to consumers in 2002. One of the few changes to the product will be that its label will warn users of the risk of toxic shock syndrome, a condition also associated with tampon use.

Also see: contraception, nonoxynol-9, toxic shock syndrome

standing positions

There's something steamy and spontaneous about standup sex. Who hasn't thought about whisking his woman into a darkened corridor, pushing up her skirt, and having his way with her?

Along with spontaneity, standing intercourse also requires some physical strength and balance. The missionary version, if you will, involves you standing with your arms wrapped around her back at shoulder height. She faces you with her hands around your neck and her legs draped over your hips. To make life easier and extend the pleasure, get wet: This is the classic position for sex in the surf when you take her on that tropical getaway she's been fantasizing about. The water's buoyancy, of course, gives you a nice load-bearing assist.

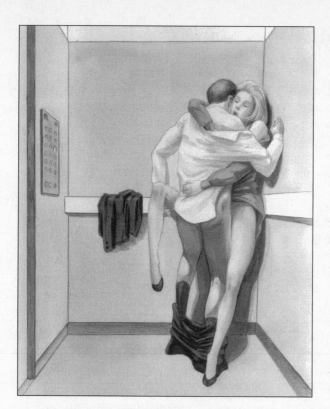

chair or places her hands on the floor. You then enter her from behind. Reaching around to stroke her clitoris, if your agility allows, will ensure that she thinks you're really a standup guy.

Also see: athletic sex, back, beds, exercise, *Kama Sutra*, planes, quickies, sixty-nine (69), zipless sex

STDs

Each year, STDs, or sexually transmitted diseases, affect more than 15 million Americans. In fact, in 1996, they accounted for 5 of the top 11 reportable diseases in the United States, 2 more than the year before. (In case you're wondering, a reportable disease is one that health practitioners must report to local, state, or national health care officials to help prevent and control its spread.) Part of the increase is attributed to people having more sexual partners than in the past, due to their becoming sexually active earlier, marrying later, and being more likely to divorce.

While the incidence of some of the diseases—such as gonorrhea and syphilis—is declining, the rates of others—such as chlamydia and genital warts, which are often asymptomatic—are rising by epidemic proportions.

Some STDs, such as chlamydia, are easily cured with antibiotics. Others, including genital warts and herpes, stay with you for life, though medications can relieve the symptoms. Of course, the worst venereal disease is one that can kill you: AIDS has already taken the lives of well more than 18 million people since the late 1970s.

As with all sexual positions, there are variations on the standard standing pose. One alternative suggested by the *Kama Sutra* is called suspended congress (and has nothing to do with what goes on in Washington—we think). You lean your back against a wall; she sits, facing you, on the "swing" of your joined hands, holding on to your neck and sliding back and forth by pushing off the wall.

Turn the tables on her to further expand the possibilities. In the standing shiva pose, the woman lies on a table or countertop with her buttocks balanced at the edge. As you enter her, she lifts her legs and rests her feet on your shoulders.

There's also a standing version of doggie style. This requires some balance on both lovers' parts, but it uses less strength since neither party is held aloft. She bends over and either leans on a

(continued on page 336)

SPECIAL REPORT
Stalking

Try winning over a woman these days with lavish gifts, love letters, and impromptu visits, and she may be more terrified than flattered. In her eyes, you could be a stalker disguised as a suitor. Welcome to the dynamics of dating in the 21st century.

While stalking is nothing new, in recent years it's been thrust into the limelight by news stories about crazed fans following, threatening, and even harming the celebrities they covet. In fact, it was the high-profile murder of actress Rebecca Schaeffer, gunned down in her apartment doorway by an obsessed fan, that prompted California to pass the nation's first anti-stalking law in 1990. The other 49 states quickly followed suit.

But the headlines tell only half of the story. In reality, regular folks are stalked far more often than the likes of Letterman and Madonna are. According to a 1997 survey by the National Institute of Justice, one million women and 370,000 men are stalked each year. In 87 percent of stalking cases, the stalker is a man. Couple these findings with movies like *Cape Fear* and *Sleeping with the Enemy*, and it's no wonder that some women confuse persistence with pathology.

We, on the other hand, can't afford to be confused. Men who pursue a love interest too ardently or try to patch things up with an ex-lover too forcefully could be fined a cool grand and thrown in the slammer for up to a year on a stalking charge.

Stop breathing into the paper bag and relax, man. Here are the facts.

• Most states define stalking as "a course of action that would place a rea-sonable person in fear for their safety." Though a true stalker, by most legal standards, means to harm or at least scare his victim, it's all too easy for even a nice guy to drift into the realm of what some might call stalking. It doesn't matter how sweet or sincere *your* intentions are. It's the way *she* reacts. If she's been finding a single red rose on her front porch every day for 2 weeks, she's probably going to feel a bit creeped out when you reveal yourself as her anonymous benefactor. Don't be surprised if she yells, "Police!" instead of "My hero!"

• Unwelcome attention is unwelcome attention, period. The nature of the attention is irrelevant. Don't count on absolving yourself with an explanation like "Your Honor, if I had really wanted to hurt her, would I have sent all those beautiful gifts?" Believe us, you won't be the first offender to have offered up such a benign-sounding rationale. In fact, you'll be exhibiting the first signs of a classic behavior pattern. The judge will probably be happy that you've been caught before the typical next step: That's when the suitor starts getting really pissed about being "ignored," and his attentions turn malevolent.

• Some guys don't take rejection well, and others have a tough time reading women's brush-off signals. Here's a clear sign to follow: When a woman doesn't respond to your persistent pursuit, take it as a no. Keep in mind that in 25 states, as few as two unwelcome acts can qualify as stalking.

• On the other end of the relationship, in those immediate postdumping days of emptiness and anxiety, heed her requests to not call or see her. Even if she hasn't explicitly said, "Do not call or stop by," proceed with caution. The next time the two of you talk, ask whether she's okay with you contacting her. Again, take a noncommittal response as a no, and back off.

• Whether you're pursuing a date or trying to reconcile with a former mate, don't pop up in places you know she frequents. She'll feel hounded if you start showing up at her Laundromat or favorite lunch spot. Even worse is parking outside her office at quitting time or strolling by her apartment late at night just to see if she's around. Can you say, "restraining order"?

• Sneakiness is spooky. If a woman at a club piques your interest, don't hover around her—not even in the background. Don't be the clod in the corner, either, who abruptly looks away each time she catches you staring at her. If you're unskilled in the mating dance, see our entries on *flirtation*, *eye contact*, and the *singles scene*, among others. In the meantime, while you're honing your skills, avoid giving women the idea that you're Hannibal Lecter.

• When asking a woman out on a date, it's only natural to want to talk to *her* rather than to her answering machine. But don't keep calling and hanging up without leaving a message. She may be screening her calls, as many telemarketer loathers do, and be freaked out by all the hang-ups. With the technology of caller ID and the *69 function, she can easily find out who's been repeatedly calling. The only date you may get is a court date.

• Some women nowadays record phone calls, save e-mails, and even snip and save instant-message communications, all for the purpose of protecting themselves should a dogged pursuer turn out to be a stalker. So be very careful

how often you contact her and what you say when you do. We know this flies in the face of romance, but you don't want to come on too strongly in the early stages of a relationship and inadvertently scare the living daylights out of her.

What's the right strategy for "safely" pursuing a woman by phone? If you get her machine, leave a clear message in which you identify yourself, provide a return number, and state your interest in a date. Watch your tone of voice. The first phone call is neither the time nor the place for a Barry White impression. (And unless you've received some *very* clear prior signal from her that she's up for some sexual gamesmanship, never say anything in that first call that you wouldn't want someone to say to your kid sister.) If she doesn't respond within a few days, it's okay to try again: Messages do get accidentally erased, and people do forget to write down phone numbers. But don't give her a third call if she hasn't taken the bait after the first two.

If, for whatever reason, she seems unreceptive when you do get in touch with her—and she has that right—be careful how you handle any ensuing conversation. Assuming that she doesn't warm up quickly, tell her you're sorry you bothered her. Say it like you mean it, without sarcasm. Tell her you don't plan to call again (in case she's recording all this). Once you get yourself off the hook, put the phone back *on* the hook and resolve to look elsewhere for romance.

Also see: begging, breaking up, compulsive behavior, desperate, masher, meeting women, no, past partners—longing for, rejection—romantic, sex offenders, unwanted advances

S

Right now, read this book's entry on *safe sex*, just in case you're one of those 15 million people who hasn't gotten that message already and therefore will get infected this year. You should also talk frankly with your doctor about your sexual history, and make sure that he includes exams of your genitals as part of your regular checkups. It's better to experience the red cheeks of embarrassment than the red rash of infection.

Also see: abstinence, AIDS, anal sex, chlamydia, condom, crabs, ectopic pregnancy, epididymitis, fears/phobias, free love, genital warts, gonorrhea, herpes, infertility, K-Y jelly, NSU, ointments, papilloma, pee—bloody, pee—painful, pelvic inflammatory disease, Pill—the, promiscuity, pubic lice, sex research, short-arm inspection, syphilis, urinary problems, urologist, venereal disease

steroids

It's true that these drugs can add 20 to 30 pounds of muscle per month to a man who regularly works out with weights. "Juice" increases not only strength but also stamina, all while reducing recovery times after workouts and injuries. Now, if only it weren't for those damn heart problems and the breast enlargement. We're not kidding. Ailments attributed to steroid use run the gamut from cosmetic problems such as acne, baldness, and breast enlargement to dizziness, infertility, rectal bleeding, shrunken testicles, liver toxicity, liver tumors, and heart disease. Happy injecting.

Another purported benefit of steroid use is an increased libido. In one study, steroid users boasted of having twice as many orgasms as nonusers. But the boost wasn't so much an increase in pleasure as it was an animalistic need to have sex. And though they may have humped like rabbits, they probably didn't reproduce like them: Another study found that bodybuilders who took large doses of steroids experienced 25 percent drops in their sperm counts that lasted as long as 6 months after they stopped taking the drugs.

Even so, the allure of 'roids remains strong. Football players can attain the superhero bulk of a lineman combined with the world-class speed of a wide receiver; cyclists can move from the back of the pack to a podium finish.

Vanity may be as much of a motivator as enhanced performance. Adolescents—who account for one-fourth to one-half of steroid abusers—admit taking them to enhance personal appearance. Many of the teens are not even athletes. They just want to bulk up to attract girls and intimidate their peers. (Who knew shriveled balls and bloody asses were desirable and daunting features?)

To make a long story short, if your woman lusts for a sterile, sex-crazed musclehead with man boobs, you should run right out and get yourself some 'roids. Otherwise, you're better off just hitting the gym more often.

Also see: athletic sex, beefcake, body fitness, body shapes, drugs, muscles

stimulation

For men, stimulation comes easy. All we have to do is lean too close to a belt sander or take a bumpy bus ride, and we're ready. Women, however, usually need a bit more than vibrating shop tools and lurching public transportation. They also need mental stimulation: They might close their eyes and imagine that they're riding the tall, dark stranger in the seat in front of them instead of just going Greyhound.

Because female arousal is as much cerebral as it is physical, there is no one surefire stimulation strategy that works on all women. What worked on your ex may not work on your latest. Even more challenging, what worked on your latest last week may not work tonight. We will tell you that you should caress her slowly and gently while professing your delight—except when she wants you to throw her down on the bed and tell her how naughty she is. But buck up, soldier: Exploring new paths to pleasure is not just a job, it's an adventure. The very fact that women want and need many different types of action is one of the most stimulating things about them.

Also see: anal sex, arousal, biting, breast fondling, breast sucking, coitus, erogenous zones, fantasies, feel up, flogging, French kiss, hickey, kiss, licking, manual stimulation, massage, masturbation, oral sex, rimming, sexual aids, spanking, tickling, touch, whispering

stress

It can make you too tired and preoccupied to have sex. It can cause a heart attack that will answer for you the question of whether there's an afterlife and, if so, whether you can have sex there. But stress can also have direct physical effects on your sexual performance. It can lower your libido by decreasing your testosterone levels, and it can cause erectile difficulties by constricting blood vessels that lead to your penis.

As you well know, it's impossible to avoid stress. But you can take steps to relieve it before it relieves you of your sex life.

Work is one of the biggest sources of stress in many men's lives. To minimize its negative effects, take occasional 10- to 15-

S

Hot Dates 1980s The VCR put porn in America's bedrooms. Between 1979 and 1990, the number of X-rated titles available on video leaped from 1,000 to 5,000.

continued from page 326

The driver of the Pontiac Grand Am said he and his brother were Pentecostal preachers in Texas. According to police reports, **the Lord had told them to get rid of their clothing** and other belongings and head to Louisiana. (And then He said, "Find thee 20 naked ladies. . . . ")

Foreign Affairs

Another reason to be glad we won: **Select diners in England feature waitresses who whip customers'** bottoms if they fail to eat all the food served on their plates. Caning has a long history in schools and clubs in that country.

In Extremis

At least he died happy: A South Carolina woman went to desperate lengths to conceal an affair from her husband. When **her lover died from a cerebral hemorrhage while they were having sex** on the floor of the woman's living room, she dragged

True or Phallus ?

The porno wing of the film industry has its own "walk of fame," where stars imprint their genitals.

BAWDY BALLADS "Tittie Man," *Drink Small*

continued on page 342

minute breaks. Go for a quick walk or sprint up a flight of stairs to recharge mentally and physically. Or simply stare off into space for a few minutes and indulge in a little sexual daydream. If you have to work long hours, try to clock in earlier in the morning rather than staying later at night. This will give you more time in the evening to spend decompressing with your partner.

But don't spend all of your downtime with her. Schedule time to yourself to exercise, read, or otherwise relax.

Sex itself is a great stress buster. When you're ready for a rendezvous, retreat to a place that is comfortable and free of distractions. Take time to enjoy each kiss, each touch, instead of gearing up for penetration and orgasm. Don't pressure yourself to perform, thereby creating yet another stressor. Enjoy the primrose path as much as the down-and-dirty destination.

Also see: fatigue, infertility, job loss, medication, performance anxiety, PMS, premature ejaculation, relaxation, rhythm method, sex addiction, sex—lack of, sperm count, thrush, workaholism

striptease

While erecting a brass pole in your bedroom may be a bit excessive (and dangerous, if you sleepwalk), performing an occasional striptease may not be. A little burlesque—by either a man or a woman—can be an effective opening act in a great sexual play.

Advance planning will definitely add to the allure. Candles work well as mood lighting; sultry music can provide the pulse for the swinging hips and playful tosses of clothing. Sophisticated dress, such as lingerie for women or tuxedos for men, is usually more enticing than peeling off a sweatshirt or flannel work shirt (though a talented stripper can make those work as well).

Instead of a haphazard undressing with clothes strewn about the floor, there should be some flair and deliberateness to the affair. The disrobing should be slow, with each button and zipper undone to provide one tantalizing glimpse of bare skin after another. Constant, riveting eye contact communicates to the lone viewer that this dance is private indeed.

Above all, no clumsy move should crash the mood. A chair or a bed is a convenient prop for maintaining balance. Feigned coyness ("Uh-oh, I'm stuck. Can you help me take this off . . . please?") or a convenient fall into a lover's arms is an effective and seductive last resort. And it certainly doesn't signal the end of the show: The climax is yet to come.

Also see: exhibitionism, fantasies, lingerie, music, topless bar, underwear, undressing, voyeurism

stud muffin

This is a man whom women want to eat up, in every sense of the term. (In gay culture, it's also a man that other men want to eat up, so avoid using the phrase among your guy friends unless you're intending to send a certain message.) He's hard, strong, upstanding, and fully capable of mounting a woman as if he were a wild stallion. But just behind this is a softer, sweet side. This juxtaposition of strength and gentleness is what women hunger for. Mel Gibson is the prototypical stud muffin: a good-looking guy with a good-natured sense of humor as well as a sense of decency.

If a woman calls you a stud muffin, she's hoping you'll eventually spend some time in her oven.

Also see: attraction, beefcake, sexual attraction, sexy

succubus

According to medieval European folklore, this evil spirit or demon assumes a female form and has sexual intercourse with men as they sleep. You say that sounds wet dreamy, not demonic? Wait, there's more. Legend has it that any man who has coital relations with such an entity will never awaken. Damn, there's always a catch.

An equally evil male spirit called an incubus was said to have sex with sleeping women, sometimes planting his sinful seed. The most famous offspring supposedly fathered by this impregnating poltergeist was Merlin the magician.

Also see: dreams, fantasies, wet dreams

supplements

Performing at your best in the bedroom requires more than just staying in shape physically. It means keeping your tank filled with premium fuel. The best way to do that? Eat lots of fruits, vegetables, whole grains, and lean meats. We heard that collective groan. The fact that most of us prefer junk food over rabbit food is the very reason why we generally don't get enough of the vitamins, minerals, and other vital nutrients that healthful foods supply.

The easiest way to remedy this deficiency is to take a multivitamin and mineral supplement. It should contain zinc, the most important element we know for boosting male sexual function. Zinc

seems to help you make stronger, faster sperm, and make them in greater numbers. It also aids in the metabolism of the mighty male hormone, testosterone.

Other crucial supplements that aid in reproduction and sexual ability are antioxidants and the B vitamins. Sperm cells rely heavily on antioxidants for protection against damage caused by the very chemicals they produce to break through barriers to egg fertilization.

The most effective way to take antioxidants is by combining vitamins C and E with more specialized antioxidants like alpha-lipoic acid and coenzyme Q_{10}. You'll have to purchase the antioxidants separately since they're not usually included in a multi.

All of the B vitamins assist in hormonal reactions. Vitamin B_6 is particularly helpful in stimulating the adrenal glands. And B_{12} is essential in sperm production.

Another way to boost your sex life is with herbal supplements. Our favorites are American ginseng (*Panax quinquefolius*) and ginkgo (*Ginkgo biloba*). Ginseng has been revered in Asian cultures for centuries as a male-potency and longevity tonic. It's been proven to build physical stamina and may stimulate testosterone production. Ginkgo is excellent for increasing blood circulation to your privates, which can help, uh, give your love life a lift.

Also see: prostate cancer, sex drive, zinc

suppositories

The facts: These are small, bullet-shaped medicinal packages that you place in the rectum or vagina to treat a range of conditions from hemorrhoids to constipation to yeast infections. There's also a pellet-size suppository form of the erection-enhancing prescription drug alprostadil (Muse) that you insert in your penis.

The rumor: Some guys like to use rectal suppositories for anal arousal. If you're one of them, listen up: Save suppositories for when you *really* need them. They may contain powerful drugs that, with overuse, can irritate or inflame your anus. And most have a mineral oil base, which will break down a condom, making anal or vaginal sex unsafe.

If you're looking for that little extra kick, flip instead to the entries on *anal beads* and *anal plug*, things we consider more, er, wholesome for anal stimulation.

Also see: anal sex, erection difficulties, klismaphilia, rectum, rimming, sodomy, sphincter, yeast infection

surprises

Our sexual motors tend to be constantly running on idle, just waiting to be shifted into gear. Not so with women. Their engines rev up more slowly.

So sometimes it's helpful—and fun—to jump-start your partner with a playful surprise. That doesn't mean (at one extreme) pushing her down on the bed and engaging in spontaneous cunnilingus, and it doesn't have to mean (at the other extreme) returning from the mall with a 2-carat gem. What you're looking to demonstrate here is some kind of spontaneity that isn't directly sexual. She wants you to present her with tickets to a play and a new dress for the occasion. (Tip: There is no end to the gratitude of a woman whose lover knows her exact sizes—blouse, dress, pants, ring, shoes—and her preferred style of clothing.) She'll

appreciate surprise rides in various modes of conveyance: limousines, helicopters, hot-air balloons, horse-drawn carriages.

The surprise doesn't even have to involve money, or at least not lots of it. She'll warm when you give her a rare orchid on an otherwise ordinary day, just for no reason at all. Bring home her favorite dessert. Or consider a picnic: Whisk her away to the woods for a quiet walk; hike to a secret pool of hot springs. Hire a mime to perform at her birthday party . . . okay, maybe not that. But basically anything else that shows you're still *trying*.

Also see: birthdays, dating, flowers, lingerie, marriage proposal, romance

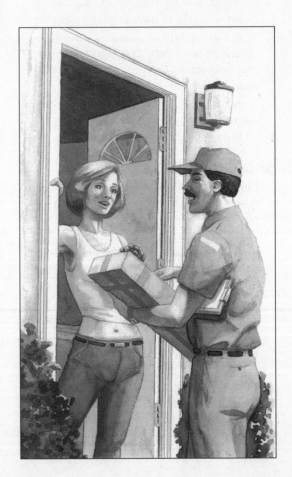

surrogate

You're probably thinking, "Isn't that just a fancy word for hooker?" The answer is no.

Here's the difference. A man pays a prostitute for what essentially amounts to entertainment. Her goal is to get him off. It's a once-and-done thing.

A man pays a surrogate partner for therapy. Her goal is to resolve his sexual problems. She offers a series of hands-on therapy sessions that enable him to have a healthy sex life on his own.

Now you're probably thinking, "Finally, a way to deal with a problem without talking it to death." Again, no.

Surrogate partners actually focus on communication as an avenue to physical and emotional intimacy. Actual genital contact, we hate to tell you, may not even be part of the therapy. What's more, a surrogate partner works with a sex therapist or psychologist, with whom the client is required to talk after each session. Certainly not the typical hooker/john relationship.

Many surrogate seekers are late-life virgins, ashamed of their inexperience and nervous about sexual arousal. Others have trouble maintaining an erection or postponing ejaculation. Women, too, sometimes see surrogates for help overcoming sexual fears and phobias.

Typical surrogate therapy can run anywhere from several months to a year and a half before most people resolve their concerns. Early sessions consist of talking and relaxation exercises. Later, they often progress to nudity, communication exercises, sensual touching, and possibly direct sexual contact, including intercourse. Because you're actually paying for two therapists at once, working with a surrogate can get pricey—anywhere from $100 to $200 a week, and that adds up by the time you're done.

For information, write to the International Professional Surrogates Association at P.O. Box 4282, Torrance, CA 90510-4282.

Also see: communication, dildo, erection difficulties, faking orgasm, frigidity, manual stimulation, performance anxiety, prostitution, sex education, sex therapy

sweating

Slipping and sliding during hot, sweaty, head-to-toe body contact is sexy to many women. They love the feel of moist skin, they dig the smell, and the heat drives them wild.

For other women, sweat symbolizes just one thing: soiled workout clothes pungent from a night spent in your gym bag. Not exactly the olfactory image that makes a woman beg, "Do me!"

Whether it's the buckets you generate from athletic sex or the "glow" that comes from kissing and touching, perspiration is a normal part of arousal. If you're lucky enough to have a partner who appreciates sweat's erotic benefits, enjoy it as an extension of the other bodily fluids you exchange during sex. Wet your fingers with perspiration from your chest or neck and massage her body with the natural lubricant.

While you can't change sweat's turn-off factor for many women, you can change its smell. Some guys notice that certain foods alter the scent of their sweat, so stay away from ingredients such as garlic, onions, cumin, and curry before a big date. And, much as we hate to admit it, the sweat of vegetarians is less pungent than that of meat eaters. So if your partner has a problem with your after-meal funk, you might want to lay off the meat.

But suppose she's made it clear that

your regular salty soaking will never make her feel much like getting it on. Pre-sex, try sprinkling your bodies with moisture-absorbing, unscented powder. Crank up the air-conditioning and keep towels handy. For maximum cleanliness, make a habit out of shower or bathtub sex.

Realize, too, that your partner may have a deep-seated reason for not wanting to sweat it out. If she was raised to believe that sex is filthy, for example, sweat may actually make her feel guilty and dirty. To lay the groundwork for a satisfying sex life—in areas that go way beyond the issue of sweat—you'll need to get such feelings out into the open.

One way to ease her into the world of sweaty sex is by smoothing fragrant massage oils or lotions over both your bodies before lovemaking. The pleasant smell and "clean" lubrication may help her associate sweatiness with feeling good.

Also see: athletic sex, body odor as an attractant, body odor—controlling, exercise, hang-ups, hygiene, latex, pheromones, pubic hair, slick, sloppy sex, yeast infection

sweet talk

This is a topic near and dear to your woman's heart, much like cards and flowers and the status of the garbage. Regardless of which one of you is doing the actual talking at any given moment, sweet talk, to her, reinforces your coupleness. It reminds her that she's your lover, even when you're not making love. It reassures her that she's special to you.

Some of us have a problem with this. There's something inside us—maybe that primal need to be looked upon as men, not as boys—that cringes just a little bit when she lapses into baby talk. Something that makes us feel uncomfortable when she comes up with some silly pet name for a body part.

Hot Dates 1981 A *New York Times* headline declared RARE CANCER SEEN IN 41 HOMOSEXUALS. Two years later, the AIDS virus was isolated. Between 1981 and 1990, more than 160,000 AIDS cases were reported in the United States.

continued from page 337

Answer:
False. The Los Angeles Pussycat theater chain did establish a tribute to porn stars, but only hand- and footprints have been cast in cement. Honorees include Marilyn Chambers, Linda Lovelace, and Harry Reems.

his limp body into the backyard, then phoned police to report a prowler. Just one problem: The pants of the "burglar" were around his ankles when police arrived.

LEGAL BRIEFS
A Wisconsin man on probation for child molestation was jailed after he refused court-ordered sex therapy aimed at spurring interest in adult erotic images. The man claimed the therapy was unconstitutional because **it required him to violate his religious beliefs by masturbating**.

Seemed like a Good Idea at the Time. . .
Linda Lovelace, star of 1972's infamous and lucrative porn classic *Deep Throat*, got the short end of the stick on payday. **She received just $75 for her efforts.** Lovelace's co-star, the celebrated Harry Reems, got not only an extra $25 but also the benefit of her considerable oral expertise.

BAWDY BALLADS "Nuts for Sale," *Chick Willis*

continued on page 353

Nevertheless, go along with it. Learn to like it. Participate. As we said, it means a lot to her.

It means a lot, also, when you tell her how pretty she looks at just-out-of-the-blue times, such as when she's preparing your favorite dinner or doing the laundry. She wants you to notice her new hairdo, her new dress (and not by saying, "Oh, you went shopping again, huh? How much did that cost?"). She wants you to call her Sweetie and Honey and, yes—if you can stomach it—Pookey-Poo.

Here's one warning: Among the many things with which God equipped women, for reasons known only to Him, is a built-in B.S. detector. She senses the difference between sincere sweet talk and pretty-sounding words that you're using to manipulate her. Context is also relevant. If you suddenly get cozy at a time when she knows you want something from her (such as sex), she'll see through you like the proverbial pane of glass. And you'll be worse off than if you had said nothing at all. That's why we said it has to be out of the blue. It's also why you shouldn't think of sweet talk as a prelude to seduction. To have any real value for her, it should be a show of affection that's free of any sexual expectations.

Oh, and if she asks you why you're being so nice, the answer, the only answer, the always answer, is: "Because I love you." We assume you mean it.

Also see: communication, courtship, making up, romance, talking dirty, teasing, voice, whispering

swinging

We don't mean those dance lessons women keep trying to drag us to. We're talking partner-swapping, plain and simple.

America's swingers-club culture originated in the 1960s. Although club memberships dropped drastically during the early 1980s, some couples—surveys suggest 2 percent of the population—attend swingers events today.

Most swingers are married or committed couples with a mutual agreement to be sexual with others from time to time. A typical swinging couple stays close together at a club or party, mingling until they encounter another couple they find interesting. Once they meet a couple they find attractive and intriguing, they may spend an evening socializing before they decide whether they'd like to swap for sex. Or they may go for it after a few minutes of small talk.

Some couples never actually switch partners when the sex starts. These "self-swingers" get pleasure watching others go at it, and they get excited putting on their own sexual spectacle.

Occasionally, couples swing with the mistaken impression that it will help strengthen their marriages. That's exactly ass-backward. Don't try the swinging lifestyle unless things at home are rock solid. After all, if your relationship is on shaky ground to begin with, do you really think having sex with other partners is the way to fix it?

If you're still curious about swinging, check out the book entitled *The Lifestyle: A Look at the Erotic Rites of Swingers*, by Terry Gould.

Also see: best friend's wife, exhibitionism, extramarital sex, jealousy, marriage—open, voyeurism

switch-hitter

Also known as batting from both sides of the plate. This term usually refers to a bisexual—someone who has sex with both men and women.

Better news: It's also a hand-job technique in which a woman strokes up and down the penis, alternating one hand with the other for double the stimulation. No need to change pitchers for this batter.

Also see: AC/DC, bisexuality, get off

sympto-thermal method

Sounds more like something Al Roker would use to forecast the weather than a form of birth control. For couples who want a more accurate form of natural birth control than the rhythm method and don't mind a week without intercourse, most family-planning centers now teach this scientific technique that determines a woman's fertile period through variations in her vaginal mucus, cervical condition, and body temperature. The presence of mucus signals that ovulation is imminent. Simultaneously, her cervix rises, softens, and opens, and her temperature drops slightly below 98°F. She can resume having sex once she's had 3 consecutive days back above 98°F and 4 days of relative dryness.

Sympto-thermal is about 85 percent effective, on average, when a woman documents her cycle diligently, which takes just a few minutes each morning.

Come to think of it, this sounds almost as complicated as predicting the weather. Our advice? Consult a natural-family-planning program such as the Couple to Couple League to learn exactly how to do this.

For the record, the sympto-thermal method and other natural methods of birth control don't stack up at all against artificial means of contraception. The Pill, an IUD, or a condom and spermicide is much more effective.

Also see: contraception, ovulation, rhythm method

syphilis

A sexually transmitted disease caused by the *Treponema pallidum* bacterium, syphilis is often thought of in connection with the profound mental disturbance it can bring on its victims if left untreated.

The illness is no longer the scourge it once was. In 1998, only about 7,000 cases were reported in the United States. Prompt treatment with penicillin or other antibiotics usually does the trick. And that's key, because without such care, syphilis can leave you institutionalized. Notable victims are said to have included philosopher Friedrich Nietzsche (famous for pronouncing God dead), painter Vincent van Gogh, and mob boss Al Capone.

During the first 2 years that a person is infected, symptoms are often so minor that they go ignored. The very first sign tends to be a painless ulcer on the penis. The woman from whom you contracted the disease may have a similar ulcer, or chancre, on her vulva or inside her vagina, where neither of you would notice it. A rash usually follows the chancre's disappearance. Though it may cover the entire body, it's certain to show up on the palms of your hands and the soles of your feet; the sores that accompany the rash harbor contagious bacteria, so be sure to keep any open wounds covered.

Other typical early-stage symptoms include low fever, headache, and sore throat. You may lose small patches of hair and feel fatigued. If left untreated, these symptoms can persist on and off for up to 2 years; but they eventually fade away, at which time you're no longer contagious.

About one-third of people who get to this point develop late-stage complica-tions: After a period (of varying length) during which the disease exhibits no ill effects whatsoever, it suddenly returns with a vengeance, damaging your bones, joints, or heart. The usual progression leads to blindness, insanity, and death.

Also see: rashes, short-arm inspection, size—nose, STDs, venereal disease

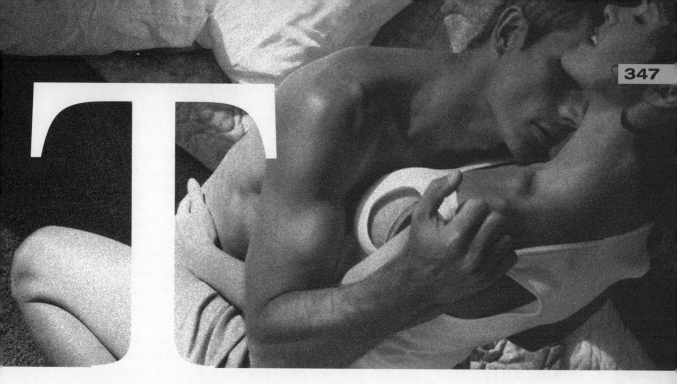

taboos

Practices prohibited within a cultural group.

For some, the more taboo the sex act, the more they love it. The prohibition of an act actually makes it more arousing.

Such people grow bored when they're not being taunted by those deliciously tempting boundaries. Continually searching for naughtier ways to "do it," they venture into darker, more forbidden forms of sex. They violate new taboos.

Exploring a taboo now and then can be healthy and invigorating. That's not to recommend breaking any laws, jeopardizing your relationship, or causing someone harm just for the thrill of it. Consequences trump pleasure. Fortunately, there's so much about sex that's been taboo at one time or another that you can

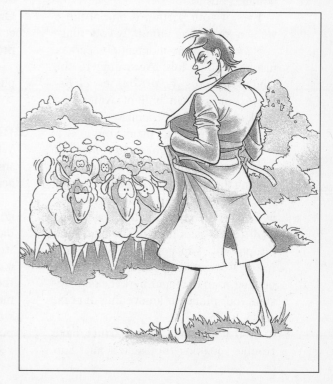

surely find something "forbidden" to exploit without getting yourself into trouble.

For example, try something kinkier than what's on your usual sex menu. Gradually introduce a few of these acts into your lovemaking. You and your lover will find that there are still some lines you are unwilling to cross, but you'll discover other taboo territories that spark the primitive passion you've been missing.

Also see: abnormal, danger, fantasies, fears/phobias, guilt, interracial sex, kinky, paraphilias, perversions, risky sex, violence, wild

talking dirty

A pastime popular enough to make those 1-900 phone sex numbers a booming business.

Even if your partner is one of those women who's a bit put off by your fondness for heat-of-the-moment obscenities, just remember this: According to the landmark *Janus Report on Sexual Behavior,* more than half of Americans think that a bit of raunchy language during sex is just fine, thank you.

In fact, when it comes to sex, many of us are more at ease using slang terms (including the more than 200 euphemisms for intercourse) than clinical, scientific words. And, for those folks who like it, dirty talk isn't just for the bedroom. Graphically whispering in your girlfriend's ear while you're, say, picking out guavas in the supermarket can jumpstart your plans for an evening of great sex.

And if you and your partner have trouble speaking the same sexual language? Here's what sex therapists suggest for bridging the great divide.

• Ask your partner if she has a pet name for her vagina. When she stops laughing, tell her about the childhood nickname you gave your penis. This may amuse her enough to reveal her own secret words or the slang terms she prefers.

• Another exercise is for each partner to make two side-by-side lists, one containing clinical words, the other, the corresponding dirty words. Exchange lists and look for words that you've both picked. Discuss which are the most mutually arousing, then try them in bed later.

• If this still sounds too silly or embarrassing for a face-to-face setting, you might experiment first over the phone or online. The relative anonymity makes it easier for some people to open up. Just don't do any of this in Willowdale, Oregon, where town fathers have enacted a law against a husband uttering profanity while having sex with his wife.

Also see: communication, dial-a-porn, phone sex, sweet talk, voice, whispering

tampon

What most dogs, and some of us, can smell in a sealed trash can from clear across the house.

These most basic of female essentials go way back. The ancient Egyptians made them from papyrus; the Romans, from wool. (That must've been really comfortable for Cleopatra and the rest of the gals.) Some cultures believed that menstrual blood had evil powers, so the women burned their soiled tampons to purge the mysterious powers and prevent harm from befalling them or their families. These days most tampons are made of absorbent cotton or rayon; and while they may be messy, they generally don't have evil powers.

Still, many guys prefer to avoid walking down the feminine-hygiene aisle at the supermarket. And some of us get downright squeamish if we happen to encounter those products while they're actually in use.

Truth is, a tampon probably won't cause her any serious damage if she somehow forgets to remove it before sex, but you'll both be uncomfortable. And the normal rigors of intercourse may wedge it in so deeply that she could have trouble removing it.

Of course, gentleman that you are, you can always offer to remove it yourself, before sex. Just give the cord a slow, steady tug. Or, if you're feeling brave, gently pull it with your teeth. Have a paper towel handy to wrap it up.

Period sex just not your game? Urge your partner to check out a product called the Instead Softcup. It fits over her cervix, diaphragm-like, and catches the blood till you're done. It can be left in for up to 12 hours.

Also see: cramps—menstrual, diaphragm, menstruation, period, toxic shock syndrome

tantra

A 2,000-year-old Hindu spiritual system whose followers all over the world use ritual sexual intercourse as a vehicle to greater enlightenment. If you're thinking of converting, know that the Tantric quest for salvation alternates the ritualistic sex with periods of abstinence—and often, even during the sex phase, practi-tioners of tantra don't allow themselves to climax. They believe that the semen they reserve gives them greater energy and increased sexual vitality.

Also see: chakras, *Kama Sutra*, orgasm, refractory period, religion, spiritual sex, yin and yang, yogi

tattoos

Back in 1950s America, they were associated exclusively with Hell's Angels, their molls, and punks with long rap sheets. Since then, body art has grown in respectability and popularity. Tattoos not only draw attention to inviting regions of the body but also make a powerful statement about sexual style. It doesn't take a lot of imagination to realize that a guy adorned with snakes and scorpions (traditionally associated with sexual power and aggression) is probably advertising a more ferocious approach to life and sex than is a guy decorated with oriental designs or other softer depictions. So, too, with women's tattoos.

Guys tend to put tattoos on their biceps, backs, and shoulders. Women prefer their hips, thighs, backs, and the area between their necks and breasts. We've heard reports that, as a penetration of the body, the tattooing experience can be sensual in itself (though given the amount of pain involved and the lack of any real "release," we suspect that anyone for whom this is true skews far toward the sadomasochist end of the spectrum).

Taking your cue from the Indian and Middle Eastern cultures that cover a bride's hands and feet in removable henna dyes as part of the marriage ritual, you can use temporary tattoos as situational decor. We know a guy who had symbols of love applied to the palms of his hands in honor of his wife's birthday. The elaborate design achieved its purpose, then disappeared within days. We assume the effect of the gesture lasted longer.

If you do go for the permanent variety, tattoo artists caution that you should give ample consideration to the design. You don't want to be one of those customers who selects his body art from the tattoo-shop wall. And be sober, or assign a friend to stop you from getting a tattoo while in an impaired state. Daffy Duck indelibly inscribed on your bicep is decidedly unsexy.

Because there is no certifying organization for tattoo artists, look for someone who at least meets the following criteria: He uses an autoclave to sterilize his equipment, wears properly fitted medical gloves, is vaccinated for hepatitis B, does not reuse inks or ointments, pulls new sterile needles from a sealed bag and then disposes of the used ones in a "sharps" container, and is willing to show you examples of his work.

Also see: piercing

teasing

Guys relate to one another through good-natured jeering. We love thinking up ingenious ways to imply that our best buds have tiny peckers, just as we delight in ripping some poor schnook for his notoriously bad luck with women. And all this is generally okay because friendly competitiveness is the way we men interact on a private, more-or-less intimate plane. We even have a sweet-sounding name for it: male bonding.

Women have different names for it— names like *stupidity* and *childishness*.

They don't get it. They think teasing is basically mean-spirited, and it often goes on far too long for their tastes. True, every now and then you'll run across a woman who goes along with the flow, especially when she's outnumbered—when in Rome, and all that. (This is often a gal who grew up with three or four brothers.) You know what, though? If *your* woman is the lone female in the group and, at some point, the give-and-take hits a nerve . . . well, she may laugh it off at the time. But believe us, you're gonna hear about it later.

Your better half is not one of the guys, so you should never put her down when you're "just kidding around." There's a difference, after all, between taking a light-hearted approach to life in general and making some wisecrack about how your wife looks in her new bathing suit.

If you keep it up, she may very well develop a thicker skin and even her own sassy style of having the last word. You just have to ask yourself whether you really want a relationship that's built on thick skin and one-upmanship?

Save the teasing for the guys. When it comes to your woman, go with the sweet talk.

Also see: communication, laughter, sweet talk

techniques

Great sex takes more than a willing partner and 3 spare minutes up against the fridge. Half of it depends on intimacy between you and your partner. The other half is technique, which is why we dedicate a good chunk of this book to describing a variety of sexual tactics. Read and learn. You—and your partner—will be glad you did.

Also see: stimulation

teddies

Items that make the Victoria's Secret catalog such great bathroom reading. If only it were easier to get the damn things off in the heat of the moment!

Popularized in the 1920s, when women's clothes became tighter and skimpier, this one-piece substitute for a bra and panties usually is made of any combination of soft, sheer, or lacy material that hugs a woman's body to curve-enhancing advantage. (S/M devotees rejoice—they're made in leather too.) The hottest teddies leave little to the imagination: They're crotchless, cupless, or fitted with thongs. That's the good news. The bad news is that the delicate process of teddy removal often brings out the Godzilla in us. Still, keeping clumsiness to a minimum doesn't require any advanced degrees.

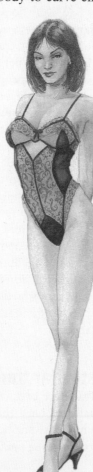

When you wriggle a woman out of her dress and find this one-piece wonder underneath, give it a quick once-over. Basically, try to determine whether to go north or south with it. Start by gliding your fingers lightly along her crotch. Though this is a fun activity in its own right, what you're really doing is looking for snaps. If you find them, release them and maneuver the teddy over her head. If you don't find them, just reach up, ease the straps off her shoulders, and pull the whole thing down over her hips.

On more complicated teddies, you'll find, oh, 4,000 tiny buttons or ties all the way down the back or front. Start at the top and see how far you get before the teddy slips off. Or, to generate excruciating anticipation, unfasten them one at a time—very, very slowly—attending to other little matters like earlobes and eyelids and toes between each individual unfastening.

Sometimes, no matter what you do, you're unable to get the thing figured out. No biggie. Ask for help. Or leave the teddy on. Move it aside as needed, and enjoy the sexy way it makes her look and feel.

Also see: lingerie, striptease

testicles

We seldom call them that, of course. To us, they're balls, nuts, jewels, cojones. And though we think of them primarily in terms of pumping out sperm cells, they also produce testosterone, our hormonal ticket to manhood.

The average testicle weighs less than an ounce. It's oval-shaped, about 1½ inches long, and 1 inch in diameter. For some reason, the left ball is usually a bit bigger, and hangs a little lower, than the right.

Most doctors and sex therapists will tell you not to worry if you don't have balls that'd be the envy of the Merrill

T

Lynch bull. Size doesn't affect your sexual endurance, sex drive, or level of fertility. Yet some studies do appear to show a link between large testicles and promiscuity or infidelity. Robin Baker, Ph.D., a biologist at the University of Manchester in England, announced in 1997 that men with big balls were likely to have more lovers and more active sex lives than their more modestly endowed counterparts. Dr. Baker's studies also suggested that when two pairs of testicles competed for one woman's affections, they were both likely to generate more sperm. Go figure.

Also see: epididymitis, gonad, infertility, prostate cancer, scrotum, sex—lack of, sperm count, steroids, testosterone replacement therapy, urethritis

T

testicles—undescended

Your testicles don't start out nestled snugly in your scrotum. They work their way down there from up in your abdomen. In about 1 in 100 male infants, one or both testicles don't make it. These undescended testicles, or abdominal genitals, are easily put in their proper place via routine surgery, but their early truancy may leave some damage that affects your fertility. It's worth noting: An undescended testicle puts you at greater risk for developing testicular cancer—even after corrective surgery.

Also see: infertility

testicular cancer

Though it accounts for only about 1 percent of cancer throughout the entire male population, it's still the most common cancer among guys ages 15 to 35. No one really knows the cause. Doctors do know that the highest single risk factor is an undescended testicle that wasn't corrected before the boy's second birthday.

Periodically check yourself for rockhard, pea-sized lumps, particularly if you're in the high-risk age group. (Or get your woman to do it for you. Ninety-four percent of women say they'd gladly check your danglers for lumps.) Before you start squeezing your scrotum, take a warm bath or a shower to ensure that the tissue is relaxed and hanging low. Then use both hands to examine each testicle thoroughly, placing your thumbs on top of the gland and your forefingers and middle fingers underneath it. Gently roll the testicle between your fingers, squeezing slightly.

See your doctor immediately if you think you feel a suspicious lump. He can perform an ultrasound or check your blood for further signs of cancer.

For years, people associated testicular cancer with the end of a guy's manhood. Cycling champion Lance Armstrong taught us differently, by not only recovering from the disease but also going on to win the Tour de France 3 years in a row. Even in its more advanced stages, the cancer is totally curable, sometimes through either radiation or surgery.

Overall, more than 90 percent of afflicted men conquer it. Still, we repeat what we said above: Don't wait to see a doctor. You don't want to be among the 10 percent who don't make it.

Also see: penile cancer, prostate cancer

testicular trauma

There are two ways to get kicked in the balls: so hard that it creates a surgical emergency and just hard enough to cause excruciating pain that doesn't last much beyond the initial moan and breathlessness. When it comes to testicular trauma, there's no middle of the road.

If your testicles start to swell immediately after a kick, a rough tackle, or some other impact, and if the pain is more than you can ride out by bending over and holding your groin for a few minutes, get thee to a hospital right away. The swelling is a sign that your testicle may have ruptured. If the problem isn't diagnosed and treated quickly, you could lose a nut. Or two.

Torsion is another testicular emergency, and it's mostly a concern for guys under 20. At some point in your life, you've probably used a hose that's gotten twisted around on itself or otherwise kinked, thus stopping the flow of water. The same kind of kinking can happen to a testicle, for a variety of reasons. The tissue can actually do a full 360-degree turn, completely shutting off bloodflow. A testicle so twisted must be untwisted—professionally—within 6 hours. So if your 15-year-old son is writhing in sudden inexplicable scrotal pain, don't tell him to buck up and be macho. Pain caused by testicular torsion doesn't cease by itself until the organ dies.

Also see: eunuch, injuries, sperm count, urologist, zippers

testosterone

The main male sex hormone. This powerful, steroid-based chemical generated by your testicles and adrenal glands reaches peak production at around 8:00 A.M. and drops precipitously by bedtime. This may explain why some of us prefer morning sex—and, since women also produce some testosterone, why many of them don't mind accommodating us.

Testosterone is often talked about as if its sole function were to enhance your more manly functions on demand:

Hot Dates 1982 The authors of *The G-Spot and Other Recent Discoveries about Human Sexuality* unveiled a "new" female erogenous zone. The book became a *New York Times* bestseller.

Foreign Affairs

Some Orthodox Jews practice *niddah*, a ritual that requires married couples to have no physical contact with each other for 10 to 14 days each month. This period commences when a woman's menstrual period begins and ends 7 days after it ceases. During this time, **a husband and wife may not sleep in the same bed together**, touch each other, or hand anything to one another.

In Extremis

Maybe he meant "bondage": Among the clients that police turned up in a prostitution probe in Wisconsin was **a 98-year-old man who had spent $7,000** over 2 years with three women. The man denied this, saying if he'd had that kind of money, he would "invest it in bonds."

LEGAL BRIEFS

A Canadian woman was charged with robbery and theft for pilfering

True or Phallus

Gangster John Dillinger's penis was of such impressive dimensions that it has been preserved in formaldehyde in a glass jar at the Smithsonian Institution.

BAWDY BALLADS "Let's Get a Quickie," *Clarence Carter*

continued on page 358

pumping up your muscles, flaring up your temper, boosting up your sex drive. In reality, the substance benefits your entire body, all day long. It keeps you strong, lean, and energetic. It helps prevent arthritis, depression, stroke, diabetes, and osteoporosis. In fact, though testosterone has long gotten a bad rap for raising blood pressure, more recent science indicates that it may actually dilate your coronary arteries, strengthen your heart, lower your cholesterol, and even thin your blood. Not bad for a hormone that for too long was linked almost entirely with erections and anger.

Also see: body odor as an attractant, chromosomes, DHEA, finasteride, marijuana, menopause—yours, nipples, oral contraceptive, oysters, pituitary gland, progesterone, stress, supplements

testosterone replacement therapy

If there's one thing that's associated with male virility and power, it's testosterone. And that's the theory behind testosterone replacement therapy: If your tank is running low, just top it off.

Your testosterone level decreases as you age, usually at the rate of 1 to 2 percent a year starting in your 30s. But here's the kicker: The "normal" testosterone range is unusually wide—anywhere from 275 to 850 nanograms per deciliter of blood. So even if your levels decline every year, depending on where you started, you may never drop into the low margin.

That's the good news. The bad news is that there are four million to five million American men with *hypogonadism*, the term used to describe the fact that their testicles have stopped producing enough testosterone and their blood levels have dropped below normal. When you have hypogonadism, your energy level and sex drive plummet. You can also come down with depression, extra belly fat, a decrease in bone and muscle mass, and erectile troubles.

Men thus afflicted are prime candidates for testosterone replacement therapy (though doctors caution that testosterone alone won't fix erectile dysfunction). Prescriptions for the treatment are surprisingly easy to get. If you're approaching middle age and you visit your doctor complaining of a reduced sex drive, he probably won't even bother testing for low testosterone levels before writing the scrip.

Maybe you're reluctant to see the doctor because you've heard horror stories about the negative side effects of testosterone replacement. It's true that when the treatment was first developed, it could be done only with needles and pills. The shots made some men aggressive and jittery, while the pills put them at risk for liver damage. Though the patch was better, its first incarnation had to be applied to the underside of a freshly shaved scrotum—undoubtedly causing stares in the locker room and adding a frightening new dimension to razor burn. Fortunately, the science has improved so that you can place the patch almost anywhere on your body. And now there's also a gel that you can apply to your shoulders, chest, upper arms, or abdomen.

Though testosterone replacement has come a long way, you need to consider a few things before you start. First off, this is a lifelong commitment: Pumping added testosterone into your body causes your system to cut its own production. That means that your testicles will shrink over time. If, after a few years, you stop taking it, your gonads may have atrophied too much to kick-start the production process anew.

As if the prospect of microballs weren't scary enough, there are also other health concerns, including baldness, increased sleep apnea, lowering of your HDL (good) cholesterol, breast enlargement, and prostate enlargement. That last side effect means that extra testosterone can be especially harmful if you have prostate cancer, so before you start therapy, you should undergo a prostate-specific antigen screen to check for tumors.

Remember, too, that your testosterone levels took decades to diminish, so it's likely that your wife also spent decades adapting to your diminishing sex drive. Testosterone replacement therapy can reverse those declines in a matter of weeks. Make sure that your relationship is up to the newer, hornier you. If your wife is happy with the sheep who walked into the doctor's office, she may not know what to make of the charging bull who comes out.

Even if she is game, cost may be an issue. Unless you have a proven testosterone deficiency resulting from disease or injury (which, remember, many doctors will not bother to test for), most insurance companies won't reimburse you. Expect to spend about $100 a month for your newfound friskiness.

Also see: eunuch, impotence, menopause—hers, menopause—yours, urologist

third-degree cleavage

There you are, suddenly face-to-chest with a woman whose jugs really are bigger than her head. Her head? Oh yeah, her head . . . you forgot to look at that.

Breasts bigger than a size DD are quite rare. Most women don't even fill C cups. Still, occasional genetic anomalies and modern surgical procedures do provide us with remarkable hooters. European porn star Eve Lolo Ferrari was listed in the 1999 Guinness Book of Records as the record holder for heaviest breasts. After numerous implant surgeries, Lolo's mammaries weighed in at 6 pounds, 2 ounces each—and she wore a size 57F bra. Examples of even bigger breasts abound on the Internet, including a photo of a woman whose boobs reportedly weigh 44 pounds—each—and measure 33 inches around.

The practical element here? Elsewhere in this book, we say that breast size per se is no barometer of a woman's sexual interest or her desire to have you fuss over her bosom. While we stand by that advice, breasts this far over the top—especially when the woman has gone to great lengths to either make them that way or show them off in tight, skimpy fashions—suggest a certain exhibitionism and pride of ownership. At the very least, tell her that you find them attractive. It shouldn't be the first thing out of your mouth; but in bed, it's something you ought to mention early on. Which we're pretty sure you will.

Also see: breast enlargement, breast reduction, implants, media, size—breasts, va-va-voom

thongs

Decades ago, thongs were known as G-strings and were associated mainly with strippers. Today, they're wildly popular even among women who don't know the first thing about dancing around poles (not brass ones, anyway).

Victoria's Secret is evidence of this. The lingerie company sold 20 million thongs in 1999, 40 percent of all panty sales.

The reason for this is twofold. Thongs are sexy as hell to men (and women know it). Plus, they eliminate something that has become a cardinal sin in women's fashion: panty lines. Because the thong's material doesn't exit the anal cleft until high on her buttocks, you can't see it under tight-fitting clothes. Such is the stuff of daydreams.

Here's your 5-second gift-giving guide: The three most popular colors are black, white, and nude, in that order.

And who's to say you can't pick up a little something for yourself while you're shopping? Several menswear companies, such as Intimo and DKNY, have introduced rump-revealing undies in styles ranging from cotton plaid to velour tiger stripes. Granted, such a fashion statement is not for all of us (especially not for those of us who still wince at the memory of high school wedgies). But if you think about it, a thong is not really that much different from a manly jockstrap. And consider: One survey showed that women thought a good gluteus maximus was a more attractive masculine feature than height, chiseled abs, or a full head of hair. So if you've got it and you're inclined to flaunt it, odds are, your lady won't mind.

Also see: booty, boxers or briefs, crossdressing, lingerie, striptease, topless bar, underwear

threesome

Allow us to take a leap here. We bet you fantasize about getting it on with two women. Your theory? If one is good, two has to be better.

The good news: Turns out your girlfriend has the same theory.

The bad news: She means two *guys*.

This illustrates one of the fundamental problems couples face when turning this potent sexual fantasy into reality. For a threesome to work, you both must agree on the gender of the third party.

Strong emotions, including jealousy and envy, also threaten the threesome dynamic. It's a rare couple who can handle their relationship after they've shared each other sexually with someone else (and watched).

And some issues are bigger than simple jealousy. If you're uncomfortable with homosexuality, watching your partner touch a woman may fill you with unexpected disgust or fear. Worse, being naked and aroused in the general vicinity of another man may be too much for you to handle.

If any of these issues applies to you, it's okay to have a threesome in mind—just keep it right there.

Also see: bisexuality, group sex, heterosexuality, homophobia, homosexuality, jealousy, ménage à trois, swinging

thrush

Inside your mouth live millions of microorganisms in balanced domestic tranquillity. These little buggers include bacteria and fungi—which is probably more information than you wanted. They actually keep your mouth healthy, at least until something upsets their native balance. Then it's another story.

Take the fungus *Candida albicans* (the same one that causes yeast infections). It's usually kept in check by normal mouth bacteria. When those bacteria are depleted by an antibiotic or hormonal changes, you can get thrush, an oral infection in which white patches form on your tongue, gums, cheeks, and palate. You can also get thrush if your immune system is weakened by poor diet, diabetes, or even stress.

Though it happens rarely, you can even contract thrush from performing oral sex on a woman who has a yeast infection. Then you can pass the infection to other people through kissing, sharing silverware, or, say, licking the same lollipop.

Thrush may cause some pain, but it's usually not serious. Try making a soothing rinse by gargling ½ teaspoon of salt in 1 cup of warm water. Your doctor may prescribe an antifungal medication like nystatin (Mycostatin).

Also see: STDs, yeast infection

tickling

Remember when you were 13 and in lust with that girl in your class? She wouldn't give you the time of day. (Let's face it, looking back, would you have given

yourself the time of day?) So as an excuse to touch her, you furtively tweaked her waist as she passed by your locker. This caused her to smile and giggle, which caused you to . . . well, you remember.

Point being, you know the sensual power of the tickle. And just so you're *in* the know, obsessive tickling is considered a fetish by some. Indeed, there are quite a few Web sites and chat rooms devoted to tickling.

For the more conventional among us, tickling is still an excuse to touch. Think of it as a pre-sex icebreaker—the ensuing laughter helps you both loosen up. Once you're naked, run your fingertips, your tongue, or a feather duster along your partner's skin.

Still, tickling is fun only if she enjoys it. This is where things get complicated. It's tough to tell the difference between a touch that's a turn-on and one that's too much, because even when tickling doesn't feel good, the natural response is laughter. In the Middle Ages, warriors reportedly used prolonged tickling as a form of mortal torture.

Since this isn't the Middle Ages and torture probably isn't what you're aiming for, learn to read her signals. If she pushes your hands away *while* she's laughing or if her body language says she'd rather be almost anyplace else, we shouldn't have to tell you what to do. But we will, because we're know-it-alls: Kiss her and move on.

Oh, and since you're no longer 13, tickling a woman in order to cop a feel isn't really good form.

Also see: arousal, licking, lips, skin

357

time

A fleeting resource. You can't touch it, hold on to it, bank it, regain it once it's spent. Statistics show that the average man spends about 140 days of his life shaving. He whiles away 6.28 years attaining his 4-year bachelor's degree. For 8.17 hours a day, your typical working Joe is holed up in his office, to which he spends an hour commuting. He manages 1.3 hours of eating, 7.34 hours of sleeping, 53 minutes taking care of his personal hygiene (not nearly enough, according to some women), and about 1 hour surfing the Internet. In a mere 2.2 hours, he squeezes in his hobbies, his housework (that's not a misprint), and his social life. Which brings us to sex.

The average male U.S. resident spends 28.1 minutes having it, thus holding out longer than his counterparts in every other nation. The Thai guy, for example, lasts just 10.4 minutes. So if you know a Thai woman who seems chronically depressed, you now understand why.

Regardless of how long he spends getting there, the average guy enjoys a mere 6 seconds' worth of orgasm, the contractions themselves unfolding at precise 0.8-second intervals. (A woman, on the other hand, wriggles with delight for up to twice as long.) Oh, and if you're having that orgasm for family-building purposes, you should schedule it for around 6:00 A.M. That's when your sperm count is highest.

Also see: biological clock, ejaculation, frequency, marathon, orgasm—delayed, premature ejaculation, workaholism

time-saving tips

You can't figure it out: The two of you used to find ample time for making love, even when you worked till midnight. Now, as you crawl into bed together, you barely manage to mumble, "I love you" before falling into a deep

Hot Dates 1984 Bombings rocked more than 24 abortion clinics.

continued from page 353

Answer:
False. The Smithsonian says it has never possessed the penis. Nor has it been proven that Dillinger even had a massive member.

wallets while fondling the genitals of elderly men. Police said the woman bamboozled more than a dozen men between the ages of 60 and 83 by approaching them as they worked in their garages and asking for a light or a cigarette. When she was near them, **she'd rub their genies with one hand** while lifting their wallets with the other. If the men got suspicious, the woman would squeeze their lemons until she found her booty, police said.

Seemed like a Good Idea at the Time. . .
When the Ripley's Believe It or Not! museum in Buena Park, California, exhibited two Ivory Coast fertility statues in 1997, **13 women who touched the statues soon became pregnant**. This should've come as no surprise to Ripley Entertainment. Four years earlier, 13 Ripley staffers at the Orlando headquarters either became pregnant or gave birth during the

BAWDY BALLADS "Back Door Man," *the Doors*

continued on page 363

sleep. (That's if you even go to bed at the same time anymore.) You wake up disappointed that you didn't get any again last night, but there's no time to complain. You have another busy day ahead.

Among couples who've built a life together, finding time for sex is seldom a matter of cutting out a few TV programs or shortening a seven-course meal to a one-bowl dish. Most sex-starved couples have already trimmed their lives to the bare minimum: work, kids, necessary chores, quick eats, a few precious hours of sleep. Sex almost starts to seem like another chore to squeeze in, time permitting.

It's possible and practical to shift your priority back to sex and get your relationship back in balance.

• If the kids are the biggest issue, don't be afraid to send them off to grandma's house or to a trustworthy sitter. Your partner may be particularly skittish here. She shouldn't be. Kids think that time away from you is an adventure.

• Invest in a couple of wireless phones so you can call one another as you commute home from work. Talking about the dirty deeds you'd like to do will make the drive time pass more pleasantly and will make you eager to slither out of your clothes as soon as you step in the door. Also, you'll be able to alert one another to sudden openings in your schedules, thus paving the way for quickies.

• Start the festivities in public. We don't want you to get busted or written up in the next day's paper. But hey, remember the days when you were nearly thrown out of restaurants because you couldn't keep your hands off each other? The days when you never got to see the ends of any movies? Now you think you're too old to be so playful in public. That's a load of crap. Frolicking with your lover is an excellent way to avoid growing old.

• Also avoid the classic mistake of always waiting until after a late dinner to have sex. That mass of food reposing in your bellies is sure to send you straight to dreamland (or cause a lot of discomfort, if you do stay awake for the deed). Have sex before your meal. Just grab some quick carbohydrates for sustenance and energy—fruit sugars are ideal—and head straight for bed.

• Spend a weekend sequestered at home. Tell friends, bosses, mothers, and all those nosy neighbors that you're going away. Pull down the shades, lock the door, and get naked. Then you and your partner can spend 2 straight days eating strawberries with whipped cream between—or during—bouts of uninhibited sex.

Also see: afternoon delight, appointments, fatigue, kids, phone sex, public places, quickies, routines

toes

Even if you rolled your eyes at that toe-nail-polishing scene in *Bull Durham*, you might want to consider that toes are one of the body's most sensitive erogenous zones. And learning to navigate these zones is key to better sex.

Toes don't usually make it onto our foreplay maps. And for good reason. They can be pretty rank after a day spent in a sweaty pair of shoes or walking on a salty beach. But this uncharted erotic territory can be the ideal sexual prelude. It's starting foreplay from the ground up, so to speak.

Fill a basin with warm water. Remove your partner's shoes and socks (or hose), and soak her bare feet for a few minutes. Then, lather your hands with scented body gel or soap, and rub the suds over her feet, between her toes, and up her ankles—not just to get them clean but also to massage away stress. When you're finished, dry her feet in a warm towel.

We've heard that some women can climax just from a well-done toe massage. To find out if yours is one of them, lube your hands with lotion (peppermint is a cooling favorite) and stroke her feet and toes. Using moderate pressure, focus on her middle toe: It's supposed to have a direct nerve connection to more traditional erogenous zones.

Sucking a woman's toes is a lot like giving her good head: The pleasure comes from your exciting small bunches of nerves. So don't slobber all over her feet, and don't shove too many toes in your mouth at once. Suck or kiss each one gently, beginning with the smallest and working your way across one toe at a time. If you don't know what she likes, follow our familiar refrain: Listen and feel for signals. Still can't figure it out? Ask.

Some foot diseases are contagious and can even spread to your mouth. Athlete's foot is one of them. Be on the lookout for redness or cracked skin between her toes, an unusual odor, or telltale scratching. And it goes without saying, don't put your mouth on anything you can't identify as harmless, such as an open sore.

Also see: body odor—controlling, fetish, hygiene, licking, rashes, warts

tongue

Consider your tongue an integral part of sex, from opening line to orgasm. Without it to help articulate the words that make a woman want you, you'd never get to experience its multitude of erotic uses.

Covered from base to tip with keen sexual receptors and sensitive tastebuds, this muscular organ combines strength and sensitivity to lick and suck, taste and be tasted, tickle and caress. It provides its own warm, natural lubrication that feels good on bare skin. Along with lips, it's the purveyor of what many women consider the most sensual of sexual contacts: the kiss.

But user beware. She'll perceive your tongue to be something other than sensual if you use it too forcefully (think Kiss front man Gene Simmons) or don't keep it fresh.

Taking the second point first, please remember to brush your tongue along with your teeth. Even if she's one of those cool gals who just loves burgers, that doesn't mean she wants to partake of the raw onions and spicy sauce remaining on your tongue from the one you ate at lunch.

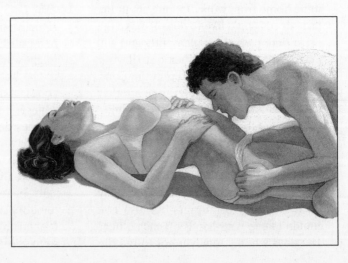

As for the first point, get her cues. A backed-away head during a kiss means, "Quit shoving it down my throat or I'll kill you." Likewise, a turned-away head when you're licking her ear says that she doesn't appreciate your slurpy probing. And if you're wondering what kind of action or pressure to use during oral sex, pay attention to the noises and movements she makes. Not sure you're hitting her sweet spot? Employ your tongue the most basic way possible: Ask her.

Also see: glans, performance anxiety, piercing, talking dirty, thrush, tickling

topless

Here's all you need to know about America's comfort level with naked breasts, even in this, the third millennium: In many states, it remains illegal for mothers to breastfeed their babies in public, regardless of whether their breasts are actually exposed. Law enforcement's reasoning? If women made a habit of being outside their homes without blouses, bras, camisoles, undershirts, or other layers of clothing securely covering them, we men—animals that we are—would be unable to control our impulses. Sex crimes would skyrocket.

Isn't it heartwarming that society has such faith in us?

Then again, think about how we tend to act upon encountering a pair of naked breasts (or even snugly clothed ones) in a public setting. We leer. We catcall. We say things we'd probably strangle some other guy for saying about our wives or kid sisters.

Where this really comes into play for you is if you travel abroad. Throughout most of Europe and Australia, female toplessness is ingrained in the culture; par-

ticularly on a beach, it's as natural for a woman to be topless as it is for a man. So if you vacation overseas, try to remember that women who go topless are not—we repeat, not—doing it just for your viewing pleasure. And they are *absolutely* not issuing a sexual invitation. They may be looking for full-body tans, or they may be making political statements. Or they may simply be more comfortable that way. In any case, if you go around spewing lewd or otherwise obnoxious comments, all you succeed in doing is making people uncomfortable and reinforcing the image of the ugly American.

Even here at home, in fact, the advice is much the same: If you find yourself on a topless beach, go ahead and enjoy. But keep your "clever" remarks to yourself. And what if your wife or girlfriend wants to go topless on a beach? First, find out if it's legal. Then, be sure you're okay with the ogling (and, potentially, the tasteless remarks) that *she'll* get from your brothers in gender.

Incidentally, while state and local "top-free" advocates pursue lawsuits that would give women the right to go topless at parks, beaches, and pools, fact is, most American women don't seem to want to bare their breasts in public. In a 1992 Gallup Poll, 93 percent of women surveyed said they wouldn't consider sunbathing topless on a public beach—legally or otherwise.

Also see: exhibitionism, nudism, ogling, outdoors, size—breasts, skin, travel as an aphrodisiac, va-va-voom

topless bar

The unofficial home office of Tony Soprano and his Mafia cronies. If only we could all work for a company with such an employee-friendly corporate culture.

Visits to strip joints have long been a point of contention between men and women. Try to look at it her way. If she gets the idea that you have a need to watch other women dance naked, she may feel insecure about her body and her ability to satisfy you. Worse, she may worry that your mind is still on the thong-strapped babe with a boob job when you're back home having sex with her. She may even think your ultimate hope is to someday be with a woman like that.

There are ways to ease her fears. Start by listening sympathetically when she voices her concerns. As we say many times in this book, this all-important aspect of good communication goes a long way in preserving and enhancing your relationship.

When you're all listened out, try sending her on a girls' night out to a club where men perform. After she and her friends spend an evening shoving dollar bills into the G-strings of lubed-up muscle-heads, maybe she'll see the fun of such entertainment and feel less threatened by it.

What's that? You say that's a bit more fun than you're ready for her to have? Okay, Hondo. Strip for her yourself. In a landmark survey, 81 percent of women described watching their partners undress as somewhat to very appealing. So she doesn't need Chippendales, nor for you to look like you could work at Chippendales, to enjoy a good bump and grind. (By the way, you do realize that your reluctance to let her partake of the same type of exotic entertainment that you enjoy makes you a big chauvinist hypocrite, right?)

If your partner is still adamantly against your frequenting such establishments, you're asking for trouble by sneaking off

to them anyway. Remember that women are generally welcome in topless bars. Invite your partner to join you; she might surprise you by accepting. If she does, she'll see that legitimate bars have no-touching rules and that dancers don't take customers home. She might even get ideas for new ways to turn you on. And believe it or not, lots of heterosexual women enjoy watching other women dance even more than they enjoy watching men.

We probably don't need to tell you this, but if you do go there together, never make audible comparisons between her and the dancers. Not unless you want to have to spend the rest of your evening reading the entry on *withholding*.

Of course, you could always just take the path of least resistance: Accept that your visits to nudie bars make her unhappy, and stop going. This is an especially effective tactic if her objections are based on a feminist opinion that strip clubs objectify and oppress women. You don't have to agree with her, but if you go to the clubs anyway, she'll hang that "big chauvinist" label on you again. And that will probably have a negative effect on how often you see *her* topless.

Also see: body image, jealousy, media, size—breasts, striptease, third-degree cleavage, voyeurism, wandering eye

touch

Believe it or not, there are women who actually think that every time you start touching them, you're trying to get into their panties. Imagine that!

Women do, in fact, love to be touched. But they need to be touched in ways that don't suggest you're merely trying to prod them into sex.

Call her silly, but a woman—especially one who thinks of herself as *your* woman—wants to believe that your sexual feelings toward her are secondary to your love for her. This is why it's important to familiarize yourself with areas of your partner's body besides her breasts and genitals. Touch her hair lightly. Brush her cheek with the backs of your fingers. Hold her face tenderly between your hands as you kiss her. Put your arm lightly around her waist as you approach to ask her a question. And don't be surprised if she's the one who starts steering you toward the bedroom.

Also see: body image, courtship, erogenous zones, sensate focus, skin, stimulation

toxic shock syndrome

A rare but potentially fatal infection caused by a strain of the *Staphylococcus aureus* bacterium that produces poisonous wastes. Toxic shock syndrome, or TSS, occurs most often when a woman uses tampons that are too absorbent for her menstrual flow or when she leaves a tampon in her vagina too long, but it can also be caused by a diaphragm, cervical cap, or contraceptive sponge. Any of these devices can allow *Staphylococcus aureus* to grow to levels higher than those normally found in the body and can act as a reservoir for the subsequent higher levels of toxins. Though it's not transmittable, men and children occasionally get TSS when the same toxins infect skin wounds and insect bites.

TSS is most dangerous when it's not caught early and treated as quickly as possible. Symptoms resemble those of the flu. If your partner develops the syndrome, she'll likely run a fever exceeding 102°F. She may act dizzy or spacey, or she may faint. As the syndrome progresses, she'll vomit, have diarrhea, and get a red rash mostly on the palms of her

Hot Dates **1987** The first condom ad appeared on TV. Between 1980 and 1986, annual condom sales soared from $182 million to $338 million.

continued from page 358

year that the statues worked their magic at that venue.

The statues have been shown in various cities worldwide. All told, more than 600 women have credited them with births. Believe it . . . or not.

Foreign Affairs
Roman men and women wore amulets or charms depicting a phallus. This was thought to **protect them against the evil eye**.

In Extremis
A man told Florida police that a woman armed with a knife forced her way into his car one afternoon, kidnapped him, **made him submit to oral sex**, and then forced him to sign a paper stating that he owed her money.

LEGAL BRIEFS
After several women phoned police regarding their suspicions about **a barber shop called Le Salon Sex**

True or Phallus?
Flip ("The devil made me do it!") Wilson had his penis surgically enlarged.

BAWDY BALLADS "Me So Horny," *2 Live Crew*

continued on page 370

hands and the soles of her feet. Eventually, she may go into shock.

The good news is that, when diagnosed and treated promptly, TSS can be cured with antibiotics.

toys

We love to play with 'em: our computers, our sound systems, our power tools, guns, and guitars. We fiddle with our fishing rods and, if we've had some luck in life, we polish our Porsches. We fondle our old, worn baseball gloves.

And, too often, we forget to fondle our women.

They often resent our playthings, and for good reason. Your partner may feel that she can't compete for your attention when her rival is a new Jet Ski or drum set. She may complain to her girlfriends that she could stand naked in the same room as you fiddle with your latest piece of video gear, and your only acknowledgment of her might be to blurt something like, "Uh, honey, could you move over a bit? You're in my light."

Now, we'd tell you to put down the video equipment and get involved with your woman's equipment, but we know that's not always going to cut it with you. So at the very least, as a sort of compromise, why not try including her in your life among gadgets? As long as she's standing there in the altogether, why not turn the camera on her?

Guys tend to think that their partners don't have much interest in changing guitar strings or cleaning shotguns. Wrong. Many women want to learn how to strum, and yes, shoot (if only to be able to take aim at you later, when they can't stand the boredom anymore). Give her a seminar on muscle-car maintenance, then invite her on a moonlight ride. And don't whine if she wants to adjourn to the backseat at some point.

Remember, there was a time when you couldn't take your eyes off her. Convince her that you can still summon that early ardor at least as often as you mess around with the new video game.

Also see: desertion, videos, workaholism

transvestism

Hard as this may be for you to take, some guys—perhaps even one of your own buddies from the softball team—enjoy dressing in frilly, silky getups; putting on lipstick; donning 6-inch heels; and cavorting about. Also called crossdressing, this behavior doesn't necessarily mean a guy is gay or dysfunctional. It merely means he gets satisfaction from feeling or looking feminine and, if he has the nerve to leave the house that way, being treated like a lady.

It can be hard to understand why a masculine man would want to go out on the town dressed like that. (And it's downright annoying to women when a transvestite looks better in panty hose than they do.) But look at it like this: Do we think twice when we see a woman in blue jeans and boots? In general, the guy who likes flowery dresses has no more of a sexual problem than the woman who wears flannel (keep your lesbian jokes to yourself, please).

Sometimes a man chooses to dress like a woman because his mother used to dress him like a girl and treat him like the daughter she wishes she'd had. She may have given him dolls to play with and let his hair grow unusually long. As an adult, then, he feels more relaxed and natural when he's wearing women's clothes. It's a comfort thing, with much the same motivation, no doubt, as that which prompts so many of us to constantly seek a return to the breast.

Occasionally, a transvestite turns out to be a guy who feels that he's a woman trapped in a man's body. That makes him a transgenderist. He may take female hormones in order to evolve more feminine characteristics. In extreme cases, he may undergo transsexual surgery.

Also see: androgyny, anima and animus, cross-dressing, drag, drag queen, fetish, gender bender, hermaphrodite, heterosexuality, homosexuality, phalloplasty, yin and yang

travel as an aphrodisiac

You whisk her away, and she tackles you the minute you step into a hotel room. At home, you're lucky if she climbs on top after you've spent an hour pawing her. What's up with that?

There's a two-part answer here. The first part is that travel frees a woman from her housewifely obligations. Usually, she's expected to be the good, efficient housekeeper; the perfect mother; and, if she works outside the home, the ideal employee. In a new environment, she's able to abandon herself to her more primal feelings—particularly to the sexual feelings that tend to get suppressed when she's obligated to, say, scrub green baby poop off the sleeve of her white sweater.

The second part of the explanation is that your woman is more naturally given to fantasy than you are. That's why she sits there spellbound by the latest of-

fering from Oprah's Book Club while you thumb through the Chilton manual trying to find the right plug gap for an Olds Cutlass Rocket 350. Travel piques her sense of escapism.

Don't fight it. Just budget a few extra bucks for some well-timed travel here and there. It'll give you both something to look forward to.

Also see: aphrodisiac, boredom, fantasies, planes, routines, sex tours and resorts, travel—planning

travel—loneliness during

You're in a strange city (or at least a different one) on business. You're pacing your drab, cookie-cutter hotel room, missing your honey and your kids, if you have them. But maybe you're also just a little bit turned on by the idea that somewhere in that very building is the quartet of comely flight attendants you met in the elevator on the way up.

Before you go back downstairs to the bar and wait for them to reappear, chew on this for a while: How would you feel if you found out your equally lonely wife was entertaining some guy she met in the local grocery store earlier this afternoon?

Doesn't feel too good now, does it, slick?

So how do you deal with travel-induced loneliness? Well, you could read a book or write a journal. Take a walk or work out. Start a hobby.

But you don't have much patience for crocheting. And how are you supposed to start a stamp collection when it's already 9:00 P.M. and the post offices are closed?

If you're going to be in the same location for a week or more, ask the concierge or a congenial front-desk clerk about any local tourist spots. You'd be surprised at some of the interesting haunts you'll find in even the most unlikely hick towns. Visit batting cages, bowling alleys, museums. Avoid bars. Liquor and loneliness are a bad combination.

As the days and nights away from home stretch on, be sure to maintain telephone contact with your partner—*contact* meaning more than "Hi, baby, it's me. Did you remember to pay the cable bill?" Make these calls as sensual as your comfort level allows. You and your woman can keep your sexual spirits alive by entertaining each other with detailed accounts of the activities you'd share if you were together at that moment.

If you're thinking, "Geez, that's only going to make me twice as horny," the solution is at hand. Maybe you and your beloved aren't quite up to full-blown phone sex, but it's something you might ease into on a trip-by-trip basis. And trust us, if things click and you wind up having sex on your respective ends of the line, you'll both feel a few precious moments of authentic physical closeness, despite the miles separating you.

One final tip: Even if you don't indulge in simultaneous masturbation, it's a good idea to do the deed after you hang up and before you venture out of the room again that evening. It'll take the edge off any temptation you might feel upon running into those damn flight attendants again.

Also see: affairs, lust, phone sex, travel ruins relationships, videos

travel—planning

It's a proven fact that a woman's level of horniness is directly proportional to the distance she happens to be from home. Clearly, then, you have a two-fold job: One, be with her when she journeys. And, two, pick a destination that enhances, rather than undermines, her natural inclinations.

First of all, stay away from phone deals. They can be disappointing and may include hidden fees and inconveniences such as slummy hotel rooms and a cattle-call atmosphere.

The Internet may be a good place to purchase airline tickets, but again, you seldom have a comprehensive idea of what you're getting into when you reserve rooms or tours on a Web site. Some of the better travel sites offer virtual tours where you can get a 360-degree idea of the "typical" accommodations, the views, the amenities. Still, what do you expect them to put online: that room out back by the horse barn? Or the presidential suite? Use common sense. For our money, and yours, your best bet is to visit a good old-fashioned travel agent. He or she has real-world experience to offer and can separate the deals from the dumps.

Travel agents need your help to plan your ideal trip, of course. You have to tell them where you want to go—and be a bit more specific than "Someplace warm"—as well as what activities your woman enjoys and what kind of ambiance she prefers: A woman who adores the coziness of a Victorian B&B will absolutely despise the steel-and-glass sleekness of a contemporary resort. (And by the way, *B&B* stands for "bed-and-breakfast," for those of you who are truly romance-impaired.)

Try to recall the articles in your partner's travel magazines that made her swoon in getaway desire. What about her other tastes? Does she love flowers? Mountain vistas? Ocean surf? Cacti in full bloom? City life? Woods and trails? Where did she grow up? Does she remember it fondly? Or could she not get the hell out of there fast enough? All of these bits of background knowledge should figure in your getaway preplanning.

And never overlook the appeal of the offbeat. We know a woman who admitted to going orgasmic when her husband took her on a N'Awlins voodoo-and-vampire tour. Another flipped for tickets to a couples dance workshop in Brazil.

New Orleans? Brazil? Sound a bit too ambitious for your wallet? Don't worry. Chances are, she'll be touched by any sort of getaway that shows you put some time and effort into it. Touched, and aroused.

Also see: appointments, atmosphere, romance, sex tours and resorts, travel as an aphrodisiac

travel—returning from

When it comes to sex, the day you get home from a lengthy business trip can be just as difficult as the day you left. In all likelihood, you're ready to ravish your wife the moment you walk in the door, if not at baggage claim. She, though, may be slower to welcome you back into her arms . . . and her other parts.

A woman often needs a day or two to reconnect with her lover. After a period of absence, she wants to be reassured about the relationship and get a chance to settle back into it. (This is not necessarily any reflection on whether your relationship is solid. It's just another one of those woman things.) Start off gingerly, with hugs, kisses, soft touches—in other words, tenderness, not groping. Take your cue from her. She'll let you know if and when she's eager for sex. And don't worry; if you've been together for more than a few weeks, you won't miss the signals.

That said, the coolness shouldn't last for more than 2 days. This, in fact, is a good way to gauge the effect of travel on the relationship. If, after your second day home, she's still pulling back (or maybe you are?), and this seems to be a chronic pattern following travel, you may want to reconsider whether your relationship is up to the emotional rigors of regular separation. A lot of otherwise-good relationships aren't.

Maybe you can arrange for your lover to travel with you. Or if worse comes to worst, you can always look for other employment. A soul mate is harder to find than a job.

Also see: communication

travel ruins relationships

When work separates you from your woman for weeks at a time, expect a certain strain on your relationship. And let's get one thing cleared up pronto: It doesn't matter that you think she's the most understanding woman in the world, a woman who supports your career 100 percent. Unless she's also the most unusual woman in the world, to some degree she's going to feel frustrated by your travel. It's in the blood. Face it, accept it, and deal with it.

Yes, she knows you love her. That doesn't mean she can handle going days on end without hearing from you. And it doesn't mean she's content with being squeezed into a 2-minute phone call from the airport before you board your connecting flight.

Nor does it matter that you're on legitimate business. Trust us here: She doesn't like the idea that you're in a strange city, out at night, in an environment that may very well involve (a) alcohol, (b) music, and (c) attractive female business associates. She sees it all as a bad combination. If the situation were reversed, maybe you would too. If your job requires you to attend business dinners or other meetings in the evening, there's nothing wrong with stealing away for a moment, most likely when you visit the john, to call your woman and let her know you're thinking about her, missing her, looking forward to seeing her again. No, this isn't the same thing as phoning her quickly from the airport. Even if the call lasts only a minute or two, she likes being a part of your evening. It helps settle her mind about what you're really up to out there.

We know what you're thinking: "But she should trust me, dammit." Yeah, and pepperoni pizza should be fat-free. Especially early in a relationship, it doesn't hurt to *demonstrate* to her that she can trust you. You achieve this by being where you said you were going to be and by including her as much as possible in your away-from-home itinerary. So always give her your contact numbers at the hotels where you're staying. When you talk to her, tell her—before she asks—about your day.

Oh, and never, ever rave to your wife about some female co-worker who's on the trip with you, not even if you're just talking about what a wonderful spreadsheet presentation this colleague made on the Bloomquist account. What your

wife thinks is "My husband is excited about another woman."

She doesn't see spreadsheets. She sees hotel-room sheets.

Also see: communication, jealousy, travel—loneliness during, trust—rebuilding, workaholism

trick

There are two related meanings here. One is a guy who patronizes a prostitute, also known as a john. The other is any given prostitutorial encounter with a john, as in, "Lola turned 11 tricks last night before her vagina fell out."

Also see: brothels/bordellos, escort services, john, prostitution

trophy wife

A luscious babe—often very blonde, sometimes constructed of silicone and cosmetics—with a wealthy, usually older, husband. In general, a trophy wife is not a man's first wife but rather a late-arriving accoutrement he attains as he climbs the ladder of success. Think Marla Maples.

We'll assume that most of you reading this aren't The Donald, but still, there comes a point in your life—maybe around 45 or 50—when you're financially comfortable. Maybe the magic goes out of your life with the woman who's been your companion all those years. And maybe you get attention from cute, younger women at the office. And you start to wonder, "Hmmm. . . . What would it be like to pull a Michael Douglas and hook up with a Catherine Zeta-Jones?"

While you're lingering over that fantasy, here are a few reality checks.

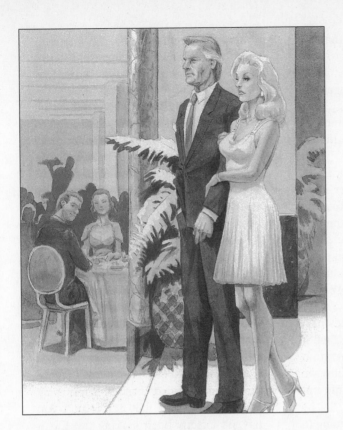

along with the joke. Just don't kid yourself. In the end, that's probably how they perceive your latest conquest: as a joke. "So, I see Ted went out and bought himself a wife. . . ." It may seem unfair, but if you have some money and she has some looks, that's how it will be.

All that said, well, if you're just lucky enough to fall in real, true love with a drop-dead gorgeous woman who's also a dynamic lover and a sensitive sweetheart—in other words, if the fundamentals of a good, honest relationship are all in place—damn the torpedoes. Go for it.

Also see: bimbo, midlife crisis, politicians, power, size—wallet, young women/older men

• Realize that you want to share your life with someone who loves *you*, not the size of your 401(k).

• Realize that young women, trophies or not, are going to hear the alarms on their biological clocks. Will you really be up for that?

• Realize that if you have to dump your existing wife in order to effect this change, it's going to cost you, maybe big-time. A woman scorned, and all that.

• Realize that most people, especially friends who enter midlife along with you, are not going to be impressed by a big-breasted young thang. Sure, they may wink and elbow you on the golf course, making sly references about how hot the sex must be, going

trust—rebuilding

If the so-called experts agree on little else, they agree on this: The most important element in a relationship (and if you're thinking "big jugs," please put the book aside for now and come back when you're ready to be serious) is trust. Lovers need to feel assured that their partners will remain honest and faithful. Without that knowledge, that trust, a healthy relationship cannot survive.

Let's assume, however, that some regrettable dalliance has broken the trust between you. You're both devastated by the betrayal, but you want to salvage the relationship, which entails rebuilding the trust.

Couples commonly assume that it's acceptable for the hurt partner to take on the role of avenger, to flog the offender with a steady stream of anger and loathing. The guilty party—okay, let's say it's you—must then grovel and beg until the wronged party feels adequately recompensed.

What we're about to say sounds self-serving, but it's true: Your partner's role as the One Who Seeks Great Retribution is just as destructive as the piggish behavior that provoked it. Yes, you must admit your mistake and take full responsibility for damaging the relationship. But yes, she must take responsibility for her part as well. For example, she may have inspired your faithlessness by withholding affection. This, in fact, is an all-too-common complaint that drives both husbands and wives into the beds of people whose names do not appear on their marriage licenses. So, by refusing to forgive you and continuing to rebuff you, the woman merely perpetuates the behavior that, just perhaps, contributed to your indiscretion in the first place.

The road to recovery is paved with a willingness on the part of both of you to relinquish your black-and-white postures of criminal and victim and begin instead a period of total honesty. Not about the gory details of the disloyalty itself but about the ways you feel about your relationship and each other. Though this may go against your natural instincts, you need to stand up for yourself in the face of her anger. Your profound sorrow and regret is one thing; your willingness to let her treat you poorly is another.

If the rift was indeed an affair, explain why you chose to sleep with another woman, even if it means admitting to your own woman that she hasn't been turning you on lately. She may retort that you haven't exactly been making the Earth

---

Hot Dates | **1980s** With sex just a phone call away, scores of Americans let their fingers do the walking. One phone sex company received 500,000 calls a day.

continued from page 363

Answer:
True. Wilson claimed that he went under the knife because his member got worn down from overuse. He displayed his new and improved model to people on Howard Stern's radio program.

Symbol, the cops initiated a 2-month probe. They arrested eight people at the hair lair, where they said stylists regularly stripped, performed exotic dances, and talked dirty as they cut customers' hair. The owner of the shop was caught naked with a client, playing with a sex toy. It turned out that one of the men who was arrested really was in the shop just to get a haircut. "They have a few clients who go just for that," a police spokesman said.

Seemed like a Good Idea at the Time. . .
One morning in San Antonio, folks working in a courthouse watched a carnival freak show that was better than anything the paying customers saw.

Atop the carnival's giant slide, a couple of carnies had sex, unaware that people could see them from the nearby courthouse. As word of the carnies' copulation spread, courthouse employees scrambled for

---

BAWDY BALLADS | "Dick Almighty," *2 Live Crew*

continued on page 379

move under her feet, either. Or she may give you a host of other reasons why she's lost interest, some of them having nothing to do with the bedroom, per se. ("You never listen to me when I talk" is a common one.)

No question, such conversations will spark a great deal of pain. The upside is, at least they get to the root of the problem that's putting distance between you. That's the only way to work toward a solution, the only way to ensure that it won't happen again. It's the only way to rebuild the trust.

Also see: affairs; communication; discretion; divorce—avoiding; Don't ask, don't tell; extramarital sex; intimacy; jealousy; love; marriage; remarriage; secrets; travel ruins relationships; wife's best friend; withholding

tubal ligation

This permanent form of contraception is actually the surgical sterilization of a woman via the blockage of her fallopian tubes.

If you and your partner choose to go this route, pay special attention to the word *permanent* above. Reversal is a very difficult, costly undertaking. Some doctors refuse to perform tubal ligation unless a woman has reached a certain age—typically 30—and has already given birth to at least three children.

The process itself is relatively simple. A surgeon stitches closed and then cuts the fallopian tubes. Thus, your sperm can no longer reach her eggs. The technique is 99 percent effective in the year following the surgery. In the years that follow, there is a small chance that the fallopian tubes will reconnect on their own. Annually, 1 in 100 women get preg-

nant after undergoing this procedure. And of the pregnancies that occur after tubal ligation, one in three will develop in a fallopian tube, as an ectopic pregnancy, and may require emergency surgery.

Simple though it may be, surgery is still surgery, and there are possible complications, such as internal bleeding or infection, injury to adjacent organs, or a serious adverse reaction to the anesthesia. Even in the best case, a woman will feel a fair amount of pain for days to weeks afterward. Emotional complications are also possible—as you may learn if you become involved with a relatively young divorcée who had her tubes tied during her marriage but now decides she'd like to have a child with you.

Also see: contraception, ectopic pregnancy, fallopian tubes, vasectomy

turn-offs

Maybe you can't understand why your partner isn't interested in resuming her riding position after a phone call interrupts the action. After all, the call was brief enough. You were gone for 10 minutes, tops. Hell, you're still hard. So why does she roll away rather than climb aboard?

Could it be that she's offended by the fact that you took the call in the first place? Or by the fact that—while you thought maybe it was your boss calling about that important account—it turned out to be your ex-girlfriend?

As any guy who's gone on more than two dates knows entirely too well, there are dozens of things we do that turn women off. Unfortunately, most of this happens beneath our radar: We don't even know we're doing it, and when they point it out to us—something they love doing—we're, like, shocked. "What? I can't scratch my balls at dinner? Geez, it was under the table and all. And your mother was preoccupied with carving the turkey. . . ."

Lots of these problems have to do with what might graciously be called a disconnect in the way men and women regard the homes they share. Maybe a man's home is his castle, but your queen doesn't like you soiling the moat or leaving the drawbridge up. The sight of your filthy, smelly socks under the kitchen table is not going to make her ravenous for sex.

So, too, in the bathroom: She doesn't want to see your beard remnants scattered all over the sink. And hey, believe us when we say we're in your corner, but flush the damn toilet. Each and every time. Okay?

Even more important than keeping the lavatory clean is washing yourself. All over. Especially if you're expecting head. If she does go down on you, don't yank her around by the ears. . . . You're sick of hearing this? Then tell all the other guys you know to stop doing it, because women still complain about it in droves.

Once you're well-scrubbed, remember that a woman generally expects a seduction to amount to more than "Uh, wanna screw?" Yes, even when she wants it too. If she's in the mood for a quickie, she'll let you know about it, have no fear.

She'll also let you know if she's not in the mood at all because she's still pissed at you for something you did or didn't do earlier. Sorry, but makeup sex is a mis-

nomer. In most cases, you should attempt it only *after* the issue has been settled and apologies have been offered and accepted. You do not delight a woman by graciously offering her the pleasure of your erection in recompense for your previous sins. You just start a brand-new fight.

If it's kinkiness you're after, don't expect to achieve it by telling her that your regular bedroom routine leaves you cold. This makes her feel very inadequate. Say instead, "I heard about this activity, and I thought you'd be very sexy doing it." Or just pick out something we discuss in this book, and bring it to her attention.

Don't ask, "Did you come?" It's annoying if she did, and it puts pressure on her if she didn't. Just ask her sweetly if she'd like you to keep going.

While you're being sweet, make sure any compliment you give her is really a compliment. We actually know a living, breathing guy who enthusiastically told his wife, "Honey, you don't look nearly as fat in that new hairstyle!"

Also see: arguing, beard burn, begging, body odor—controlling, boredom, breast pain, breath, clumsiness, communication, desperate, farting, guilt, hangups, hygiene, job loss, Madonna/whore complex, marriage—lack of sex in, masher, micropenis, midlife crisis, monotony, no, ogling, pee—bloody, premature ejaculation, rashes, rejection—romantic, rejection—sexual, rug burn, scratching, sex—lack of, shyness, sickness, smegma, smoking, spectatoring, STDs, stress, sweating, talking dirty, teasing, topless bar, unwanted advances, violence, wandering eye, wet spot, workaholism

turn-ons

Turn-ons are as individual as your woman herself. What gets your gears revving may just seize her motor.

Understanding what turns her on is an exploration into the myriad aspects of sexuality. And that's what you'll find throughout this book, listed under a fistful of entries.

Also see: aphrodisiac, atmosphere, body odor as an attractant, communication, dressing for bed, dressing you to look sexy, erogenous zones, fantasies, fetish, flirtation, food, foreplay, kiss, laughter, male body, masturbation, music, pornography, power, public places, quickies, romance, rough sex, seduction, self-esteem, sexual aids, sexual attraction, sexy, shaving, smiling, stimulation, striptease, sweating, taboos, threesome

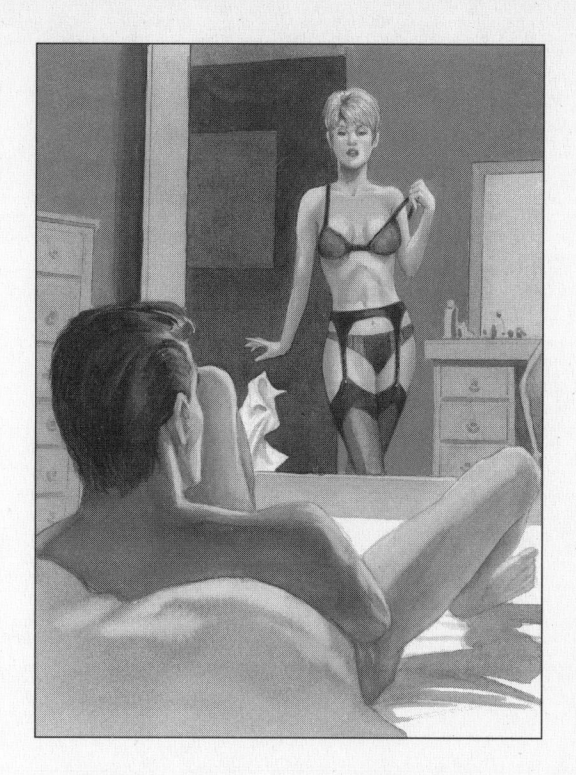

T

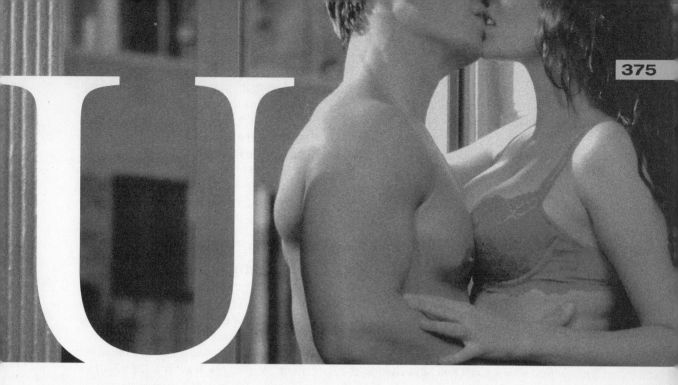

underage

She struts into your house in a leather skirt that barely covers her backside and a blouse with a neckline that dips almost low enough to meet the skirt. You don't have to study her very long to know she's wearing one of those bras that's not quite a bra. Her makeup is carefully, seductively applied. She smiles at you, parts those perfect, pouty, glistening lips, and says, "Hi, Mr. Slobotnik. Is Jenna, like, ready?"

She's your daughter's best friend. She's 13. And you're suddenly more sympathetic than ever to the quandary your single friends face.

Drive past any high school in America, and you'll see flocks of girls approximating the above description. They paint their faces to disguise their children's features. They strut around in daring stiletto heels. They make you think thoughts you can't believe you'd think, despite your best efforts to regard them as just kids.

Today's teens and preteens are growing up fast. Say what you will about the judgment of parents who let their kids out that way, the bottom line is, it can be damn hard to tell a sexy 13-year-old from a woman of legal age. Throw in the fact that many of them carry around fake IDs, and you have the makings of a life-altering mistake.

Most states draw the line at 18, the so-called age of consent. Intercourse with a woman younger than that—no, let's get it right, a *girl* younger than that—can land you in jail for statutory rape. Even if the encounter was completely consensual. Even if she made the first move, which a fair number of these nymphs are fully prepared to do. Oh, and if an excursion that culminates in sex takes you across state lines, congratulations, you have just committed a federal crime.

Following are a few pointers for getting a more reliable handle on a woman's age.

• Be aware of time limits that sound like curfews. Does she have all sorts of reasons for wanting to end the date early? Could be that it's a school night, and Mommy and Daddy have told her to be back by 10:00 P.M. or else.

• Draw her out about her past: her schooling, her job experiences, and so forth. Try as much as possible to get a time context from her—"Oh, so you graduated from college in '97?"—and then ask yourself (a) whether she seems to stumble through it and (b) whether it all adds up.

• Try to maneuver yourself into a situation where you'll meet her friends, especially male friends. This can be a dead giveaway because guys have a much harder time hiding their youth. Remember what you looked like at 13? Would anyone have mistaken you for 23?

• Explore her tastes in music. What does it tell you when her car is full of CDs by the Backstreet Boys and Britney Spears?

• If you have the slightest doubt about whether she's "legal," don't have sex with her. You're better off going without for a night than telling a jury why you shouldn't go to prison.

Also see: Lolita, pedophilia, young women/older men

underwear

If you're too busy wondering what she's wearing under her dress to think about the condition of your own skivvies, know this: A woman judges your fitness for sex, at least in part, by the appearance of your underwear.

When you expect to undress in front of a woman, you should avoid wearing undeniably *un*sexy undergarments, be they saggy, baggy, dingy, dirty, torn, gray, or worst of all, smelly. Heed us well, or it may be the last time you get to get naked in front of her.

Also see: boxers or briefs, dressing for bed, dressing you to look sexy, fig leaf, hygiene, lingerie, thongs

undressing

From our perspective, this tends to be a nonissue. The prevailing mentality is "Just get out of those damn clothes and we'll take it from there. . . ."

Women don't see it in quite the same light. And if the way you undress her doesn't gibe with the circumstances or the mood, you get things off on the wrong foot.

Helping her unclothe herself doesn't always mean going slow. If she's not wearing her favorite dress, she may be just as likely as you are—well, almost as likely as you are—to want it quick and even a little forceful. Don't purposely tear fabric, but don't be all that careful about it, either. And don't worry about getting her tangled up in her clothes: That has a certain fiery sexuality all its own. Just be prepared to replace anything you actually rip.

The quickie-minded woman may find it extremely sexy if you leave most of her clothes *on.* Just get yourself out of your pants, get her underpants out of the way, get under her skirt, and get to it.

Generally, though, slow is the most sensual and seductive speed for disrobing a woman. Take your time removing each inch of each garment, luxuriously caressing the skin below with your fingertips, lips, and tongue. Yes, this demands a certain amount of physical maneuvering—leaning and kneeling and contorting yourself around her as needed to reach each newly exposed area of flesh. She won't think you look foolish. And you'll like the response you get.

Creativity is a plus. You can open zippers and pull down panties with your teeth. You can each take turns removing one another's shirts and socks as you enjoy an almost excruciatingly drawn-out session of foreplay.

Herewith, let us share *the* key point about undressing yourself: The socks come off before the pants. There's nothing less sexy to a woman than the sight of you standing there buck naked except for a pair of black dress socks (unless it's you standing there buck naked except for a pair of striped sweat socks). Okay, maybe there's one other thing: when you're obsessive about where your clothes end up. What do you expect her to think as she waits there nude and ready while you carefully fold and hang your garments? We'll tell you what she's thinking: "LOSER." (And yes, she's thinking it in all capital letters.) Even if you're not all that smooth about integrating undressing into your sexual repertoire, don't ever turn your back on a naked woman to brush lint off your coat and tie.

Also see: boxers or briefs, dressing her to look sexy, dressing you to look sexy, foreplay, lingerie, quickies, striptease

unwanted advances

It's the stuff of romantic comedies: A guy is attracted to a woman who's not the least bit interested. He spends the entire film either secretly pining for her or pleading for just one date. After 2 hours or months or years of this (in movie time), he finally gives up, a beaten man. Whereupon, due to some magical serendipitous circumstances, she falls into his arms, realizing they were meant for each other all along. They live happily ever after.

Unfortunately, this happens only in Hollywood. In the real-world version of the same scenario, you get fed up with being ignored or rebuffed so often, or she gets fed up with your coming around so much. Or maybe she meets somebody else and gets married before she has a chance to realize that you're Mr. Right.

Which brings us back to these advances. So how often do you make a move? When does no mean no?

We're told these days that no always means no, but you know better. For instance: You offer to buy a woman a drink. She says, "No, thank you. I'm really sorry; I'm seeing someone." But she says it in a forlorn way that seems to imply she's really sorry that she's seeing someone. It's a classic mixed message. You wonder whether there's a chance she'll say yes, with a bit more coaxing. So you hang around for a while and casually strike up a conversation. She doesn't seem to mind the company.

What do you do next? And what don't you do?

You don't become a pest. (She did turn you down once, after all.) Perhaps the most face-saving tactic at this point is to tell her you're available if she ever wants to get to know you better. Either say that explicitly or drop hints about how she can find you: not just where you work but also social places that you visit. If you have a business card, this is the time to give it to her. Then tell her you've enjoyed talking to her, and leave.

If a woman doesn't call you or return your messages, that's a pretty clear signal that she's not interested. Sometimes. There are women who just do not call guys. It goes against some sort of programming, or maybe they just read that book *The Rules* one too many times. In any case, understand that there really are women—nice ones—who'll let a perfectly good relationship slip away simply because they've been taught that the man is supposed to take the initiative.

If you do manage to reach her by phone, try the following: "Look, I really like you. I don't want to just go away. But if I'm bugging you, let me know, and I won't call again." If she gives you no opening whatsoever at this point, put her behind you and move on. Bear in mind that many states have stalking-via-telephone statutes.

Also see: begging, date rape, desperate, masher, no, opening line, pickup lines, rejection—romantic, sexual innuendo

urethra

A tube, about 20 centimeters long, that runs from the neck of your bladder to the pinhole at the tip of your penis. The urethra serves double duty: It carries urine out of your body and also serves as the route that semen follows on its way to ejaculation.

Also see: cystitis, ejaculation, labia majora and minora, pee after sex, pee—painful, reproductive system—yours, short-arm inspection, NSU, urinary problems

urethritis

Inflammation of the urethra, usually caused by a bacterial or fungal infection. Chemical irritations and sexually trans-

mitted diseases such as gonorrhea and chlamydia can also cause irritation and swelling of the urethra.

If you notice a clear, milky, or creamy substance dripping from your penis, if you have pain when you pee or ejaculate, or if there is blood in your semen, you may have urethritis. Other common symptoms are a sore groin and swollen testicles.

If an infection is irritating your tube, your doctor usually can cure it with an antibiotic. However, some men with urethritis who go untreated for too long experience strictures, which occur when the urethra narrows in a spot, causing a slow stream of urine or a constant urinary drip. It's no picnic, either way. To relieve this condition, a doctor has to insert thin metal rods into the penis or cut through the strictures with an endoscopic knife. All of which leads us to this advice: See your doctor as soon as you notice any symptoms.

Also see: NSU, STDs

urinary problems

An umbrella term for a variety of conditions involving the urinary tract, which is made up of the kidneys, ureters, bladder, and urethra. The most common disorders affecting men include urinary tract infections and obstructions. In older men in particular, incontinence and prostate enlargement tend to become more common. Alas, more to dislike about aging.

Urinary tract infections (UTIs) affect millions of men each year; only respiratory infections are more common. You may not have realized that they're so prevalent, because infections in individual organs have different names: an infection of the urethra is called ure-thritis, a bladder infection is cystitis, and a kidney infection is pyelonephritis.

UTIs usually stem from a urinary blockage caused by an enlarged prostate, a kidney or bladder stone, or a medical procedure involving a catheter. As a re-sult of the blockage, your body can't flush out bacteria and other microorganisms the way it normally would when you pee. The result is an overgrowth of these nasty buggers that causes an infection.

Symptoms usually include cloudy or reddish urine, a painful burning sensation during urination, and the need to go fre-quently and urgently. The good news is that most infections can be taken care of with antibiotics. (By the way, women also get these infections, and they can be transmitted sexually. So if you or your partner has one, it's a good idea to steer clear of sex until the UTI has cleared up.)

Urinary obstructions can wreak havoc in more ways than those we describe above, especially if the blockage is a kidney stone. Roughly one in seven men will develop a kidney stone in his life-time. A stone occurs when substances in the urine form small, hard crystals that prevent urine from passing through the urethra. The feeling of a stone passing through your urinary tract can be excru-ciating (some folks liken it to the pain of childbirth). While most guys are able to pass stones on their own, stubborn cases require medical intervention. And once you've had a stone, you also have a fifty-fifty chance of a recurrence. Some easy preventive measures? Drink lots of fluids, cut back on meat and salt, and eat foods high in potassium, such as baked potatoes, bananas, cantaloupe, and steamed clams.

We know. Just reading this entry is painful in and of itself. And we're not done yet. Although rare, bladder cancer is a particular concern for guys, affecting three times more men than women. Aside from problems urinating, the hall-mark symptom is blood in the urine. The most important way to help prevent it? Quit smoking. Your body gets rid of

U

Hot Dates **1989** AIDS was the second-leading cause of death among men between the ages of 25 and 44. The virus killed more men in this age group than did heart disease, cancer, suicide, or homicide.

continued from page 370

choice spots by the windows, cheering and applauding the show (and you thought justice was blind). When the lovemaking was finished, the woman dressed and slid down the slide to even more cheers.

One local judge, who apparently has yet to develop the wisdom of Solomon, wondered why **no one had called the sheriff's department**, lo-cated right in the courthouse.

Foreign Affairs
The unkindest cut: The Skopzis, members of an 18th-century Chris-tian sect that began in Russia, urged male followers to castrate them-selves. They believed that **Jesus was sent to castrate men**, thereby making it impossible for them to sin. The sect's leader castrated himself by baptism with a red-hot iron and convinced others to follow suit.

True or Phallus ?
In Philip Roth's 1969 novel *Portnoy's Complaint*, Portnoy masturbates with an apple pie.

BAWDY BALLADS "Get Up (I Feel like Being a) Sex Machine," *James Brown*

continued on page 388

cancer-causing smoke toxins via urine. If you smoke, your bladder literally soaks in these chemicals.

Prostate cancer is the second leading cause of cancer deaths in men, with one in five Americans developing it.

Okay, we've saved the best for last. Six million men in the United States suffer from incontinence, or lack of bladder control. Causes include a weak bladder muscle, an enlarged prostate, nerve injuries, surgery, and diseases like diabetes. Cold medications, antidepressants, and muscle relaxants can also affect your urinary control.

If you have any problems urinating or experience any of the symptoms listed above, be sure to consult with your doctor as soon as possible. Take it from us, this stuff isn't anything to fool around with.

Also see: cystitis, prostate cancer, prostate enlargement, prostatitis

urologist

You should be very familiar with your local urologist by the time you reach the age of 50. Plan to meet with him at least once a year for digital rectal exams and prostate-specific antigen screens to check for prostate cancer, the leading cancer in men. A urologist isn't someone to fear. He's actually a hero of sorts: the guy we turn to for help in steering clear of problems with our reproductive parts before they turn catastrophic.

Aside from giving you annual prostate exams, your urologist can help you cope with erectile difficulties and premature ejaculation. He can also treat kidney stones, urinary tract infections, sexually transmitted diseases, tumors, testicular trauma, and other troubles in the male genital region.

One situation that definitely calls for a trip to the urologist, even if you otherwise feel fine, is when you spot blood in your urine. It could have relatively benign causes, but it could also be a sign of something serious. Don't take the chance.

Also see: erection difficulties, erection—firmer, menopause—yours, pee—bloody, pee—painful, penile cancer, penile enlargement, Peyronie's disease, phalloplasty, premature ejaculation, priapism, prostate cancer, prostatectomy, prostate enlargement, prostatitis, reproductive system—yours, sperm count, STDs, testosterone replacement therapy, urinary problems, vasectomy, vasectomy reversal

uterus

The fabled womb, where embryos develop into infants. This hollow, triangular, muscular organ weighs a little more than 1 ounce and is normally about the size of a plum. It lies suspended in the center of her pelvis, between her rectum and bladder.

Its muscularity is a double-edged sword: The same tendency to spasm that intensifies her orgasms also figures in her menstrual cramps as well as in the legendary, wracking pain of childbirth. To imagine the strength of uterine contractions powerful enough to expel a 5- to 10-pound baby through a 10-centimeter opening, think of the effort it would take to push a bowling ball through a 4-inch-wide fire hose. (Then go thank your mom.)

Throughout a woman's menstrual cycle, her uterus fills with blood and other fluids, preparing to nourish a fertilized egg. Most months, conception doesn't happen, so the uterus sheds these fluids. Pregnancy, however, brings about a thickening of the layers of the uterus. The organ's walls also take on a greater blood supply with which to nurture the tiny fetus.

Also see: abortion, cramps—menstrual, ectopic pregnancy, hysterectomy, IUD, pituitary gland, pregnancy, progesterone, reproductive system—hers, womb

uterus—tipped

The fundus, or top portion of the uterus, usually points forward, toward the bladder. In about one-quarter of women, however, it's tilted backward at about a 45-degree angle. A tipped uterus seldom creates any sexual problems (although some women complain about pain when the penis rubs against the cervix).

Also see: size—penis

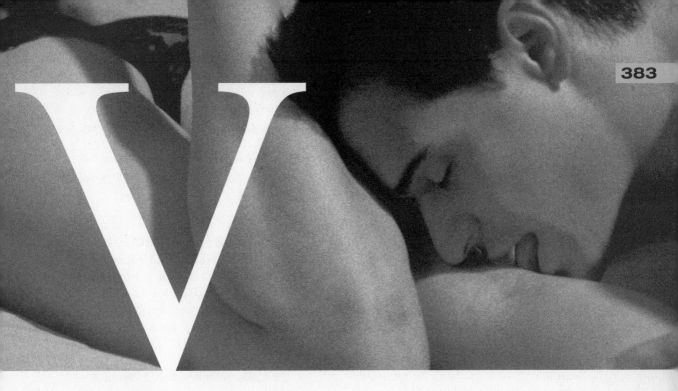

V

vacuum devices

Ever since man's first encounter with fellatio, he's been looking for a way to experience the same sensation even when there isn't a willing woman handy. Enter vacuum devices: pumps and sleeves that provide pleasurable penis sucking. They can also serve as erection aids for those times when willy isn't quite willing.

A pump is simply a tube from which the air is pulled out while your penis is inside. You get a pleasant tugging feeling. A vacuum sleeve is slightly different. It's not as rigid, and it sheathes your penis, rather than surrounding it like a tube. Similar to a blood pressure arm cuff, this toy has a pressure balloon that pumps it up. Some sleeves are made of firm plastic, while others—such as the Good Vibrations Cyberskin Sleeve—are crafted from a soft material that closely resembles skin.

You don't have to slide the sleeve up and down your shaft (thankfully); just hold it stationary with one hand while you use the other to pump. The fruit of your efforts resembles an untiring blowjob. Some vacuum sleeves vibrate as they slurp; others are coated with soft, flexible, fingerlike strands that add an extra tickle.

One word of caution: Just because these systems operate by vacuums, that doesn't mean any old vacuum device will do. One unfortunate fellow from New Jersey found that out the hard way: He almost bled to death when he tried to attach *his* hose to the part of the vacuum cleaner body where you normally attach *its* hose. Little did he suspect that the machine had a whirring blade hidden just out of sight. Its presence was made evident when it lopped off the top half-inch of his penis.

Neither will the long hose of a shop vac suffice. The vacuum is too powerful and can burst blood vessels and bruise your penis.

Also see: horny, penis pump, sexual aids

vagina

Ah, the vagina. Source of endless bewilderment, amazement, and many a good locker room joke. And the ultimate in female symbolism.

But don't get too caught up in the idea of a vagina as a symbol of womanliness—you have one too. Yes, you read right. It's called the *vagina masculina*, or male vagina. It could have been a "real" one, but when you were bouncing around in your mother's womb, testosterone kicked in and turned you into a boy. But your vagina is still there, a piece of tissue dangling uselessly from your bladder. And your would-be hymen is by your prostate.

If you don't have access to someone else's vagina these days, you're not alone. Throughout history, men have found creative ways to satisfy sexual longings when actual women's vaginas were unavailable. For example, imprisoned heterosexual men often turn to their fellow prisoners. The landmark studies by sex researcher Alfred Kinsey found that 17 percent of farmers had sex with their livestock. And even such foods as apple pie and raw liver are among the diverse substitutes made famous in movies and books. Poetic license? Maybe. But we think art imitates life.

Those options don't float your boat? Consider a vaginal substitute to help you release some of that mojo you have bot-tled up. See our entries on *vacuum devices* and *vibrating sleeve*.

Also see: anima and animus, bestiality, chlamydia, clitoral orgasm, douche, feel up, lubrication, nipples, Pap test, pregnancy, prison, reproductive system—hers, sponge, talking dirty, whipped cream, yeast infection

vaginal diseases/infections

Warning: Before reading on, please put aside anything you may be eating, your partner included. (Hey, we know guys who take our books to bed with them as helpful tools. Rocker Tommy Lee admitted as much on MTV.) Done? Good. Proceed.

The most common sign of a vaginal infection is an abnormally thick, sticky discharge (though the definition of *abnormal* differs depending on the woman and the current phase of her menstrual cycle). In the case of trichomoniasis, for example, the goo is green and frothy. You may also sniff a strange odor, ranging from the smell of bread dough to the stench of rotten fish, depending on whether the culprit is a foreign bacteria, a parasite, or a fungus.

Even a woman's natural bacteria may cause problems when they grow rampantly, often because her pH level has changed; the result is known as bacterial vaginosis. In this case, along with a fish-scented discharge, you'll notice a thin, white or colorless substance that's most fragrant right after sex. Antibiotics will do the trick here.

An overgrowth of *Candida albicans* causes a yeast infection. Symptoms include itching and a white, cottage cheese–like discharge. It's easily treated with over-the-counter medications.

Although uncomplicated vaginal infections aren't life-threatening or as serious as most sexually transmitted diseases, you should refrain from sex with an infected woman, as some of these bugs can easily spread to men.

Now, feel free to continue eating whatever you were eating.

Also see: cystitis, STDs, toxic shock syndrome, urethritis, yeast infection

vaginal injuries

Don't flatter yourself. No matter how impressed you may be with the size of your johnson, it's almost never too big to fit into the vagina of an adult woman who's been properly prepared through foreplay. The difficulty arises when you're using your tool like a jackhammer, especially when your partner isn't as lubricated as she ought to be.

It's always a good idea to go slow in the beginning, all the more so if you feel there's a slight mismatch in size. Make sure she's wet, or use sufficient amounts of artificial lubrication. If you're with a new partner, don't get too rough or rigorous until you know how she (or more specifically, her vagina) is going to react.

A second trouble source is the uneducated use of sex toys. Yeah, we know that guys don't need to stop for or read directions. But when you're introducing toys that penetrate her vagina, you owe it to her to know what you're doing.

Any vaginal pain during sex indicates that something is wrong. Infections aside, the most likely cause is vaginismus, in which her vagina contracts spasmodically, making intercourse uncomfortable and difficult if not impossible. This very real

psychological disorder is best treated by a sex therapist.

Here's one last tip that we mention elsewhere but that bears repeating: A woman's vagina is not a wind instrument. Don't blow into it during oral sex, as you run the risk of causing a fatal embolism (an air bubble that prevents blood from moving through a vein or artery). The risk increases if your partner is pregnant.

Also see: cervix, hung, injuries, lubricants, lubrication, missionary position, packing, rear entry, rough sex, sex therapy, sexual aids, size—penis, size—vagina, uterus—tipped, virginity—hers

vaginal moisture

She tells you that she's turned on, but when you slip your fingers between her legs, you discover that she's almost bone-dry. Why wouldn't a sexually aroused woman be wet?

Many women experience a period of dryness right after they menstruate. It's probably nothing that a little extra foreplay, vitamin E oil, or a good artificial lubricant won't fix. (Use water-based lubricants with condoms. Anything else—including vitamin E oil, but excluding extra foreplay—could cause rubbers to break.)

Sometimes, if a woman is just a little drier than usual, saliva will get her juices flowing. Saliva is *not* an acceptable substitute for vaginal wetness in extreme or chronic cases. Such severe habitual dryness is common in women who are nursing, past menopause, on antidepressant medications, and with conditions like incontinence, which tend to dry out everything—the eyes and mouth as well as the vagina. Aside from discomfort, such dryness creates the unhappy prospect of vaginal tearing during sex.

Take the extra time to make sure your partner is sufficiently lubricated for intercourse. A woman who learns to associate pain with sex is not apt to be a partner who looks forward to getting naked with you.

If your woman is postmenopausal, she should know that other midlifers have reported good results from prescription estrogen creams. You might also show off your newfound knowledge of the vagina by informing her that women experiencing vaginal dryness shouldn't douche, because such cleansing products just increase internal irritation. She should steer clear of bath oils as well.

Also see: arousal, female ejaculation, K-Y jelly, lubricants, lubrication

variety

Mention this word in the same sentence with sex, and we men—being, after all, men—tend to think of it in pretty much the same way Frank Gifford thought of it. (And you see how well that worked out for him.) Don't beat yourself up. The problem isn't morality; it's biology. Turns out there's a factual, scientific basis for women calling us hounds. In an animalistic sense, we're hardwired to propagate the species. And since it takes just one of us to impregnate a whole harem of females, even those of us who've come a long way since the caves still have our instinctual urges—such as when that new intern from accounting walks by.

If you're in a committed relationship you'd like to keep, variety doesn't have to mean—and really shouldn't mean—other women. It just means keeping things interesting. It means new positions, new venues, new timing (something other than her on top in the bedroom every Saturday night). It means spontaneity. It means—you're going to hate us for this—little romantic gestures that get her in the mood. It could mean sex toys. It could mean erotic videos, books, and poetry. It could mean role-playing. It could mean—you're going to hate us again—dance lessons.

You get the point. It *is* possible to sustain a varied, exciting sexual climate with the same partner, through the years, just by making little adaptations here and there—by keeping each other guessing. Plus, you'll never have to explain yourself to Barbara Walters on national television.

Also see: affairs, boredom, cars, couch, extramarital sex, games, group sex, kinky, marriage—open, monogamy, monotony, outdoors, planes, public places, role reversal, romance, routines, sexual aids, travel as an aphrodisiac

vascular disease

Another term for problems with bloodflow through your ticker and related arteries and veins—including those in your penis. We've covered it all under *heart conditions.*

vas deferens

Without the vas deferens, your sperm would be all dressed up with no place to go. These narrow, muscular tubes attach to each testicle, providing an exit portal for sperm. The little swimmers travel along the 2- to 3-foot-long vas deferens and end up in the seminal vesicles and prostate, where they mix with the other fluids that make up semen.

They're also known by several other equally unglamorous names: ductus deferens, excretory duct of testis, spermatic duct, and testicular duct.

Also see: male pill, reproductive system—yours, vasectomy reversal

vasectomy

Mention this to most men, and we react as if we'd just been kicked in our jockstraps. We're just not too thrilled with the idea of sharp and burning objects coming at our most sensitive of areas.

The procedure is, of course, a "permanent" form of male birth control in which the tubes that carry sperm from your testicles are severed and cauterized. That may sound painful and terrifying, but the procedure is actually safe, quick, relatively cheap, and highly effective. It is also quite common. About half a million of our fellow men in the United States have vasectomies each year—and the procedures are usually covered by health insurance.

There are two ways to go about the surgery: with scalpel and without. A scalpel vasectomy involves two small incisions in the scrotum, through which the doc reaches in, cuts out a piece of each vas deferens, and ties off or cauterizes the ends. In the no-scalpel version, he makes a single puncture in the scrotum and uses a special tool to do the same thing. Either way, it's a simple outpatient procedure, and you'll be done in less than a half-hour.

Which should you choose? Your choice, really—but some doctors think the less complicated, no-scalpel vasec-

tomy should become the method of choice.

A couple of things to bear in mind: Although a vasectomy can be reversed in some cases (that's why we put *permanent* in quotes, above), you need to consider it a lifelong decision. Any good urologist will spend some time counseling you to make sure you're ready for this. Among the things he should ask: Are you old enough? (If you're single and in your 20s, a responsible doc won't snip you. There are just too many reasons for you to change your mind down the road.) Have you sown your seeds? Do you have children, and are you sure you're done?

If all systems are still go, make an appointment for a Friday. You'll need the weekend to ice your twins to make sure there's no undue swelling. And don't expect to hop right back in the saddle: You'll need a few days before you'll feel like having sex. Even when you do feel like it, you'll need to wrap your willy. It takes about 20 ejaculations to clean out any residual sperm.

And forget the myth that your ejaculations will be any different in volume. Sperm make up a microscopic amount of semen. The bulk of it comes from your prostate and seminal vesicles, which are unaffected by the surgery.

Also see: contraception, tubal ligation, urologist, vas deferens, vasectomy reversal

vasectomy and prostate cancer

Medical researchers once warned men that vasectomy was connected to an increased risk of developing prostate cancer. That theory has been blown out of the water by more recent research that has shown no link between the two.

So it would appear that, while there are many things to take into account before considering this particular form of birth control, cancer isn't one of them.

Also see: contraception, prostate cancer, tubal ligation

vasectomy reversal

Microsurgery that returns sperm flow to vas deferens that were previously taken out of the reproductive loop via vasectomy. One form, vasovasostomy, reconnects the cut ends of the tubes, while another, vasoepididymostomy, stitches the vas deferens directly to the epididymis of each testicle.

If you want to have this done, prepare to spend an (uninsured) $6,000 to $15,000 as well as 1½ to 3 hours under a microscope. The success rate is near 90 percent if (a) fewer than 10 years have passed since you had your vasectomy, (b)

V

you're under age 40, and (c) you have a sperm granuloma (a marblelike collection of sperm that indicates a leakage at the original vasectomy site). Absent any one of these factors, don't be too optimistic.

Bear in mind that the restoration of sperm flow does not automatically guarantee the renewed ability to procreate. Overall, only half of men who undergo a vasovasostomy are able to impregnate their partners. That drops to 20 percent for a vasoepididymostomy.

Following a vasectomy reversal, wait at least 3 weeks before you resume any sexual activity. And don't waste money on home pregnancy kits for at least a year; even in the best of cases, conception is unlikely before then.

Also see: contraception, fertility, tubal ligation, urologist, vasectomy

va-va-voom

An outdated exclamation of strong approval of a voluptuous female. The term

Hot Dates **October 1991** The name "Long Dong Silver" entered the congressional record when professor Anita Hill testified that U.S. Supreme Court nominee Clarence Thomas had sexually harassed her.

continued from page 379

Answer:
False. Portnoy masturbates with raw liver. A character in the 1999 movie *American Pie* took liberties with an apple pie.

In Extremis
On his yacht, *Christina*, Aristotle Onassis had **bar stools covered in the penis skin of a whale**. He reputedly liked to tell guests they were sitting on the biggest penis in the world.

LEGAL BRIEFS
A Georgia jury awarded a woman $2.4 million in damages, accepting her contention that **the 1997 Miss**

Nude World International pageant **had unfairly disqualified her** from the competition. The woman said pageant organizers dumped her after she refused several of their requests, which included allowing one of the coordinators to lick whipped cream off her naked breasts, allowing herself to be auctioned off to a group of drunken golfers, and doing lap dances on a tour bus equipped with wet bars and beds.

BAWDY BALLADS "Soft and Wet," *Prince*

continued on page 393

was common during the 1950s, when muscle cars and glamour girls occupied the largest portion of a guy's gray matter. It seems to have been derived from *vroom*, a term originally associated with the mean sound of a powerful V-8 engine. Thus, presumably, it was applied to women who could really "get your motor going." The term also had adjectival uses, as in, "She's a va-va-voom lady," or simply, "She's voomy."

Also see: ogling, opening line, pickup lines, third-degree cleavage, sexy

venereal disease

Until about the 1960s, venereal disease (or VD, a shorthand popularized in military circles) was the common expression used to refer to five diseases contracted through genital contact: gonorrhea, syphilis, granuloma inguinale, lymphogranuloma venereum, and chancroid.

It wasn't till the advent of free love that medical researchers began to catalog a host of maladies spread predominantly through sex. And by the 1980s, the phrase *venereal disease* became outdated in favor of the term *sexually transmitted disease*, or *STD*, which officially classified the greater universe of diseases, including AIDS and hepatitis—illnesses that are sometimes contracted by nonsexual means. This more inclusive definition also acknowledged transmission via sexual contact with body parts other than genitalia, such as the mouth and rectum.

Also see: safe sex, short-arm inspection, STDs

Venus butterfly

Imagine that you and your partner are attending a private cocktail party or a chic art gallery opening. She's mingling elegantly across the room, looking quite the sophisticate. You reach into your pocket and press a button. Suddenly, she shivers slightly. She glances over at you, her lips curling into a sly smile that only you can read. You've put a fluttery feeling in her panties, tingling her little labia with a secret, remote-controlled device called a Venus butterfly. Now she wants you to sneak off with her for further gratification.

This pretty and delicate sex toy is designed to give a woman hands-free clitoral stimulation. The device can be worn under her panties for discreet clit-tickling in public, or it can be used during sex play when she's wearing nothing at all. Some versions, intended primarily for a woman's solo use, have attached remotes or built-in dildos. Others, meant to be used with a partner, operate via a wireless remote from as far as 15 to 20 feet away.

The typical version stays put thanks to elastic straps that encircle a woman's waist and run down between her legs (something like an old-fashioned sanitary napkin belt, for those of you who grew up with teenage sisters during, say, the 1950s).

The butterfly does have a few minor downsides. Most women find that its vibration is good for getting them aroused, but too mild to bring on an orgasm. And its hum may be a bit too obvious for quiet public places. ("Um, Ms. Jones, what's that buzzing sound? And why are you breathing so hard?")

Also see: dildo, sexual aids, vibrator

vibrating sleeve

No, it has nothing to do with your suit coat. It's a device that slips over your penis and provides a certain tingly stimulation. It can be placed at the head of your penis or slid down around the base. Generally, you don't need to slide the sleeve up and down your shaft in order to get off. You just hold 'er steady and plug 'er in.

A lot of guys who think that mechanical devices are for women develop a newfound appreciation for the breed once they happen upon the vibrating sleeve.

Also see: ahhh, masturbation, vacuum devices, vagina

vibrator

A sex toy that can either offer external stimulation or serve as a faux phallus that penetrates the vagina or anus. Otherwise known as a woman's best friend.

Vibration causes genitals to engorge, or fill with blood, which intensifies sexual arousal and may lead to orgasm. Because the genitals and all surrounding areas are exquisitely sensitive

to vibration, an external vibrator can be placed just about anywhere except the toenails to produce pleasure. And even the toenails might work on the right person. More commonly, women place vibrators on their clits and let them buzz away.

You can find vibrators in a variety of sizes and shapes: from rocketlike dildos to small egg-shaped devices to tiny ones meant to be worn on a fingertip and held in a pleasant place.

Vibrators have traditionally been thought of as something women enjoy using solo. You're going to be wiser than that. Adventurous lovers report excellent results from incorporating vibrators into their lovemaking routines. You can use a vibrator to get your partner off if you come first during intercourse. It sure reduces the pressure to last forever. Or use a vibrating dildo for anal stimulation during oral sex to enhance the sensation of orgasm. As always, here's our anal-activity mantra: Use a water-based lube, and wash the device thoroughly or slip a latex condom on it before you use it anywhere else.

Never feel competitive with a vibrator or feel that you've failed if your partner suggests using one. Be glad that she's cool enough to use it in front of you. To be sure, a vibrator allows you to do certain things that you couldn't accomplish with your hands or penis alone. Why limit yourself to a few simple appendages?

Also see: cock ring, dildo, manual stimulation, masturbation, pregnancy, vacuum devices, Venus butterfly

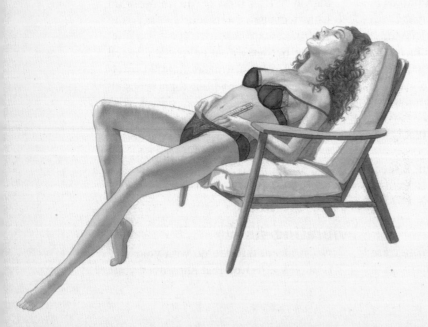

videos

As much fun as it is to use your video camera to document your toddler's progress at potty training, you may be able to find spicier uses for the device. You're not unusual, after all, if you get pretty hot while watching sex on film. Wouldn't you get even hotter if it were you and your partner in the leading roles?

Videotaped sex actually serves several purposes. First of all, as we said, it's a huge turn-on. Many couples use it as a form of, or a complement to, foreplay. (It's as if there were twice as many of you going at it at the same time!) But it's also affirming of your relationship. There's something about watching yourselves go through your sexual paces together—caressing each other's bodies, bringing each other to orgasm—that helps cement the bond of couplehood more firmly than could a million quick pecks on the cheek before you both run off to work. A videotape could come in, uh, handy for you on a lonely business trip or when your partner is away. And years from now, you might like having documentation of the days when you were young and beautiful, to show the grandkids. (Okay, we're kidding about the grandkids.)

If you decide to go this route, understand that you're not going to get it right the first time. Or the second. In fact, your first performances may even be comical because, to some degree, you'll probably play to the camera instead of just being yourselves. You'll do goofy stuff, make unusual noises, have overly theatrical climaxes (or maybe even be too self-conscious to climax). And so forth. After a while, though, you'll both forget about the camera. You'll relax and do what comes naturally. That's when the real fun begins.

Now for the disclaimer: Before making erotic tapes, you and your partner must agree on whether and where to keep them. You should also decide whether anyone besides the two of you will be permitted to watch them. Finally, though it's not a fun prospect but a necessary one, determine what will happen to the tapes if you ever go your separate ways. We don't need to tell you how embarrassing it could be to have such recordings fall into the wrong hands or to have outtakes from your lovemaking sessions become the featured event at your ex's next get-together with the girls.

Also see: discretion, erotic films, exhibitionism, mirrors, movies, pornography, voyeurism, X-rated

violence

Assuming your father wasn't an abuser himself, there's a good chance that when you were still quite young he told you something that you remember to this day: "Son, you don't hit a woman. Ever."

Unfortunately, you don't have to look very hard for evidence of the fact that either some guys' fathers didn't tell them this or it just didn't take. The network newsmagazines brim with stories about abused women. Ever since Farrah Fawcett's compelling performance in *The Burning Bed*, a stock theme in made-for-TV movies has been the battered wife who finally turns on her monster of a husband in a moment of apocalyptic fury. The statistics supporting all these grim depictions are just as grim: They tell us that between two million and four million women are victims of domestic abuse and that one out of every four or five women will be raped in her lifetime (rape having been defined as a crime of violence, rather than one of sex).

Some of this is misleading. Violent men are frequently serial offenders who repeat their disturbing behavior with one woman after another. Thus these bad apples skew the overall figures on the incidence of violence, making all men look bad. And some of the stats—the ones on rape in particular—may in part be a product of urban legend, generated by overeager political groups. Still, we're told that the statistics do represent, if anything, just the tip of the iceberg: It's estimated that two-thirds of rapes and sexual assaults go unreported.

We shouldn't have to tell you that violence has no place in sex. Rough, energetic lovemaking, if it's consensual, is one thing. Actual violence—meaning a man's unilateral decision to "have his way" with a woman and to do it in a belligerent, physically hurtful manner—is always wrong. And illegal.

But let's, for a moment, back out of the bedroom and examine the general landscape of your relationship with your woman or with women in general. Have women told you that you have a "dominant" personality? When you argue, do you frequently yell at the top of your lungs or throw or break things? Are you inclined to bare your teeth or raise your hand in a threatening manner if a domestic debate isn't going your way? Is grabbing, holding, or shaking your woman a standard part of your argumentative repertoire? Does your woman sometimes seem to cower in your presence, like a hand-shy puppy? Do you run her life, where she goes,

who she sees? Do you make her punch the equivalent of a household time clock?

Collectively, these are symptoms of a controlling, brutish personality. There's intimidation and implied violence in your demeanor. And even if you want to look at the subject in the most self-serving terms, you can't expect loving, gratifying sex from a woman who fears you—not unless she has deep-seated problems of her own.

Sure, women can be frustrating. They'll taunt you and even assault you. (Yes, Virginia, there are male victims of domestic abuse—sadly, a forgotten minority.) But know this: Whatever your rationalization—even if you think she "asked for it"—there is no justification for abuse, ever. Violence is wrong. If you can't resolve a conflict without losing control, leave the situation, and try to deal with things later, once you've both calmed down.

So if too much of the above sounds like you, get help from a psychologist or other licensed mental health professional. Or else get arrested.

Also see: arguing, divorce—issues that lead to, fantasies, gang rape, pornography, rape, rough sex, sex offenders, sex therapy, X-rated

virginity—hers

You're ready, and considering the eager way she's kissing you, you suspect that she's ready too. She's crouched in your lap, loving the way you stroke her face and neck. There's no question she wants to go further, but just as you reach for the zipper of her leopard-print catsuit, she pulls back slightly and whispers..."I'm a virgin, you know."

Stay calm. Take a deep breath. The emotions you're feeling are apt to be overwhelming and contradictory. You're aroused, you're terrified, you're incredulous. You haven't met a virgin since you were 16 (and still a virgin yourself). And in a corner of your brain, you wonder: Do virgins really wear catsuits?

Yes, a woman can behave like a tigress and still be hanging on to her hymen. She's probably not afraid of sex, but she may be afraid of disease and disappointment. Or—you may want to take an extra gulp here—she might just have been waiting for that special someone.

So, Mr. Special Someone, make it a special memory, for both of you. After all, what's wrong with being the guy who introduced a woman to the splendors of good sex?

Proper defloweration requires a certain amount of gentleness and sensitivity. You must move very slowly, taking note of her responses to each of your touches; you must be willing to put her pleasure and her comfort ahead of your own. Look at it as a mission, of sorts. Take your time, and think about what you're doing.

Spend extra time on foreplay. The body is full of erogenous zones—at full arousal, it may be one big erogenous zone—and you should explore them all with patience and grace. Start with her face, ears, and throat; try a variety of touches and pressures with your fingers and mouth. Move down toward her waist, caressing her breasts, her back, and her abdomen. Monitor her reactions, and pay close attention to her emotions. If she seems anxious or threatened, pause your seduction and talk to her.

If you think she's ready to take the next step, whisper sweetly in her ear, "Would you like me inside you?" If her answer is yes, put on a condom, lubricate,

Seemed like a Good Idea at the Time...

Shortly after the turn of the 20th century, masturbator hater Albert Todd received two patents for devices he created to stymie self-abusers. The first was a wire-and-coil cage worn over the penis and testicles. Todd vowed that the contraption was tough enough to "resist any reasonable effort on the part of the wearer in an attempt to break or cut" his way to phallic freedom. It also featured a belt with zinc and copper plates that generated a current of electricity. The current was activated when the belt was dipped into acid before it was cinched around the masturbator or when it came into contact with bodily secretions. Ever humane, Todd said that **the device could be insulated to prevent too severe an electric shock.**

Todd's second contrivance was a penile cylinder fitted with an internal detector that would sound an alarm in the unfortunate event of an erec-

True or Phallus
Napoleon's penis was removed and sold after his death.

continued on page 402

and slide in *slowly*, watching her carefully for cues that say, "This hurts." She probably expects a certain amount of discomfort—and she may not want you to stop anyway—but you should go slowly enough that she can blurt out the word before you've achieved full penetration. Increase the speed and strength of your thrusts gradually. Keep watching her face for winces.

Don't be a dictator. Don't tell her what to do or how to feel. Don't expect a lot of creativity on her part, and frankly, this is not the time for you to get very creative, either. In the back of her mind, she may feel a little bit of guilt about finally letting go. You don't want to do anything that makes her feel slutty.

This next bit of advice should be obvious, but our feedback from women over the years tells us that guys routinely manage to sidestep the obvious: Don't compare your virgin to other women you've been with. You say you'd never do that? Well, that's precisely what you accomplish when you goad her into performing the sexy tricks that others have used to rock your world. What this makes her think is "I stink at this. I'll never catch up to other women."

Do ask her to tell you what feels good, and give her plenty of positive feedback when she makes *you* feel good. Don't assume she can read your body language and your sounds. Use the actual words *Mmmm, that feels wonderful.*

As you move along in the act, don't get so carried away with your own pleasure that you forget to check in with her. If the flinching gets worse or if her face seems contorted into one big grimace, stop moving and ask if she'd like to take a breather. It's the gentlemanly thing to do. And—this is important—after you

ask that question, you can't betray any irritation if she says, "Yes, I'm sorry, can we please stop?" Comfort her and let her know it's okay.

Even if things go well, don't expect her to have an earth-shattering orgasm thanks to intercourse alone. (Many women never reach the stage where they can climax reliably through standard intercourse.) You may very well have to finish the job with your hands or your mouth. Or, she may tell you not to bother, because she's sore.

However the sex act itself ends, end the experience with a long session of cuddling. Even if it didn't go well, let her know that you're willing to do a lot more practice. Success as a lover has a big impact on a person's self-esteem, so do the lady a favor by enhancing her self-image. Tell her how much you enjoyed making love to her. Tell her that you enjoyed experiencing her body and that you can't wait to explore it further, as soon as she's ready again.

Also see: abstinence, afterglow, celibacy, clumsiness, communication, cystitis, first lover, first time with a lover, innocence, morning after, vaginal injuries

vixen

A true beauty who also happens to be contentious and quarrelsome. She has a temper as short as her skirt and a tongue that, when it's not sending shivers up your spine, can bite like dry ice. She knows all of your sore spots and seems to love nothing more than poking at them. A vixen also delights in using her sexuality to get to you, tantalizing you with her charms and then withholding sex for the very purpose of driving you nuts and showing you who's boss.

Since a vixen may be skilled at hiding her ugly side until she knows that she has you where she wants you, be on the alert for occasional slipups, which tend to occur, oddly enough, in restaurants. She's the type who treats a waitress like a dog: no "please" or "thank you" or other polite touches. She just sits there looking down her nose at your server (especially if it's another woman). But you'll see her wicked tongue move into high gear if, God forbid, her spoon is missing or she doesn't get her drink pronto.

The vixen doesn't like to order off the menu; she wants dishes created especially for her. And she loves sending meals back and complaining in general: The wine stinks. The soup is too cold. The salad is wilted. The meat is too rare. And so on. When the check comes, she won't make even the barest pretense of reaching for her pocketbook. Not this lady. She expects to be pampered all the way.

Dealing with a vixen requires something that a lot of us don't have in abundant supply, especially around beautiful women: self-discipline. She's the high that's not worth the risk of addiction; the rich, delicious meal that will give you heartburn. You need the willpower to just say no—*before* she gets under your skin, drives you crazy, and breaks your heart.

Also see: bimbo, boss's wife, danger, pussywhipped

voice

Here's a depressing truth that you probably already know if you've paid attention to the outgoing message you put on your answering machine: Your voice never rings as rich, deep, and full to others as it does to you. The wonderful resonance you hear through the bones and cavities in your head creates not only an auditory sensation (one that also tends to provide additional bass tones) but also a tactile one. You literally *feel* yourself talking.

Women are probably more sensitive to male voices than we are to theirs. You may not be fond of a woman's high-pitched squeal (and if you haven't seen Steve Martin's film *The Man with Two Brains*, it's worth renting just for the one relevant scene; it's a classic), but you'll probably overlook it, at least for a night, if she has certain other attributes. Women, however, tend to evaluate you as a total package—and not necessarily as the package you're thinking of. No matter how good-looking you are, she may have a hard time getting past a nasal, Woody Allen whine. Similarly, if you mumble, whisper, scream, talk in a monotone, or are chronically hoarse, she may be nodding on the outside but cringing on the inside.

To find your ideal voice, you first need to have healthy vocal cords. If you have a lousy voice but you also seem to have an unusual number of sore throats, a persistent nasal drip, or similar afflictions, you may want to consult an otolaryngologist (also known as an ear, nose, and throat specialist, or ENT).

You also need to be able to focus your tone, meaning that your voice should sound like it emanates from the center of your mouth, not from one side or the other. (You'd be surprised by how often the latter is the case, especially with smokers.) The middle of the mouth also implies a point not too far forward and not too far back. Too far forward?

V

You're nasal. Too far back? You're garbled and throaty.

You can find your natural pitch range through this easy exercise: Think of something positive—the sexiest woman you saw today?—and say, "Mmmmmm hmmmmm!" The range of pitches you hear are those that should be present throughout most of your regular, modulated speech.

If you're still not happy with what you hear, biofeedback (or perhaps "soundofeedback") can help. Some men with irritating speech patterns have been able to retrain their voices by talking into a tape recorder until they sound more like what they want to hear. Or look for a professional speech-language pathologist licensed by the American Speech-Language-Hearing Association.

Many actors, disc jockeys, and broadcasters hire voice coaches to help them tune their pipes. How do you find one? Call the drama or speech department at a local university, a TV or radio station, or a talent agency.

Also see: communication, dial-a-porn, grunting, hypnosis and seduction, moaning, phone sex, sweet talk, talking dirty, whispering

voyeurism

Though accurate statistics on sneaky peekers are hard to find, the true peeping Tom is believed to be a rare fellow. The crime of voyeurism—that is, when a person slinks under windows, hoping to catch a glimpse of a woman undressing or a couple making love—is seldom reported, probably because most peepers are sly enough to avoid being noticed. Clinical voyeurs can't stop their secret behavior; they have a psychological disturbance that calls for therapy.

That doesn't mean you're a mental case if you find yourself craving live visual stimulation. Both men and women, of course, commonly are excited by viewing nudity and sexual activity. The easiest legal way to satisfy such harmless urges is to visit a cybersex Web site, where you'll be treated to performances right on your screen.

Some couples get the same thrill from watching themselves engage in steamy sexual activity that they would get from watching others. You and your partner can make your own erotic videos, or you can simply install mirrors around your bedroom. As you view yourselves making love, you may find that, along with heightened sexual arousal, the mirrors give you the urge to go the extra

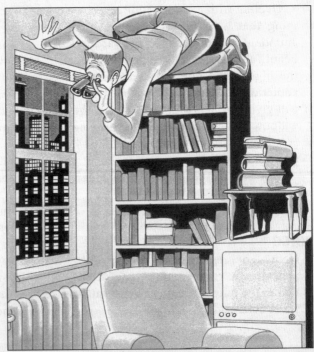

mile—to perform with more gusto and improve your sexual style.

If none of that satisfies your voyeuristic drive, you might try hard-core swingers clubs. Or go to a strip joint that features women poking each other with strap-ons or having sex on stage with male customers. Bear in mind that much of this activity crosses the border into illegality; that's almost certainly the case when couples engage in genuine sex acts on stage. If the place gets busted, you may go to jail along with the performers.

Also see: compulsive behavior, cybersex, exhibitionism, fantasies, mirrors, ogling, paraphilias, perversions, pornography, sex offenders, spectatoring, striptease, swinging, topless bar, videos

vulva

Add a whole bunch of female genitals together, and you get a vulva. Basically, *vulva* is the collective term for the entire area that you can see between her legs. It's made up of things like the labia majora and minora, the mons pubis, the clitoris, and the vaginal opening. Wander farther in, and there's her vagina.

Also see: cunnilingus, pudenda, reproductive system—hers

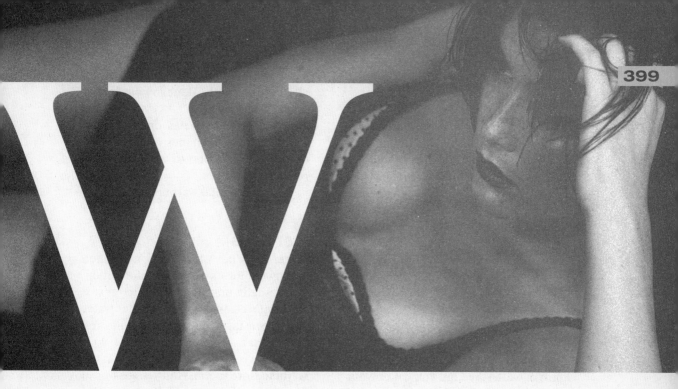

wandering eye

Here's the scenario: A scantily clad, sweet thing strolls by on the beach. There are two people staring hard—you, at her, and your woman, at you.

We'd be the last ones to condemn you. Your gal and all her sisters around the globe will be the first. This scenario has been played out for as long as there have been scenarios. That's because men are simply more aroused by visual stimuli than the women in our lives would like. Since the dawn of man, our primary way of assessing the opposite sex has been visual.

Stone age though our programming may be, that doesn't mean our manners have to dwell in a damp cave. Discretion, friends, is a good thing. The key is to avoid an

obvious, lengthy stare, even when your partner isn't around. The woman being

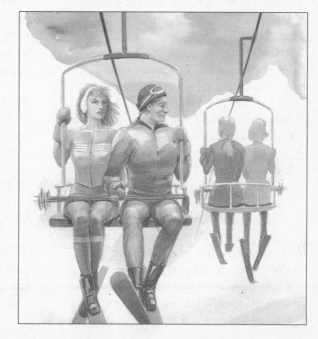

observed likely enjoys an appreciative look, but not a boorish leer.

It also helps if you simply follow the subject at hand with your eyes, without moving your head. (And keep the grunts and moans to yourself.) As your relationship progresses, your mate may allow you an occasional glance, as long as you show some self-restraint; it's a matter of respect for her.

Also see: affairs, bimbo, eye contact, fantasies, jealousy, legs, ogling, sex symbols, third-degree cleavage, topless bar, va-va-voom, voyeurism

warts

When it comes to sex, there are two kinds of warts: the kind you get on your genitals and the kind you don't. And never the twain shall meet.

A woman with a wart on her hand cannot give you genital warts if she caresses your penis. Likewise, if she has a plantar wart on her foot. (Did you think that only hands could caress your penis?)

That's the good news. The bad news is that warts are still warts. Even worse, not all warts are visible to the naked eye. You *can* transmit a wart from your hand to her hand, even if you can't see the little lesion. And not too many women appreciate that.

A doctor can remove warts for you. Or, if you want to try getting rid of them at home, a good over-the-counter wart remover to try is Wart-Off. It contains 17 percent salicylic acid, a compound that knocks warts flat. If after 2 weeks of this treatment your wart has not gone away, see a doctor. Plantar warts require a more aggressive treatment like cryosurgery, laser excision, or a few treat-

ments with a dilute nitric acid solution, all of which can be done in your podiatrist's office.

If you have diabetes or circulation problems in your hands or feet, see a doctor before trying to treat any warts on your own.

Also see: genital warts, papilloma

water beds

Water beds have long been associated with two things: sex and misinformation. And usually misinformation about sex. First, let's clear up the myth that water beds devastate your sperm count. Yes, your gonads are located outside your body for a reason—because 98.6°F is too warm to store sperm. And yes, soaking in blazing 104°F hot tubs kills sperm. But nobody heats their water beds that high nor do they soak their testicles in them.

That said, sleeping on a water bed *can* lower the number of tadpoles in your semen by a mere 10 percent. That's not enough to affect a normally charged man, but it can make a difference if you already have a low sperm count. If a fertility specialist tells you your troops are depleted and you're trying to conceive a baby, switch to a regular mattress.

Now let's get to the recreational-sex part. If you don't want to act out the part of a hockey player slamming the boards, make sure your bladder is filled correctly. That's the one on your water bed. A bed that's low on juice sloshes like a half-swigged 12-ouncer. Also, be diligent in maintaining a comfortable temperature. Most people like to stop sweating after sex. Likewise, no one wants to wake up shivering after the heat of a sexual encounter has subsided. A good temperature is anywhere between 85° and 95°F. Regularly check the thermostat to make sure the dial wasn't bumped or unplugged while you were riding the swelling waves.

The ability to tweak traditional sex positions is one of the great benefits of a water bed. Here are a few to get you started: In a variation of the missionary position, alter the pushup use of your hands and arms and instead slide them under her back, hold on to her shoulders, and go with the flow. The side-by-side, or spoon, position also works well on water. Get into the rhythm of the waves, and you may find that you never want to go back to dry land.

Also see: athletic sex, beds, lovemaking, sperm count, variety

water sports

This ain't tossing water balloons. Rather, it's the street term for urophilia, the use of urine for sexual fun and games.

Urine has long been a source of fascination for men, whether or not in a sexual context. How many times did you have distance-pissing contests as a kid? Write your name in the snow? Have you ever peed on your mate in the shower? Gotten kicked in the jewels for peeing on your mate in the shower?

For the most part, urinating on someone during sex—the so-called golden shower—is part of the fetish scene, a form of humiliation popular in domination practices. But not always. Some people find the dribbling stream to be a source of warmth and comfort. That's not so surprising when you realize that for centuries urine has been thought to have medicinal properties. Therapeutic urine drinking dates back to the Holy Roman

Empire, when great urinal troughs were erected in public squares so residents could both contribute and partake.

Even today, there are organizations for the advancement of urine therapy, but from a hygiene point of view, we don't recommend you drink the stuff. Urine can transmit diseases such as HIV and urinary tract infections.

Also see: klismaphilia, paraphilias, pee—her—during orgasm, sloppy sex, urinary problems

weight loss

We're going to go out on a limb here. We're going to assume that you like sex.

We're also guessing that you want to keep liking it for a long time to come. Then do yourself a huge favor: lose some weight. No, we haven't seen you, but typically, men between the ages of 30 and 55 gain a pound a year, so you're likely sporting more of a Goodyear gut than you should be.

For every extra pound of pudge, you increase your risk of developing diabetes, high blood pressure, and poor cholesterol counts. That's bad enough by itself, but those three conditions also happen to be prime factors in impotence. A Harvard study showed that men over age 50 who had 42-inch-plus waists were almost twice as likely to be unable to hoist their mizzen masts as men with waists under 35 inches.

On top of that, there's the aesthetic impact of being fat. Like it or not, we're a society that treasures slimness. One of the reasons you're not getting as much sex as you want may simply be that few women lust after—or enjoy being crushed beneath—a Ralph Kramden–size gut. Finally, multiple studies confirm what people who exercise and maintain their weights have known all along: Fit folks with positive body images think about sex more often and have sex more often than do sofa spuds.

So put down this book for a bit, and get out for a workout. Here's one to get you started: A 200-pound man engaged in moderately energetic sex will burn around 118 calories per hour. If he cranks it up a notch to vigorous sex, he'll burn 136 calories per hour. See you at the "gym."

Also see: abs, beefcake, body fitness, body image, body shapes, cervical cap, diaphragm, erection, exercise, impotence, male body, muscles, sexual attraction, size—penis

wet dreams

Ejaculating is like flying a plane. Sometimes your hand is on the stick, and sometimes you're on autopilot.

Wet dreams are the latter. Virtually all boys mark their entry into adolescence with a startled discovery in their shorts one morning. Why it happens is anyone's guess. Some think it's simply a pressure-relief valve being triggered when your system is highly charged. Others think it has more to do with the dream itself.

But don't think that wet dreams are reserved exclusively for the skateboard set. You can have one at almost any stage of life, if the conditions are right. (In what could be considered divine intervention, even monks have them.)

If you have sons, do yourself and them a favor: Explain wet dreams to them before they hit puberty. That way, they won't be traumatized by the experience or mortified by the thought that they've wet the bed.

Also see: come, dreams, ejaculation, fantasies, heterosexuality, puberty, sexual thoughts, succubus

---

Hot Dates **1994** President Clinton signed a bill that made prior conduct of an accused sex offender admissible in court. The law allowed Paula Jones to name Monica Lewinsky as a witness in her sexual harassment suit.

continued from page 393

Answer:

True—we think. An object purported to be the little leader's peter was sold at Christie's in 1968. It was auctioned again in Paris in 1977. The current reputed owner is said to be a New York urologist.

tion. It also zapped the wearer with an electrical charge. Todd created a top-of-the-line version of this erection detection device that included metal points and brads "of sufficient length to cause considerable annoyance and pain to the patient should any attempt be made to manipulate the penis by means of the tube."

Foreign Affairs

Women in several African tribes used to stretch their inner labia so

that they would hang 2 inches or more below their vaginas. These women were highly sought by male tribal members, in part because **the men liked the feeling of having the labia envelop their penises** during intercourse.

In Extremis

Philip Bondy's sexual quirk cost him his life. Bondy, 79, was an apotemnophiliac—somebody who gets sexual pleasure from the re-

---

BAWDY BALLADS **"Sugar Walls,"** *Sheena Easton*

continued on page 409

wet spot

You've probably been blamed for the wet spot since you've been old enough to make one. No more. You're not the only one who's gushing. The pool of passion has some, if not more, of her in it too, ranging from vaginal lubrication to outright female ejaculation.

Even though it's not all your fault, some women are turned off by the mess associated with sex. That's why it's wise to keep a towel or moist cloth handy. She can snug it between her legs afterward to keep her cup from runningeth over. Or you can even make a game of cleaning her up post-coitus.

In all seriousness, arguing over who sleeps on the wet spot—like similar flare-ups over how toilet paper should be hung or the way toothpaste should be squeezed—may signal a general unwillingness to compromise or some other, deeper issue in the relationship. But if this is the only trivial argument you ever have with your lover . . . well, be a man. Suck it up, as it were, and take the side with the wet spot. (Throw a towel over it if it bothers you that much.) We're confident that your small sacrifice will pay ongoing dividends.

Also see: afterplay, arguing, beds, female ejaculation, dry hump, gusher, klismaphilia, lubrication, menstruation, sexual etiquette, sloppy sex, water sports

whipped cream

Is there anything edible that's as synonymous with sex as this? (We're talking, here, about things you find in the fridge, not in your lover's panties.)

You should know that true connoisseurs prefer hand-whipped cream over chemical-laden offerings from pressur-ized cans. The flavor is richer, the scent more alluring, the texture more sensuous. But don't let culinary snobbery completely oust the nozzle-tipped cans from the bedroom. They can be a lot of fun when it comes to creating erotic sculptures on one another's bodies.

Here's a truly erotic way to whip your partner into a creamy frenzy: Use her naked body as a sundae dish, sculpting little swirls of the topping all over her thighs, abdomen, breasts, and neck. Then, slowly and playfully kiss, lick, and nibble the cream away. You can, of course, bring chocolate sauce, honey, fresh fruit, and other delectables into play. The sensations you'll provide her will be rapturous. And you'll save yourself a trip to Dairy Queen afterward.

One caveat: *Never* spray or spoon whipped cream into your partner's vagina. The sugar could give her a yeast infection, and the pressurized gas from a can could cause an embolism—a potentially fatal air bubble in her blood.

Also see: aphrodisiac, erogenous zones, food, games, licking, lubricants, ointments, oysters, sexual aids, sloppy sex, yeast infection

whips

These are a symbol of bondage and discipline rivaled only by chains. The irony is that both the traditional bullwhip and chains are rarely employed in today's bondage scene. For one, a 6-foot bullwhip is too long to be used indoors. Oh, and there's one other downside: These tools can be quite lethal, able to slice through flesh and down to the bone. That's undesirable even for the most ardent sado-masochists.

In pain-and-pleasure recreation areas, known as dungeons and playrooms, the bullwhip usually is reserved for decor. Whip masters opt for smaller whips, like carriage whips, riding crops, and the dressage whips used in horse racing.

For some, the mere crack of the whip is enough to induce pleasure. Others crave the welt-raising pain of being struck. Among enthusiasts, the isolated strike makes skin more sensitive to the touch, thus making erogenous zones, well, more erogenous. One psychotherapist compares the love of pain to losing baby teeth: Once children notice loose teeth, they push and pull with their tongues and fingers, drawn to the sensation despite the pain.

Still other sadomasochism fans use whips to participate in pony play. The "ponies" don horse costumes and shuttle their "riders" with specially designed saddles or carts. The riders then use whips to encourage the faux animals to go faster or to simply behave if they're being especially naughty.

Also see: bondage and discipline, dominance and submission, flogging, kinky, leather, Sade—Marquis de, safeword

whispering

If you want your lover to hear you loud and clear, whisper. Lowering your voice actually grabs her attention more than raising it does.

Think about it for a second. Like you, your partner spends her days in a loud, loud world. She copes with roaring cars, screaming jets, bellowing children, and barking dogs. Not to mention barking bosses. And then, in the middle of all that, you whisper her name. Imagine the impact.

Whispers are also one of the sexiest things you can bring to bed. Such coital communiqués can range from sensual to outright saucy, from "I love you" to "I want you, you uncaged tigress." Whispers, too, can convey likes and dislikes, what's working and what isn't. These soft suggestions should be just that, though—more requests than critiques. Most of us want to learn to better please our lovers, but who wants to be reprimanded during the act itself?

Also see: ahhh, communication, grunting, laughter, moaning, sweet talk, talking dirty, voice

wife's best friend

A female, we hope. A female you must leave alone. This is not a case of "Look, don't touch"; this is "Don't even get caught looking." And never, ever tell her anything that you wouldn't want your wife to hear. Anything you say may be repeated in exaggerated and sarcastic tones. And saying or doing anything that you shouldn't will come back to haunt you in the bedroom, one way or another.

Just be friendly and caring and an all-around good guy. Treat her like a nice sister. Let her see that you love and respect your wife. Never, ever hit on her, no matter how tempted you are. Not even if she seems to be suggesting it. She is apt to be around a lot, so it's not unusual that you may fantasize about taking a turn or two with her. Fantasy is okay. But never confess that you have this fantasy. And don't let the lust show in your eyes.

Here's some harder-to-follow advice: Don't worry about what she and your wife talk about. You really don't want to know all the details. And don't let the ones your wife shares with you bother you. That your wife can vent with this friend helps keep your marriage alive and healthy. Be grateful for this. This friend is, very likely, your wife's number one marriage counselor. And, if you're up to no good, she's probably one of the few people in the world who really could blackmail you if she wanted to. Pretend that you don't know that she knows things about you that you wouldn't tell your own best friend, and life will be easier.

Also see: best friend's wife, discretion, fantasies, trust—rebuilding

wild

There's something thrumming deep down in your veins. You might not always recognize it, acknowledge it, or permit it to surface, but it's there nonetheless. It's your wild side.

Getting wild means different things to different people. For the faint at heart, it may mean having sex with the lights on. For others, it may mean a raunchy night filled with hot tubs, exotic lubes, and live-stock. Whatever your definition, getting wild has one common thread: pushing the limit of what you've done before. In essence, it is embracing the idea of sexual exploration.

A healthy sex life should always have room for moments of wildness. These times can be experimental, playful, and solely pleasure-oriented, as opposed to pregnancy-oriented. Contemplating a wild act should spur one of three thoughts: "I've got to try that," "I'd never do that," or "I've got to find someone who will do that to me."

Before donning your loincloth, you need to initiate a discussion with your partner on taking a safari into the sexual wilds. It's unfair and unrealistic for you to assume that your desire to try X should be followed automatically by her shouting, "I can't wait!" Don't badger or browbeat her. If you feel awkward bringing up something you want to try, frame it as a dreamed desire: "Honey, it was the weirdest thing. I dreamt of you and me naked in a bathtub full of cold cuts last night." Gauge her reaction, and if she seems amenable, immediately walk hand in hand to the nearest deli.

Also see: athletic sex, communication, danger, dreams, fantasies, kinky, play-acting, risky sex, surprises, sweating, taboos, zipless sex

wild women

Be honest, you've either had it or fantasized about it: an experience with that elusive creature known as a wild woman . . . a chance encounter that turns into a night filled with more steam than Robert Fulton himself would know what to do with in his wildest dreams. (And if you don't get the reference, read up on your history, fella: Women find knowledgeable men very sexy.) Other women with a streak of the vicious in them call such a woman easy. We call her manna. Whatever your term, she's a woman who doesn't hesitate to go to bed with a guy she likes. And she doesn't hesitate to do things to that guy that he's only read about in books like this.

Compared to her less demonstrative sisters, a wild woman has far more sexual experience under her belt and far fewer inhibitions. And after you have her, you'll do more than inventory all your parts to see if everything still works.

You'll ask yourself a very valid question: Is this a one-night stand or the beginning of a long-term orgasmic odyssey?

It depends.

Some wild women simply aren't ready to settle down. That's why they're out there being wild in the first place. You'll know pretty quickly by the way she ends the evening. If she's interested in seeing you again, she'll make sure you know it. If not, thank your lucky stars she wandered your way, then forget her and move on. Don't try to coerce a serious relationship out of a wild woman who's not yet ready to be tamed.

But if you catch her at the end of her oat sowing, buddy, you secure yourself a lifetime of adventurous, satisfying sex. Treasure it. And don't let jealousy or excessive thoughts of her sexual history get in the way. The last thing she needs is you condemning the very characteristics that attracted you to her in the first place.

Also see: commitment, dating, first date, free love, lust, Madonna/whore complex, nymphomania, one-night stand, past partners—longing for, promiscuity, succubus, zipless sex

winking

Imagine a single word that meant the following: "Hey, nice game." "How's it going?" "I'm here for you if you need me." "You're cute." "I'd like to lay you like a roll of vinyl." Imagine now how incredibly difficult it would be to decipher what somebody meant when he used that word on you. Winking is a lot like that. The hundreds of primary and secondary meanings of winking would fill a small textbook.

But therein, too, lies its charm. A wink from a close friend is as good as a hug—better, if he has stinky pits. A wink from your boss means check your pay stub for additions. And a wink from a lover means buckle up because you're going for a ride.

But in today's litigious workplace, a wink sent as a salutation could easily be misinterpreted as a sexual come-on. Don't try it with women co-workers with whom you're only casually acquainted.

What if a woman sends a wink your way? Don't just assume it's an invitation. Interpret it as a congenial greeting, and take a little time to glean the intent of the glint. If verbal contact hasn't yet been made, make it. If you've spoken with her before, use this opportunity to strike up another conversation. But again, don't ever rely on a wink alone in drawing a conclusion about her interest in you. A single gesture from a woman can never be counted on for that.

Unless maybe she lifts her skirt at the same time.

Also see: best friend's wife, communication—nonverbal, eye contact, flirtation, sexual innuendo

witch's milk

Milky drops may issue forth from your woman's nipples at the most unlikely of times—like when she's not breastfeeding or even a mother. Yet there they are, sweet and exotic pearls of liquid that have inspired connoisseurs of the erotic to borrow an old folk term for them: *witch's milk*. Actually, witch's milk also comes out of the breasts of many newborns—male or female—who have absorbed their mothers' hormones during pregnancy.

The adult version (galactorrhea) is harmless in and of itself, but it may signal other problems, so a visit to the doctor is in order. A common cause is a tiny, benign tumor on the pituitary gland that increases secretion of the lactation-stimulating hormone prolactin. Witch's milk may also be a reaction to drugs, including antidepressants and oral contraceptives.

We think, by the way, that this is an unduly sinister term for what can be a very pleasing phenomenon. For if she's a witch, she's a good one, indeed.

withholding

The very idea of withholding sex baffles most men. Why would anyone ever want to withhold *sex*? It's like voluntarily giving up air. Or pizza.

The thing is, when a woman in an active relationship withholds sex, it boils down to a straight, old-fashioned power struggle. In passive-aggressive fashion, she typically does it (or *won't* do it, as the case may be) to communicate that something is amiss. She's playing her trump card, getting your attention in the only way she thinks will work.

This keeps you wanting, panting, threatening, maybe even pleading. That's not healthy. And it's damn sure not dignified. While her refusal to put out may solve a short-term problem once in a great while, you're quickly going to tire of the "Guess what I'm mad about now" game.

The two of you need to address the built-up resentment that's causing her to close the barn door. If she withholds sex routinely just to get her way, she needs a therapist, and you need to decide if you want to live with a bully. More likely,

though, it's a sign that the rest of your relationship isn't so hot, either. A well-worn adage says that sex begins in the kitchen, and it's true, at least for women. How she feels about your time together outside the bedroom has much to do with her willingness to play inside the boudoir.

In other words, withholding, to her, may be shorthand for "I need to talk to you." She's trying to get your attention. Give it to her so both of you don't have to continue going through this.

One final warning: Be careful not to confuse intentional withholding—that is, the sort of gonadal gamesmanship described above—with other, legitimate reasons why she may just not be in the mood for sex. Generally speaking, you should be able to tell the difference. But it never hurts to broach the subject in a tactful, nonthreatening way.

Also see: arguing, begging, communication, desperate, fatigue, frequency, making up, marriage—lack of sex in, mood, no, power, pussywhipped, quality versus quantity, rejection—sexual, trust—rebuilding, vixen

womb

The old joke is that we spend 9 months trying to get out and the rest of our lives trying to get back in. And why not? The womb—another term for uterus—was the comfortable, warm, nurturing surrounding that brought us into the world.

Also see: hysterectomy, uterus

women

We have just a single observation to make here, but it's a deceptively large one: Women aren't men. No, we're not just being glib. They aren't men biologically, and they aren't men in countless less tangible ways that complicate our attempts to deal with them in and out of bed. We could argue all day about whether this is due to nature or nurture; we could argue about whether we could minimize gender differences by raising both sexes "the same." That wouldn't change the fact that the next woman you meet has already been raised and is far more likely to resemble her biological sisters than to resemble you.

The upshot? Don't expect your woman to react to life the way you do, and don't project your own expectations onto her. Don't expect her to explain why she feels the way she does (or at least, don't expect to be able to decipher or identify with her explanation). Don't expect to understand why she's more inclined to lead with her heart than her head. In short, don't argue with reality. The battle of the sexes is what it is. Sigmund Freud himself, for all his investigation into the workings of the human psyche, finally threw up his hands in exasperation and cried, "What do women want?"

For more detailed info on women, see, well, the rest of this book.

workaholism

If you've ever uttered the phrase "Hold that orgasm; I have to take this call," we need to talk.

For true workaholics, life at home can't compete with life at work. There are a bunch of theories on why this is so—fear of commitment being one of them. But whatever the cause, the end result is the same: Workaholics would rather be at work than anywhere else. Including bed.

There are plenty of guys out there who successfully balance work and play. Ask them their secret, and they'll tell you work can rarely, if ever, replace the gratification and fulfillment of a good private life. Yes, being obsessed with your job allows you to take the corporate bull by the horns. Yes, you make more money and gain more power. But none of it means a damn thing if you don't know the caress of a woman who loves you, the hug of a child who adores you, or the pulsations of a sexual experience that redefines your belief in God.

We don't have enough space to cover all of what you need to do if the "workaholic" label seems to fit you. For that, we recommend a good therapist.

For a therapy jump-start, think through some of this stuff beforehand. First, realize that working until all hours is likely not the real problem; it's your attempt at a *solution* to a different problem. Try to figure out what you're hoping to avoid by working so much. Is it your relationship, commitment, boredom? Heavy-duty soul searching is hard work in and of itself. So treat it as an investment of sorts—the time you spend working through your underlying problems will offset time spent working yourself to the bone.

Next, make a list of the things that your dedication to work forces you to sacrifice. If you decide you don't want to live without one or more of those items, you may be ready to take bigger steps. Here's one to try.

Find 1 day in the coming week when you can get to work late or cut out early. (Hey, don't sweat it. What's early or late for you is probably a normal time for most workers.) Make a date with your partner, to say, watch a video, curl up on the couch, or yes, have sex. Next, get out your ever-present pocket planner and schedule 5 minutes each day leading up to your rendezvous to look forward to it. Then, when you're with her, shift your priorities from work to tenderness. See which truly feels better. Finally—and this is important—recognize that you've created this pleasure by setting limits on your time at the office.

Try this each week, and with luck, gradually (we mean this—it won't happen overnight) you'll see a change in your work outlook. In all likelihood, you'll also be having a whole lot more sex.

Also see: afternoon delight, appointments, commitment, fatigue, stress, time, toys, travel ruins relationships

wrestling

Does the WWF have a place in the bedroom? Maybe not to the extreme of smack downs. But your lover may be pleasantly surprised if you bed her with a gentle takedown that places her in a submissive position.

The cradle pin, for example, can be toned down and employed in frisky fashion. Move deftly and thoughtfully, thus avoiding an errant hair pull or elbow to the jaw. With her lying on her back, approach the right side of her body on your hands and knees (or you can lie on your stomach). Lean over her so your upper body is above her chest. (Hey, nice view.) Your body should be perpendicular to hers, so that together, your bodies form a lowercase *t*. Then slide your left arm under her shoulders while simultaneously slipping your right arm under her left thigh. Slowly lift her head and leg toward one another until you can clasp your hands. It's virtually impossible for

Hot Dates **1996** The U.S. Supreme Court voted unanimously to overturn the Communications Decency Act, a law passed in 1995 to control obscenity on the Internet.

continued from page 402

moval of a limb. He had **a lifelong sexual fantasy to have his leg amputated.** Finding a reputable doctor to amputate a healthy limb is no easy task, so Bondy paid $10,000 to John Brown, 77, whose medical license had been revoked 20 years earlier for performing second-rate sex change operations.

The ex-doc did the surgery on Bondy in Tijuana, Mexico. Bondy died 2 days later from gangrene poisoning. Brown was convicted of second-degree murder.

LEGAL BRIEFS

A Brazilian man admitted to police that he was so wracked with grief over the death of his fiancée that, **3 months after her burial, he unearthed her corpse**—which was still clad in her wedding dress—and had sex with it.

"I was desperate and needed her," he explained.

True or Phallus

The custom of illuminating a house of ill repute with a red light originated in Amsterdam.

BAWDY BALLADS "Nothing Sure Looked Good on You," *Gene Watson*

continued on page 414

her to escape from this hold. Now you can kiss her to your heart's content. Or until she threatens to lace your morning coffee with strychnine if you don't release her, pronto. (In fact, we recommend agreeing ahead of time on a safeword that signals when either of you is ready to quit.)

Playfulness is definitely the key. Just as light pinching and spanking have a place in the bedroom, so can wrestling. A mean-spirited quest to pin down her arms and legs, though, isn't lovemaking. If you intimidate or hurt her—and "I swear it was an accident, honey" doesn't cut it—you'll kill any sense of passion. Match over.

Also see: athletic sex, body oils, dominance and submission, games, rough sex, safeword

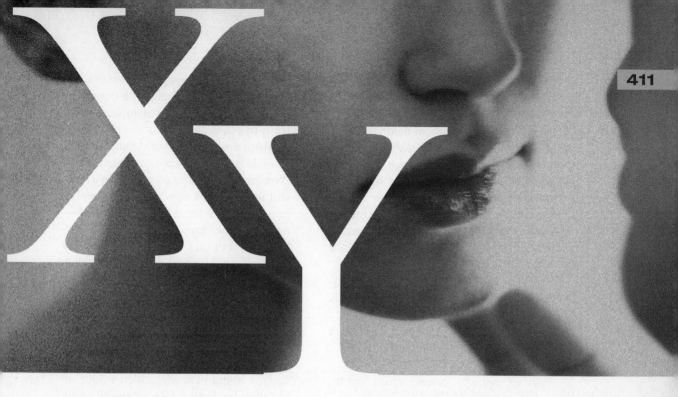

X-rated

Although it now screams of sweaty sex scenes and cheesy soundtracks, the original X rating wasn't devised for hardcore porn. It was intended to warn parents that a mainstream Hollywood release had too much violence, adult language, and lust to be acceptable for folks under age 17.

In the 1960s, the Motion Picture Association of America (MPAA) began to notice that as social codes became looser, so did the content of films. The first mildly profane phrase to enter the cinema—"hump the hostess"—caused a stir during the 1966 release of *Who's Afraid of Virginia Woolf*. A few months later, *Blowup* got another rise out of the organization as the first wide-release movie to put naked bodies up on the big screen. After that, the MPAA decided it

was time to crack down and create a rating system that let parents know when to keep their children out of the theaters.

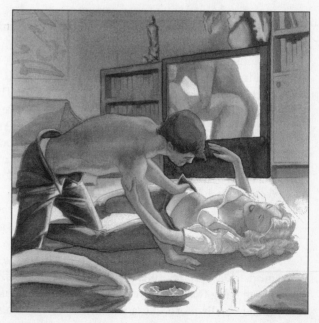

Late in 1968, the motion picture industry adopted the following letter guidelines: G, or general rating, for all audiences; M, for mature audiences; R, for restricted audiences, wherein theaters barred unsupervised children under 16; and the infamous X for those films that could be viewed by no one under 17. The association trademarked all of its ratings except the X, which any company could affix to its film without undergoing the rating process.

By 1990, the rising pornography industry had successfully swiped the X rating, adding XX and XXX, thereby giving the original label even naughtier connotations. The MPAA then changed its X rating to NC-17.

Also see: cybersex, erotic films, movies, pornography, violence

yeast infection

A vaginal overgrowth of the yeast organism *Candida albicans*—and yet another reason to be glad you're not a woman.

But before you get too thankful, consider that you can contract candida from an infected woman if she doesn't stop you from getting too close. You're more likely to pick up a case if you are obese, have diabetes, are uncircumcised, or take a lot of antibiotics.

So before you take the plunge, pay special attention to the appearance of her vagina. If it's unusually red and sore (or you catch her scratching down there), think twice. And if she's oozing something that looks a lot like cottage cheese, you'll want to put your pants back on.

If you're still not sure—and as humorist Dave Barry likes to say, we are not making this up—take a quick whiff: If she smells more like a warm loaf of sourdough than like a pleasant seashore, she may have the fungus. The odor of a yeast infection strongly resembles that of fresh-baked bread.

More unsettling news: If you do catch candida, you'll likely notice white fungus growing on the head of your penis. And still more: It can appear anywhere else that your skin folds and traps sweat—under your elbows, behind your knees, between your toes. You can even get it in your mouth. The oral version of a yeast infection, called thrush, is sometimes contracted through cunnilingus.

Yeast infection sometimes ping-pongs back and forth between partners. To break the cycle, pick up an over-the-counter anti-yeast cream, like Micatin antifungal cream, usually found near the athlete's foot or jock itch medications. Don't use the athlete's foot preparations on your penis, as they can be irritating. If you need a more potent prescription, or if the infection appears in your mouth, see your doctor.

Also see: douche, monilia, STDs, suppositories, thrush, vaginal diseases/infections, whipped cream

yin and yang

The female energy and the male energy, respectively. You have both within you. Also spoken of as the dark and the light, according to Asian traditions, these sexual energies must remain in harmony for you to experience optimum health.

As the ancient Chinese discovered, there is no better way to keep yin and yang balanced than to have good sex, and plenty of it, thus frequently joining your strong yang with your lady's tantalizing yin. (We knew we had a reason for liking those ancient Chinese.) In long-ago China, sage folks considered sex a natural, guiltless activity. Sexual pleasure led to a healthy populace.

Sex was also a spiritual activity. During the Tang dynasty, from 618 to 907, Taoism was the state religion and preached that immortality could be achieved through sex. Taoist sexual theory was then taken to India, where it evolved into Tantrism.

Also see: AC/DC, androgyny, anima and animus, bisexuality, chromosomes, gender bender, hermaphrodite, *Kama Sutra*, tantra, transvestism

yogi

No, not the celebrated baseball figure. Not the picnic-snatching bear, either. A yogi is a person who practices yoga breathing and stretching exercises to experience a sense of peace and spirituality. It's also someone who studies Yoga philosophy.

What does that have to do with sex? Well, one form, tantric yoga, calls for an abundance of sex (no argument here) in ritual form with experienced women who are worshipped not just as sexy creatures of the flesh but as authentic goddesses. This method of yoga sees orgasm as a portal to deep spiritual realms. Or as baseball's Yogi might put it, "Fifty percent of sex is 90 percent spiritual."

Also see: chakras, *Kama Sutra*, spiritual sex, tantra

yohimbine

The pharmaceutical answer to the herb yohimbe, once considered a botanical godsend by those in search of greater sexual potency. Derived from the bark of the African yo-

himbe tree, the herb was commonly prescribed to men suffering from impotence. Medical history links it to high blood pressure, headaches, anxiety, insomnia, and nausea—all of which tend to take the fun out of any erection the remedy might prompt.

Today, drug companies are involved. They found a way to extract the active compound from the bark to treat erectile problems with fewer side effects. Bear in mind, that's *fewer* side effects, not necessarily none, so check with your doctor if you have a history of any of the health problems associated with the original herb.

Also see: aphrodisiac, erection, impotence, priapism, Prozac, refractory period

young men/older women

Although it's not the most common relationship configuration, you shouldn't discard the idea of dating a woman just because she's got a few years on you.

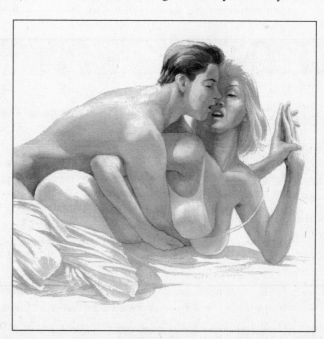

Some wise men actually prefer to date mature beauties. Part of the reason is that older women bring an air of confidence into the bedroom. They have years of practice under their garter belts and have learned not to complicate sex with all sorts of issues about "commitment." And they tend to be less clitorally focused, which can make the actual sex act more fun and rewarding for both partners. Some also tend to climax more easily than their younger counterparts.

Women, understand, have a hard time learning to be sexual. Even in this day and age, they're not taught to enjoy their sexuality. While society applauds sexually active young men for their prowess, we still label lusty young women with insulting terms. As a result, many women begin their sex lives timidly and with guilt.

By the time they've reached middle age, however, many women have shed their fears and are ready to have some fun. Perhaps they no longer feel pressured to find serious relationships and bear children. Been there, done that. Now they want to play.

It's cool to note that the essence of a good woman—*essence* defined as intelligence, elegance, sense of humor, and charm—does not diminish with age. In fact, it gets better. A more mature woman is also much more likely to be forgiving of your minor flaws. Many young women covet a man with flashy wheels, a body beautiful, and a full head of hair (preferably his own). Many older women have abandoned those idealistic expectations.

Here's one reason not to date an older lady: You're looking for a surrogate mother. In an equal partnership, an older woman may indeed have a lot to teach you, in and out of the bedroom. But she's probably not interested in mothering you. Chances are, she already has kids. She wants to be your lover, not your babysitter.

Hot Dates **1998** An estimated four million prescriptions for Viagra (sildenafil) were filled in its first year on the market.

continued from page 409

Answer:
False. It's believed to have originated in China, where red silk lamps were placed outside bars where illegal prostitution flourished.

Seemed like a Good Idea at the Time. . .

God bless Ellen E. Perkins. She received a U.S. patent for her invention of "Sexual Armor" that equipped the mentally ill to do battle against the horrors of playing with themselves. "It is a deplorable but well known fact that one of the most common causes of insanity, imbecility, and feeble-mindedness, especially in youth, is due to masturbation or self abuse," she wrote to the U.S. Patent Office.

Perkins's apparatus consisted of a lockable metal compartment that covered the crotch. Leather straps for connecting the device to the deviant could also be secured with padlocks.

The metal crotch section of the contraption did feature a hinged "gate" with holes for urinating, and it could also be swung open to permit defecation. Perkins claimed that **her armor could be worn with little or no discomfort** and that, when properly covered by clothing, it was not noticeable.

BAWDY BALLADS "Slow Ride," *Foghat*

And keep in mind that age differences do place certain endemic stresses on a relationship. The older the couple, the fewer problems they encounter. A 35-year-old man dating, say, a 55-year old woman will probably have an easier time of it than a 20-year-old man dating a 40-year-old. Career questions and child-rearing issues can make it hard for a young man to feel comfortable with a more established, family-oriented woman.

Also see: commitment, death of a partner, Freud, menopause—hers

young women/older men

Women your own age will scorn you. Other men will cheer you. Casual bystanders may offer to snap a photo of "you and your daughter." But a younger adult woman just may be the right partner for a man who wants to be with her for reasons deeper than her smooth complexion.

Many young women today are independent, ambitious, dynamic creatures who are well-rounded in ways other than their figures. They aren't searching for sugar daddies; they have their own agendas. It's not hard to see why many of them prefer older men. Remember being a young whelp? If you were like most guys that age, you were an immature, self-centered putz. Those are the pickings, among her male contemporaries. You've outgrown and outclassed them. Kudos to you.

For the record, there may be more than just the obvious reasons why you're willing to risk injuring your neck (as well as other body parts, if you're married and your wife is with you) by gawking at some nubile 20-year-old. One theory leads us back to primitive times. Males

of yore picked their mates on the basis of which females were best suited for propagating the species. That meant young and fertile. Though times have changed, old habits die hard. What's more, many men don't feel emotionally ready to start fathering kids until they're in their late 30s or early 40s. Unfortunately, women in that same age range are no longer as fertile as in their earlier years and may have trouble getting pregnant.

Problems can nevertheless arise if you, Mr. Graying Temples, find yourself entering a series of unsuccessful relationships with twentysomething women and persist in that pattern while you continue to get older. At that point, in all likelihood, you're seeking relationships based not on the person but on the age and *image* of the person. It's akin to having relationships only with large-breasted women or women with trawlers or whatever. The point is, you're not getting past the surface to find the human being underneath.

No matter how young a woman is when you first meet her, eventually she's going to get—and look—older. The deeper bonds that develop between longtime partners should more than offset the superficial ravages of aging. And we suspect, if you look in the mirror, you'll see that you're not exactly Matt Damon yourself these days.

Also see: aging, biological clock, Electra complex, erection difficulties, innocence, *Lolita*, menopause—yours, midlife crisis, pedophilia, trophy wife

Your place or mine?

A question that, when posed by a woman, translates to "pay dirt." The innuendo became popular in the early 1970s with the rise of casual sex. During that decade, a guy could whisper, "Your place or mine?" into the ear of a woman he'd met in a club just 30 minutes earlier. And he stood a decent chance of her actually answering him with a smile instead of a stiletto to his groin.

That was then, this is now. AIDS, hepatitis, and common sense—not to mention sexual harassment lawsuits—all have combined to cool things down. Right-thinking men and women alike are more selective about whom they sleep with.

Not that the phrase has lost all its charm. Try it on your wife or girlfriend, for instance. You may find that she has just the *perfect* place for you.

Also see: affairs, first time with a lover, one-night stand, pickup lines, zipless sex

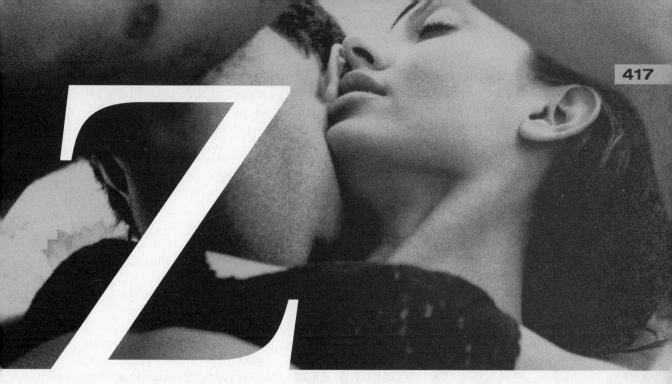

zinc

One of the most important nutrients for proper sexual function. Low levels of this mineral can weaken the reproductive system, dampen sex drive, and even delay sexual maturation in prepubescent males.

Studies show that 10 to 15 percent of infertile adult males have low zinc levels. Such deficiencies seem to wear down the swimming strength of sperm—the little guys just don't have enough gusto to rocket up the fallopian tube and penetrate the egg.

Since semen contains high concentrations of zinc, frequent ejaculation can make you lose too much of the mineral. Your body may even respond by reducing your sexual drive.

Prolific sex *is* good for prostate health, not to mention mental health. So go ahead and let it fly on a regular basis—just make sure you think zinc. Eat foods like oysters, liver, steak, crab, wheat germ, black-eyed peas, chickpeas, and miso. Also, check the labeling of your multivitamin to see if it's fortified with zinc. Some are, some aren't.

Also see: ejaculation, food, impotence, oysters, prostate, prostatitis, sex drive, sperm count, supplements

zipless sex

Picture it: A beautiful woman comes up to you during a train ride. She pulls off your pants, climbs atop you, and introduces you to the warmth of her body. She finishes, gets up, smoothes her skirt. You don't know her name; you never said a word to her, nor she to you. Then she winks, smiles devilishly, tosses her hair, and is gone.

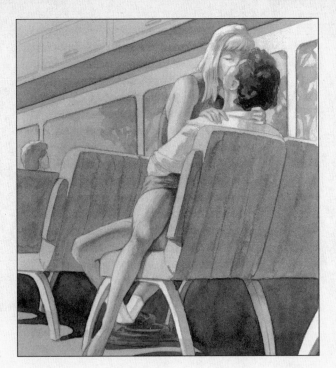

many of us still harbor fantasies of such encounters. Yet sexually transmitted diseases, legal concerns, and shyness are just some of the impediments that often prevent us from attempting to fulfill these fantasies with the proverbial stranger in the night. Fortunately, there are other, safer ways of making it happen, as with someone who agrees to act out such fantasies with you, via phone sex, cybersex, or role-playing.

Also see: blind date, cybersex, first time with a lover, one-night stand, phone sex, playacting, quickies, risky sex, wild women

Congratulations. You've just had zipless sex—passionate, unbridled lovemaking with a partner you just "met" and will never see again. It's enough to make even the one-night stand seem like a commitment.

According to *Fear of Flying* author Erica Jong (whose actual term in the racy 1973 novel was *zipless fuck*), this is the purest form of sex. It is, she writes, the ultimate expression of sexual freedom, so-named because "when you came together zippers fell away like rose petals, underwear blew off in one breath like dandelion fluff. Tongues intertwined and turned liquid. Your whole soul flowed out through your tongue and into the mouth of your lover."

Though changing mores have made such purple prose sound anachronistic,

zippers

The metal-toothed closure became fashionable for men's flies and ladies' dresses in the late 1930s.

That vintage dress in your honey's closet, from the 1940s or '50s, has a metal zipper under the left arm, along the side seam. On a newer dress or skirt, a nylon zipper is usually found at the center back seam, sometimes hidden under folds of delicate fabric that will get snagged if you undo it too quickly. So don't. The lustful exuberance of the moment will fade instantly when she realizes that you've trashed her $800 designer getup.

What to do with a stuck zipper? Don't rely on brute strength. Rub a candle stub across the teeth for lubrication, pull the slide up to free the caught fabric, then try to unzip again.

Our flies are notorious, of course, for snagging old long john. This painful predicament is best solved with petroleum jelly. Try rubbing the lubricant across the zipper to free your trapped skin. If that fails, snip the zipper slide in half with a pair of metal cutters—using the obvious and appropriate care—and take the zipper apart. (If you need to, go to your local emergency room, where they usually have experience in this area.) Wash and dry the damaged skin thoroughly, and apply an antibiotic ointment like Neosporin to prevent infection.

Also see: striptease, undressing

zoophilia

Perhaps this is what the Captain and Tennille had in mind when they sang their classic "Muskrat Love." Zoophilia—sexual and emotional interest in animals, also known as bestiality—has appeared in folklore and myth throughout recorded history. Take the Greek legend of the Minotaur: He was the offspring of Pasiphaë, queen of Crete, and a bull with whom she dallied.

Of course, zoophilia has also appeared in fact: All those jokes about shepherds and sheep didn't come out of nowhere. Though some argue that sex-capades with pets and other animals are quite rare, the landmark Kinsey sex studies posed that 8 percent of adult males and 3 percent of adult females had given zoophilia a try. Not surprisingly, these encounters tend to occur in rural settings, where chosen partners include sheep, burros, horses, dogs, cats, and even poultry.

Prurient interest in animals often stems from sexual trauma or even severe sexual frustration. Because it may well indicate a troubled past, you should consider seeking psychiatric help if you find yourself with overpowering urges to do the zoo.

Also see: animals, bestiality, compulsive behavior, fantasies, paraphilias, perversions, pets, sex offenders, sex therapy, sodomy

zygote

When one of your sperm completes its victorious swim up a woman's fallopian tube by bursting into her egg, this first cell of pregnancy is produced.

You can't make heads or tails of the one-celled zygote before it divides into many other cells and develops into an embryo, which looks a lot more like the start of a baby. But the zygote, incredibly, holds all the genetic information that a baby needs to inherit half his good looks from you and half from your partner.

Also see: chromosomes, ectopic pregnancy, genetics, pregnancy

Z

Index

A

AA, 11, 23
Abdominal muscles. *See* Abs
Abnormal, 1. *See also*
    Paraphilias; Perversions
  kinky sex and, 162–63
Abortion, 1–2
  Hot Dates in, 9, 267, 358
  pelvic inflammatory disease
    and, 238
Abortion pill, 2–3. *See also*
    Morning-after pill
Abs, 3, **3**. *See also* Male body;
    Weight loss
  body fitness and, 32–33
  body image and, 33
  body shapes and, 35
  exercise and, 98
  muscles and, 209
  sexy, 314
  thongs and, 356
Abstinence, 3–4. *See also* Sex,
    lack of
  celibacy as, 48
  in rhythm method, 289
  sex education about, 163,
    306
  tantra and, 349
AC/DC, 4
Acquaintance rape, 70. *See
    also* Rape
Acquired immunodeficiency
    syndrome. *See* AIDS

Adultery, 4, **4**. *See also* Affairs
  affairs and, 5–6
  French attitudes about,
    117–18
  open marriage vs., 188
Advances, unwanted. *See*
    Unwanted advances
Affairs, 5–6. *See also* Adultery;
    Extramarital sex
  adultery and, 4, **4**
  Don't ask, don't tell about, 80
  In Extremis, 337, 342
  Legal Briefs about, 136, 143
  lust and, 177–78
  monogamy and, 202
  politicians and, 254–55
  rebuilding trust after, 369–71
  with
    best friend's wife, 26–27, **27**
    boss's wife, 37–38
  variety vs., 386
Afterglow, 6
  afterplay and, 7
  communication during,
    57–58
  of massage, 190
Afternoon delight, 6–7, 129
Afterplay, 7
Aging, 7–8. *See also* Young
    men/older women;
    Young women/older
    men
  biological clock and, 29
  delayed orgasm and, 222–23

empty-nest syndrome and,
    90
  erection difficulties and,
    91–92
  firmer erection, 92
  frequency and, 119
  and longing for past
    partners, 232
  midlife crisis and, 199–200
  multiple orgasms and, 208
  prostate enlargement and,
    270–71
  testosterone replacement
    therapy and, 354–55
  urinary problems and, 378
  your menopause and,
    197–98
Ahhh, 8
AIDS, 8–10. *See also* HIV
  fears/phobias about, 105
  gonorrhea and, 128
  herpes and, 137
  Hot Dates in, 342, 379
  in prison, 266
  STDs and, 333
  venereal disease and, 389
  Your place or mine? and, 416
Airhead, 10
Alcohol, 10–11
  Alcoholics Anonymous and,
    11, 23
  as aphrodisiac, 14–15
  bars and, 22–23
  beer, 25

Underscored page references indicate boxed text. **Boldface** references indicate illustrations.

Alcohol *(cont.)*
breath and, 44
drugs and, 84–85
erection difficulties and, 91
gang bang and, 122
gang rape and, 122
infertility and, 148
as issue that leads to
divorce, 79
and loneliness during travel,
366
lust and, 178
klismaphilia and, 165
rape and, 281
and talking about past
partners, 234
Alcoholics Anonymous (AA),
11, 23
Anal beads, 11
Anal plug, 11–12
Anal sex, 12–13. *See also*
Lubricants; Sexual aids
AIDS and, 10
as compulsive behavior, 59
dildo and, 75–76
klismaphilia and, 165
lubricants and, 176
Madonna/whore complex
and, 179
necrophilia and, 211
no in response to proposing,
213
ointments and, 219
packing as, 227
pederasty and, 235
perversions and, 245
piercings and, 250
rear entry, 282–83
rectum and, 283–84
rimming, 289–90
role reversal and, 292
safe sex and, 298
sodomy, 328
sphincter and, 331
suppositories and, 339–40
vibrator and, 390

Androgyny, 13
latex and, 168
Anger. *See* Arguing
Anima and animus, 13
Animals, 13–14. *See also* In
Extremis; True or
Phallus? about, animals
bestiality and, 27–28
courtship among, 64
flirtation among, 113
food and, 114
as Kokigami in Japan, 249,
256
mating among, 193
monogamy among, 202
pets, 245–46
pheromones of, 247
positions among, 258
sodomy and, 328
zoophilia and, 419
Anticipatory anxiety, 14
Aphrodisiac, 14–15
courtship, 63–65
danger, 69
oysters, 224–25
power, 262–63
seduction, 301–2
sexual attraction, 309–10
Spanish fly, 329
travel, 365
yohimbine, 413
Appointments, 15–16
rituals and, 291
time-saving tips for,
358–59
variety and, 386
Arguing, 16–17
avoiding divorce and, 78
communication and, 57
jealousy and, 154
making up after, 182–83
violence and, 392
about wet spot, 403
withholding while, 407
Aromatherapy, 17–18. *See also*
Fragrances

Arousal, 18
atmosphere for, 19
erection, 91
excitement phase of, 97–98
foreplay and, 115–16
horniness and, 140
lubrication, 176–77
stimulation and, 336–37
Ass size, 320–21, **321**
booty and, 36
buttock implants and, 203
Athlete's foot, 360
Athletic sex, 18
exercise and, 98
standing positions, 332–33,
333
sweating during, 341–42
wrestling, 409–10
Atmosphere, 19
arousal and, 18
flowers for, 114
food for, 114–15
fragrances for, 116–17
mood and, 204
music for, 209–10
relaxation and, 285–86,
286
travel and, 366–67
Attraction, 19
dating and, 70–71
meeting women and, 195–96
preference and, 263
self-esteem and, 302
sexual, 309–10

B

Back problems, 21–22
body fitness and, 32–33
exercise and, 98
sixty-nine (69) and, 320
Baldness, 109–10
B&D. *See* Bondage and
discipline
Bars, 22–23
alcohol and, 10–11
eye contact in, 100

Underscored page references indicate boxed text. **Boldface** references indicate illustrations.

<u>Underscored</u> page references indicate boxed text. **Boldface** references indicate illustrations.

Underscored page references indicate boxed text. **Boldface** references indicate illustrations.

Underscored page references indicate boxed text. **Boldface** references indicate illustrations.

Underscored page references indicate boxed text. **Boldface** references indicate illustrations.

<u>Underscored</u> page references indicate boxed text. **Boldface** references indicate illustrations.

Underscored page references indicate boxed text. **Boldface** references indicate illustrations.

Underscored page references indicate boxed text. **Boldface** references indicate illustrations.

Underscored page references indicate boxed text. **Boldface** references indicate illustrations.

Underscored page references indicate boxed text. **Boldface** references indicate illustrations.

<u>Underscored</u> page references indicate boxed text. **Boldface** references indicate illustrations.

Underscored page references indicate boxed text. **Boldface** references indicate illustrations.

Underscored page references indicate boxed text. **Boldface** references indicate illustrations.

Underscored page references indicate boxed text. **Boldface** references indicate illustrations.

The Book of Sex **Staff**

EXECUTIVE EDITOR: Steve Salerno
ASSOCIATE EDITOR: Kathryn C. LeSage
CONTRIBUTING WRITERS: Jami Attenberg, Layne Cameron,
Kelly Garrett, Larry Keller, Cynthia Miller,
Deanna Portz, John Thompson
ART DIRECTOR AND DESIGNER: Charles Beasley
ILLUSTRATORS: Dærick Gröss Sr., D. W. Gröss
RESEARCH MANAGER: Leah Flickinger
RESEARCH EDITOR: Deborah Pedron
SENIOR RESEARCHER: Deanna Portz
EDITORIAL RESEARCHERS: Deborah Dellapena, Anne Dickson,
Jennifer Goldsmith, Karen Jacob,
Staci Ann Sander
LAYOUT DESIGNER: Keith Biery
PRODUCT SPECIALIST: Jodi Schaffer

Rodale for Men

VICE PRESIDENT, WORLDWIDE PUBLISHER: Edward J. Fones
MARKETING DIRECTOR: Bob Keppel
ASSOCIATE CUSTOMER MARKETING MANAGER: Matt Neumaier
CONTENT ASSEMBLY MANAGER: Robert V. Anderson Jr.
DIGITAL PROCESSING GROUP ASSOCIATE MANAGER: Thomas P. Aczel
OFFICE MANAGER: Alice Debus
ASSISTANT OFFICE MANAGER: Marianne Moor
OFFICE STAFF: Pamela Brinar, Susan B. Dorschutz

Advisors for *The Book of Sex*

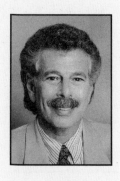

Kenneth A. Goldberg, M.D., is the founder and
director of the Male Health Center in Lewisville, Texas.

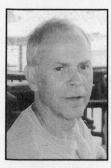

George Hartlaub, M.D., is an associate clinical
professor of psychiatry at the University of Colorado Health
Sciences Center in Denver.

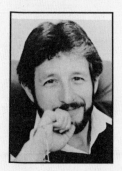

Marty Klein, Ph.D., is a licensed marriage and family
therapist in Palo Alto, California; a certified sex educator; and
the publisher of the monthly e-newsletter *Sexual Intelligence*.

Sources for *The Book of Sex*

Gloria Allred is a Los Angeles attorney who specializes in matters of sexual harassment, employment discrimination, and family law; the founder and president of the Women's Equal Rights Legal Defense and Education fund; and a radio talk show host with KABC.

Doug Anderson is a voice coach in Philadelphia and has a Web site at www.yourvoicecoach.com.

Teresa Archuleta-Sagel is an aromatherapist and the owner of TAS Touch in Espanola, New Mexico.

Audrey Ashby is senior director of public relations at Wyeth-Ayerst Laboratories, an international pharmaceutical company in Boston.

Larry Clapp is the president of Prostate90 Education and Research Foundation, the founder of the Web site www.prostate90.com, and the author of *Prostate Health in 90 Days*.

Deborah Corley, Ph.D., is a clinical psychologist at the Family Psychology Institute of Dallas.

Michael R. Cunningham, Ph.D., is a professor of psychology at the University of Louisville.

Joe Ann Demore, Ed.D., is a sex therapist and staff member at the Institute for Sex Education, Treatment, and Research in Ft. Lauderdale and a diplomate of the American Board of Sexology.

Michael of Destiny is a St. Louis–based gigolo.

Linda DeVillers is a licensed psychologist and certified sex therapist in Marina Del Ray, California, and the author of *Love Skills*.

John DuMont is certified in the sympto-thermal method, a natural family-planning option, and is the Eastern field director of teachers and promoters for the Couple to Couple League in Cincinnati.

Allen Elkin, Ph.D., is a clinical psychologist, the author of the 1999 edition of *Stress Management for Dummies*, and the director of the Stress Management and Counseling Center in New York City.

Paul Elsner, Psy.D., is the president of the Personology Foundation of the Pacific, is in the National Register of Health Service Providers in Psychology, and is a certified sex therapist and licensed psychologist in Albuquerque.

William Fitzgerald, Ph.D., is a marital and sexual therapist at Silicon Valley Relationship and Sexuality Center in Santa Clara, California, and the author of *What Every Young Woman Needs to Know: An Aid to Dialogue between Parent and Child*.

Megan P. Fleming, Ph.D., is the director of the Sexual Health and Rehabilitation Program at Beth Israel Medical Center in New York City.

Jean L. Fourcroy, M.D., Ph.D., M.P.H., is the past president of the National Council on Women's Health and an assistant professor at the Uniformed Services University of the Health Sciences F. Edward Hébert School of Medicine in Bethesda, Maryland.

Wendi Friesen is a certified clinical hypnotherapist in Folsom, California, and the author of *Hypnotize Your Lover*.

Sandor Gardos, Ph.D., is a clinical sexologist in San Francisco and the director of the advisory board of the Xandria Collection sex-product retailer.

Barbara Gillis is the editor of *The Florist* magazine.

Adam Glickman is the CEO and founder of Condomania, a condom and other sexual-products retail store in Los Angeles and New York City.

Gregory J. P. Godek is a relationship expert in La Jolla, California, and the author of *1,001 Ways to Be Romantic.*

Sue Gould is the owner of Club Adventure, a private social club for couples interested in swinging, in Vernon Hills, Illinois.

Sharon Granskog is the assistant director of public information at the American Veterinary Medical Association.

Lila Gruzen, Ph.D., is a relationship and marriage and family therapist in Sherman Oaks, California, and co-author of *10 Foolish Dating Mistakes That Men and Women Make and How to Avoid Them.*

Debra W. Haffner is a sex educator and the author of several books, including *Beyond the Big Talk: Every Parent's Guide to Raising Sexually Healthy Teens, from Middle School to College.*

Dian Hanson is the editor of *Leg Show*, the largest-selling fetish publication.

Noel Paul Hertz is a certified sex therapist in Chicago and a member of the American Association of Marriage and Family Therapy.

Alan R. Hirsch, M.D., is the neurological director of the Smell and Taste Treatment and Research Foundation in Chicago and the author of *Dr. Hirsch's Guide to Scentsational Weight Loss, Scentsational Sex,* and *What Flavor Is Your Personality?*

Irvin Hirsch, M.D., is a urologist at Thomas Jefferson University in Philadelphia.

Penelope Hitchcock, D.V.M., is the chief of the sexually transmitted diseases branch at the National Institute of Allergy and Infectious Diseases.

Martha Hopkins is a partner at Terrace Publishing in Waco, Texas, and co-author of *InterCourses: An Aphrodisiac Cookbook.*

Susan Dickes Hubbard is a certified sex therapist in Boulder, Colorado, and the author of *Spicing Up Your Sex Life.*

Frederick Jacobsen, M.D., is a clinical professor of psychiatry and behavioral sciences at George Washington University School of Medicine in Washington, D.C.

David Knox, Ph.D., is a counselor in marriage and family living in Greenville, North Carolina, and the host of the Sexual Intimacy Web site at www.heartchoice.com.

Nancy Koreen is a skydiver and the managing editor of *Parachutist* magazine.

Lavanya is a tattoo artist at the Domain of Pain in Santa Fe, New Mexico.

Carol Leigh, also known as Scarlot Harlot, is a prostitute activist and artist in San Francisco and the founder of the Web site www.bayswan.org.

Tom Liesegang is the manager of DeMask, a fetish company in New York City.

Marlene M. Maheu, Ph.D., is the editor of *SelfhelpMagazine* in San Diego and the author of *Infidelity on the Internet.*

Jason Mahnke is a trainer for the Los Angeles Dodgers baseball club.

Wendy Maltz is a certified sex therapist; a licensed marriage counselor; a licensed clinical social worker with her own firm, Maltz Counseling Associates, in Eugene, Oregon; and the author of *Private Thoughts: Exploring the Power of Women's Sexual Fantasies* and *The Sexual Healing Journey.*

Eliezer Margolis, Ph.D., is a licensed clinical psychologist and sex therapist in Evanston, Illinois; is certified by the American Board of Professional Psychology in rehabilitation psychology; and is a consultant to the amputee program at the prosthetic-orthotic certificate program at Northwestern University Medical Center in Chicago.

Commander Wayne McBride, Ph.D., is the former deputy director of preventive medicine and occupational health at the U.S. Navy Bureau of Medicine and Surgery.

Ted McIlvenna, Ph.D., is the president of the Institute for Advanced Study of Human Sexuality in San Francisco.

Marnie McLaughlin is the public relations manager at the Victoria's Secret corporate office in Columbus, Ohio.

Michael Milroy, M.D., is a urologist in Santa Fe, New Mexico.

Mary Jane Minkin, M.D., is a clinical professor of obstetrics and gynecology at Yale University School of Medicine and the author of *What Every Woman Needs to Know about Menopause*.

Glenn Mones is the director of media relations at Planned Parenthood in New York City.

Monica Moore, Ph.D., is a professor of psychology at Webster University in St. Louis.

Jack Morin, Ph.D., is a sex therapist and psychotherapist in San Francisco, a diplomate of the American Board of Sexology, and the author of *Anal Pleasure and Health* and *The Erotic Mind*.

Lewis Nemes, Ph.D., is an American Board of Sexology–certified clinical sexologist in Albuquerque; a diplomate of the International Academy of Behavioral Medicine, Counseling, and Psychotherapy; and a board-certified fellow with the American College of Advanced Practice Psychologists.

Norman J. Nemoy, M.D., is a urologist in Los Angeles.

Margery M. Noel, Psy.D., is a sex therapist and board-certified, licensed clinical psychologist in Santa Fe, New Mexico.

Richard L. Ogletree, Pharm.D., is the pharmacy coordinator and clinical assistant professor of pharmacy at the University of Mississippi Medical Center in Jackson.

Timothy Perper, Ph.D., is an independent researcher and writer in Philadelphia and the author of *Sex Signals*.

Tina Pieraccini is a professor of communication studies at the State University of New York at Oswego.

Mary Lake Polan, M.D., Ph.D., is the chair and a professor of the department of gynecology and obstetrics at Stanford University School of Medicine.

Carol Queen, Ed.D., is the director of continuing education at Good Vibrations sex-product retailer in San Francisco and the author of *Exhibitionism for the Shy*.

Mike Ramone is the editor in chief of *Adult Video News* magazine.

Candida Royalle is the creator and president of New York City–based Femme Productions, which creates erotica from a woman's point of view.

Howard Ruppel is a former executive director of the American Association of Sex Educators, Counselors, and Therapists.

Linda Savage, Ph.D., is a licensed psychologist and sex therapist in Vista, California; a diplomate of the American Board of Sexology; a member of the Institute of Marital and Sexual Therapy in Chula Vista, California; and the author of *Reclaiming Goddess Sexuality*.

Alan Schragger, M.D., is a dermatologist in Allentown, Pennsylvania.

Arthur G. Schwartz, Ph.D., is a microbiology professor and DHEA researcher at Temple University's Fels Research Institute in Philadelphia.

Jonathan A. Segal is a law partner at Wolf, Block, and Solis-Cohen in Philadelphia, specializing in counseling, policies, and training to avoid employment litigation.

Kathryn Sellers is the director of public relations for the Carpet and Rug Institute in Dalton, Georgia.

Phillip R. Shaver, Ph.D., is the head of the doctoral program in personality and social psychology and a professor of psychology at the University of California, Davis; and co-editor of *Handbook of Attachment: Theory, Research, and Clinical Applications*.

Michael Sheinberg, M.D., is an obstetrician and gynecologist in Allentown, Pennsylvania.

Josephine Sinclair, also known as the Mistress Moth, is a professional dominatrix and the founder of Club Dominion in Muncie, Indiana.

Devendra Singh, Ph.D., is a professor of psychology at the University of Texas in Austin.

Julian Slowinski, Psy.D., is a certified sex therapist, a senior clinical psychologist at Pennsylvania Hospital in Philadelphia, and co-author of *The Sexual Male*.

Michael Smolensky, Ph.D., is the director of the chronobiology center at Hermann Hospital in Houston and the author of *The Body-Clock Guide to Better Health*.

Frederick Snoy, M.D., is a urologist in Albuquerque.

Gary Storkan, D.C., is a chiropractor in Alamos, New Mexico, who specializes in nutrition and metabolic diseases.

Kathleen Strimple is a speech-and-language pathologist in Sante Fe, New Mexico.

Kenneth Ray Stubbs, Ph.D., is a psychologist and the editor of Secret Garden Publishing in Tucson and the author of *Erotic Passions*, *Erotic Massage*, and *The Essential Tantra*.

Joan C. Sughrue, R.N., is a certified sex therapist in Atlanta.

John Sughrue Jr., M.D., is a certified sex therapist in Atlanta.

T. Joel Wade, Ph.D., is an associate professor of psychology at Bucknell University in Lewisburg, Pennsylvania, and a researcher on interracial relationships.

Melinda Walker is a psychotherapist and relationship counselor in Santa Fe, New Mexico.

Louanne Cole Weston, Ph.D., is a certified sex therapist, a sex-advice columnist for Onhealth.com, and a licensed marriage and family therapist in Fair Oaks, California.

Beverly Whipple, Ph.D., R.N., is a professor at the College of Nursing at Rutgers University in Newark, New Jersey; a past president of the American Association of Sex Educators, Counselors, and Therapists; and the author of *The G-Spot and Other Recent Discoveries about Human Sexuality* and *Safe Encounters: How Women Can Say Yes to Pleasure and No to Unsafe Sex*.

E. Douglas Whitehead, M.D., is a urologist and the director of the Association for Male Sexual Dysfunction as well as the New York Phalloplasty, both in New York City.

Wade Wilson is the author of *Fantasy Island: A Man's Guide to Exotic Women and International Travel* and the Web master of www.fantasyisles.com, a Web site for meeting international women.

Susan Young is the owner of the Santa Fe Sewing Studio in New Mexico.

Matt Zinicola is the owner of Ravedata Project, a database collection of rave flyers.